T0136796

Beyond Method

Interpretive Studies in Healthcare and the Human Sciences

VOLUME IV

Beyond Method

Philosophical Conversations in Healthcare Research and Scholarship

Pamela M. Ironside

Volume Editor

THE UNIVERSITY OF WISCONSIN PRESS

This book was published with the generous support
of the Evjue Foundation, Inc.,
the charitable arm of *The Capital Times.*

The University of Wisconsin Press
1930 Monroe Street, 3rd Floor
Madison, Wisconsin 53711- 2059
uwpress.wisc .edu

3 Henrietta Street
London WC2E 8LU, England
eurospanbookstore .com

Printed in the United States of America

Library of Congress Cataloging-in-Publication Data
Beyond method: philosophical conversations in healthcare research
and scholarship / edited by Pamela M. Ironside.
p. ; cm.–(Interpretive studies in healthcare and the human sciences; v. 4)
Includes bibliographical references and index.
ISBN 0-299-20820-6 (hardcover: alk. paper)
ISBN 0-299-20824-9 (pbk.: alk. paper)
1. Medical care–Research–Philosophy.
[DNLM: 1. Health Services Research–methods.
2. Philosophy. 3. Science. W 84.3 B573 2005]
I. Ironside, Pamela M.   II. Series.
R852.B49   2005
362.1'072–dc22   2004025719

ISBN 978-0-299-29823-4 (e-book)

To John and Nancy Diekelmann
who, for the past 13 years,
have gathered researchers and scholars
from around the globe by creating a place
for listening and responding to phenomena
in healthcare and the human sciences.
*Nursing Institutes for
Heideggerian Hermeneutical Phenomenology
University of Wisconsin–Madison*
1992–2004

Contents

Introduction

Thinking Beyond Method

to think beyond the concept of method in the human sciences . . . is to ask
the question of the "possibility" of the human sciences

Gadamer, 1960/1989, p. 512

Issues of method and practice continue to take center stage in discussions
of research and scholarship in the human sciences. The work, or product, of researcher-scholars, communicated in written or spoken forms, is
shaped by delineations of method. As the detailed specification of the procedures utilized in a given inquiry, discussions of method are assumed to
provide readers and listeners with detailed descriptions of the approaches
to the analyses reported.

From the ontic perspective, detailing method as a rational, logical,
and linear procedure allows for the verification of a particular proposition
or hypothesis or for the quantification of an object or action such that
subsequent practice decisions can be made, supported, and defended.
The rigor of inquiry as well as its use or application reflects the degree to
which the scientific community judges the method to be credible, repli-
cable, and valid, or in the case of interpretive scholarship, warranted
(Baker, Norton, Young, & Ward, 1998; Browne, 2000). Understood in this
way, discussions of method are the basis upon which the veracity of the
researcher's claims can be ascertained. That is, discussions of method
legitimize the findings and delineate the context within which results are
utilizable. For example, in scientific studies the sampling procedures a
researcher employed in a particular study are delineated such that the
reader or listener can decide the extent to which the study sample is

representative of the population being studied, whether or not the findings are generalizable to other groups, and whether competing explanations for the findings have been controlled for (i.e., internal validity) in the study design. Likewise in interpretive studies, the philosophical texts or frameworks used to interpret study data are explicated, excerpts from the textual data are provided so the reader or listener can participate in the analysis (Diekelmann & Ironside, 1999), and audit trails (Morse, 1994) may be constructed by the researcher to document changes in his or her thinking during data analysis.

Such considerations of method are philosophically tied to the realist/idealist and interpretive traditions (J. Diekelmann, 2005) such that the inquirer seeks to uncover the epistemological/ontological "thatness" of a thing or action (*that* a thing or action exists), "whatness" (what the thing or action exists *as*), or "howness" (how a thing or action *is* a particular way) (Sheehan, 2001). However, science, as in the scientific method, predominates contemporary thinking about what constitutes method (Honderich, 1995). Method in this sense is linked to the *object* of inquiry (as something other than the inquirer or things "out there") and as such necessarily reinforces the subject/object split (the object of inquiry is an independent entity that I, as an independent subject, can study). Although significant advances in the health and human sciences have occurred as a result of such methods, the thinking that underpins method in the ontic sense cannot escape the realist/idealist tradition. Even in interpretive scholarship, method is perhaps too often claimed by idealist/realist concerns. That is, from a realist/idealist perspective, "improvements" in method are obtained by enhancing their persuasive power (idealism) by devising methods that move closer to revealing the truth of what *is* in the metaphysical realm (e.g. providing ultimate explanations for *what is*) or by enhancing the certainty of their claims (realism) through devising methods that are increasingly abstract, precise, warranted and accurate (measurement or description of the "actual"). In contemporary scholarship method itself becomes a matter of concern for both scientific and interpretive scholarship and is claimed by efforts to develop better methods ("super-methods" that become ever more comprehensive, extensive, inclusive, warranted, precise and accurate) with which more can be known or understood and with more certainty.

The method of science, in the scientistic sense, *controls* for the context (as a way of establishing the veracity of the study—what I am studying is X and nothing else), it establishes in advance what will be studied (X and nothing else), the evidence that will count as determining some property of X (X-ness) and how such evidence can be understood (as X and nothing else). The ground of such assertions, since the time of Descartes, has been the assumption that the world is knowable by the knower (Gadamer, 1983/1998). In other words, all that is to be known is "out there" (as an idea or entity) and methods will continue to be improved for use *by* humans until all that is to be known is known *by* humans.

One problem with this approach, despite its epistemological contributions, is that what one takes as an object of inquiry is never a historically or temporally neutral position. That is, *that* a phenomenon (X rather than Y) emerges as interesting or concerning (or fundable) reflects how the researcher currently understands the phenomenon—how he or she is already engaged with the phenomenon (Gadamer, 1983/1998). Similarly, how the researcher currently understands the phenomenon makes some aspects (and uses) emerge more saliently than others, and again, this is neither a given, objective, "out there" characteristic nor a mere cognitive insight by the researcher but part of an always already *givenness* of world as an unquantifiable totality of meaning and significance involvements (Heidegger, 1927/1962).

Interpretive approaches to method, specifically those elucidated by continental philosophers beginning with Heidegger, emphasize not what shows up as salient but how it is that salience occurs at all (Sheehan, 2001). For example, in the health and human sciences the hand is not merely a hand but is always already bound to the context (the ways in which) in which it is confronted. The hand can be *taken as* an object to be examined, *a part* of a human body made up of particular configurations of bones and muscles. The hand can be *taken as* a site or location within which treatment can be introduced (infusing intravenous therapy) or monitored (pulse oximeter). The hand can be *taken as* a biomedical tool with which a healthcare worker assesses peripheral pulses, holds pressure on a punctured artery, performs chest compressions, or monitors changes in warmth or can be *taken as* an alternative modality for restoring a patient's energy via "therapeutic touch" (Krieger, 1979; Quinn, 1989). The hand can be *taken as* caring presence when laid upon a frightened patient's shoulder during a painful procedure or as a concerned but aggressive, controlling presence when used to subdue or restrain a combative, confused patient. Understood in this way, the "object" of inquiry is not *the hand* (properties of the hand or effectiveness of the hand as a tool or presence) *per se* but how one becomes engaged with the hand that matters. But engaging with the hand (as this or that) always already also requires that the hand is already there to be engaged *with*. This contention reflects a significant contribution of Heidegger's thought. There is no objective "out there" into which we, as researchers or care providers inquire. Rather, world shows up through human engagement and humans engage with world because the world always already worlds (Sheehan, 2001).

In this way, Heidegger's thought provides new possibilities for thinking beyond method (as a tool or procedure), by questioning (listening and responding to) phenomena as phenomena. Diekelmann (2004, p. 1) states:

[Heidegger] opened up for questioning the basic assumptions that have driven the research paradigms that have reached every corner of the globe. His work is an attempt to bring language to the heretofore unarticulated forces driving the methodologies that we find ourselves placed/drawn into. It was not his purpose to deny all human agency but to approach the phenomenon of our comportment from its ownmost ground, wherein grounding becomes a play that turns on participatory "being-with" rather than the centrality of human cognition. The practice of splitting the world into subject and object *by* humans *for* humans as an 'in-order-to' which is claimed by a will to control . . . can only obtain as a will-to-will.

Thus, for Heidegger, the meaning and significance of phenomena are inextricably linked to this *taking-as* in which humans are necessarily always already engaged. Isolating phenomena for study (the hand as object or entity) reifies the anthropocentric conceptualizations of the world in which "method" becomes the "in-order-to" of scientistic assumptions of and commitments to knowledge generation and certainty. Such approaches cover over new possibilities for "method" that emerge in the play of listening and responding to phenomena.

Considering the brief comparison between the methods of science and interpretive methods above, what becomes clear is that although methods are, in common parlance, used in the service of inquiry—as procedures or perspectives—what becomes equally apparent is not only how a particular method is used but what grants or grounds methods, that is, how methods shape and are shaped by researchers' understanding of phenomena. Taken in this way, methods are not only tools or procedures but *ways of thinking about phenomena*. Converging conversations of philosophy, methodology and epistemology are possible ways via which such thinking can be encountered—thinking in which what is otherwise overlooked or forgotten (Heidegger, 1927/1962), and new possibilities for the human science (Gadamer, 1960/1989), can be revealed.

The Hermeneutic Circle of Understanding

Many interpretive methods overturn the common conception of the world as "things out there" to be studied by the researcher and rather provide ways to think through how things are *taken as* X or Y. In order to take something *as* something, however, requires a practical familiarity (fore-having) with the thing (Heidegger, 1927/1962). That is, because I am familiar with the world in which I am engaged, my practical familiarity with hands allows me to use hands in particular ways because I understand hands as suitable for giving care and comfort or for monitoring patient progress. Such understanding, while allowing me to engage in the world in a seamless way, can also serve to limit and direct the nature of questions to be asked, establishing, as Gadamer contends, the "horizon of the question" (1960/1989, p. 370). The horizon of the question is the coming-into-language (Gadamer, 1960/1989) of the researcher's thinking. That is, the very questions a researcher asks in a particular study reflect how phenomena are understood—how the researcher thinks about (speaks) the phenomenon. This is an important departure from the scientistic conception that questions emerge from a "gap in the literature."

Similarly, researchers (being finite human beings) always approach "things" from a particular perspective (fore-sight) and with an anticipated sense of what the inquiry will reveal (fore-conception) (Heidegger, 1927/1962). Fore-sight and fore-conception are intimately connected to discussions of method. That is, when embarking on a particular project, researchers determine the perspective from which the inquiry will be conducted. For example, am I interested in studying physiological determinants of chronic illness or how chronic illness is experienced? Because this fore-sight shapes our understanding it is important to consider how our perspective allows us to see particular aspects of a phenomenon (cellular level changes accompanying arthritis) while necessarily covering over others (the meaning and significance of arthritis in the lived world). *The point here is not to argue for the ascendancy of one kind of question (or method) over another.* Clearly the complexity of current problems facing researchers in the health and human sciences require that multiple methods inform our understandings (Browne, 2000). Rather, the point is to emphasize Heidegger's contention that with every revealing there is also a concealing (Heidegger, 1927/1962, 1967/1998). Our finitude prevents us from seeing/understanding the world in an "all-at-once," complete or eternal way. Thus, even when multiple methods are employed (or triangulated) (Foss & Ellefsen, 2002) what is revealed necessarily conceals something else.

Closely linked with fore-sight, fore-conception is our anticipated sense of what our inquiry will reveal. Our fore-conception allows us to recognize findings as findings because they "fit" with our practical familiarity with the phenomenon and the perspective undertaken in the study. That is, understanding (interpreting) our "results" or "findings" relies on our familiarity with the phenomenon (fore-having) and with the perspective we are taking (fore-sight) in our inquiry. And our "results" or "findings," become part of how we understand the phenomenon (fore-having) of inquiry and the perspective from phenomena are considered. The hermeneutic circle circles.

From this perspective, there is no opportunity for humans to step "outside" the hermeneutic circle of understanding to consider a phenomenon in its "objective," essential or eternal sense. That is, recognizing an object as "an object" requires a priori familiarity with the object and a particular engagement within which the "object" is taken as this or that. To ask a question about the object or phenomenon is to have in advance an anticipated sense of the answer. Thus, Gadamer contends *new possibilities lie in questioning* (rather than answering). To think beyond method is not to create new methods that ensure more certain or defensible answers (findings) or to replace current methods with a single, universal, unfailing method, but to persistently question the possibilities of method for the health and human sciences.

Yet, questioning requires an openness in thinking that acknowledges that answers are always tentative, fallible, and indeterminate (Ironside, 2003). Gadamer contends the "essence of the *question* is to open up possibilities and keep them open" (1960/1989, p. 299), or to understand the questionableness of what is being asked. Thought of in this way, persistent questioning prevents researchers from imposing their perspectives or opinions on the inquiry (seeking to prove or demonstrate this or that), and requires them to "recognize the full value of what is alien and opposed to them" (Gadamer, 1960/1989, p. 387), what is confusing, seemingly incongruent or unknown. Løvlie, Mortensen, and Nordenbo maintain that "alienation is inescapable if one is genuinely to remain open to things [*sic*] that are different from what one has known and from that to which one has become accommodated" (2003, p. vii). Thus, the willingness to listen and respond to diverse perspectives of phenomena is fundamental to questioning (Ironside, 2003).

Thinking Toward Possibilities: The Play of Methods

The departure from the traditional (realist/idealist) sense of methods as tools to derive findings for answering clinical questions, then, calls for reconsideration of the primacy of questioning. Questioning, in this sense, is not merely *posing* a question but persistently questioning what is confusing, seemingly incongruent, and unknown as well as what is familiar, taken-for-granted, and assumed. Similarly, such questioning is not the deconstructive questioning in the postmodern sense, questioning that seeks to persistently challenge the structure of extant systems of knowledge (Stevenson & Beech, 2001). Rather, when thought of phenomenologically, questioning is being open to phenomena in ways that let phenomena show themselves *as* phenomena (Gadamer, 1960/1989). This questioning is not an experience of seeking an answer but one of thinking toward possibilities that self-possibilize and obtain as *play*.

Gadamer (1960/1989, 1986) explicates play to describe the dialogical and dialectical human relation to understanding the world. That is, humans seek to understand the world through interpretation, but the relationship is more fundamental than the Cartesian conception of the human subject in a world of objects. That which is to be understood presences itself, becoming an experience for and changing the person who experiences it. Play cannot be described then as a mere object or as the "subjectivity of the person who experiences it" (Gadamer, 1960/1989, p. 102). Play is characterized by the to and fro movement between the interpreter and that which is to be interpreted. The movement of play is not toward a goal or telos but toward the constant repetition of the movement of play, which Gadamer exemplifies using the metaphors of the play of light or the play of the waves. Put more simply, the repetitious back and forth movement *is* the play—"play is the self-representation of the movement" (Gadamer, 1986, p. 23).

However, the movement of play cannot be separated from the players. That is, to understand the play requires that one "plays along" (Gadamer, 1986, p. 23). "Play fulfills its purpose only if the player loses himself [or herself] in the play . . . play merely reaches presentation . . . through the players" (Gadamer, 1960/1989, p. 102, 103). To make play an object, to impose order on the movement of the play is to distance play from the experience; thus the movement of play is lost. Gadamer further describes play by relating his notion of play to the common understanding of playing games.

The particular nature of a game lies in the rules and regulations that prescribe the way the field of the game is filled. This is true universally, whenever there is a game. . . . The playing field on which the game is played is, as it were, set by the nature of the game itself and is defined far more by the structure that determines the movement of the game from within than by what it comes up against—i.e., the boundaries of the open space—limiting movement from without.

Apart from these general determining factors, it seems to me characteristic of human play that it plays something. That means that the structure of movement to which it submits has a definite quality which the player "chooses." First, he [sic] expressly separates his playing behavior from his other behavior by wanting to play. But even within his readiness to play he makes a choice. He chooses this game rather than that. Correlatively, the space in which the game's movement takes place is not simply the open space in which one "plays oneself out," but one that is specially marked out and reserved for the movement of the game. (1960/1989, p. 107)

Considering the play of methods in Gadamer's (phenomenological) sense reveals new possibilities for thinking and questioning methods in the health and human sciences. That is, the nature of inquiry is determined more by researchers' pre-given understandings than by the rules or guidelines detailing "proper" methodological procedures for epistemological development. Methods are not directed to an end (an answer) but constantly self-renew as questioning continues. The play of methods, then, is not primarily directed toward solving a problem or completing a project (although in the ontic sense this may occur) but toward preserving the movement of the play—the play of methods (questioning) in interpretive scholarship.

The studies in this volume each reflect the play of methods, that is, the movement of questioning within and beyond methods in which new possibilities for understanding in the health and human sciences emerge.

This is not to say that scientistic or "traditional" conceptions of methods are useless and insignificant and should be assigned to oblivion. Rather, the chapters in this volume, by illuminating the play of methods, reveal multiple paths to thinking beyond methods via converging conversations of philosophy, methodology and epistemology.

In Chapter 1, "The Retrieval of Method: The Method of Retrieval" John Diekelmann brings the thinking of Martin Heidegger, Hans-Georg Gadamer and Jean-Luc Nancy into converging conversation in exploring the granting of method in human understanding. Moving beyond the realist/idealist conceptualizations of method that end in particular transcendental or cognitive assertions, Diekelmann explicates a phenomenological view of methods as listening and responding to phenomena in ways that overcome the claims of metaphysical investigation of presence.

Kathryn Hopkins Kavanagh, in "Representing: Interpretive Scholarship's Consummate Challenge" (Chapter 2) unsettles the contemporary practices of representing participants in interpretive research. Exploring both the limits and uses of representation, Kavanagh reveals the significance of language in codifying outside-in conceptualizations of participants and problematizes the interpretive practices therein.

Chapter 3, "Socratic-Hermeneutic Interpre-viewing," Christine Sorrell Dinkins describes how examination of the Socratic dialogues provides new possibilities for interviewing participants in interpretive research. Challenging the common yet artificial separation between interviewing participants and interpreting data, Dinkins delineates how the Socratic dialogues (as presented in Plato's works) provide a new model for contemporary interpretive researchers to co-collaborate with participants in inquiry thereby enriching research endeavor.

Rosemary McEldowney challenges the researcher-centered prespecification and use of methods and offers an alternative wherein, working collaboratively with participants, methods are developed, employed and refined as the phenomenon becomes increasingly understood. In "Revealing Shape-shifting Through Life-Story Narrative" (Chapter 4), McEldowney illustrates how inquiry into methods is intertwined with and reflective of researchers' and participants' understanding of the phenomenon of interest.

Phillipa Seaton examines multi-method research from within the interpretive paradigm in "Combining Interpretive Methodologies: Maximizing the Richness of Findings" (Chapter 5). Seaton explicates how, through challenging and extending familiar models and methods of triangulation, interpretive researchers can be true to the philosophical and epistemological commitments of diverse interpretive methods while allowing multiple interpretive methods to coalesce around specific topics, revealing facets of experience obscured by the rigid adherence to single methods.

In Chapter 6, "The Thinking of Research," Elizabeth Smythe hermeneutically analyzes the thinking of researchers to overcome the split of analytic thinking of scientific studies versus the situated thinking of interpretive studies. Her study reveals how within the hermeneutic circle of understanding both kinds of thinking are necessary for all forms of research and neither is sufficient. By revealing how the thinking and the phenomena both shape and are shaped by the thinking of the researcher, Smythe interweaves the voices of new and experienced researchers across academic discipline and methodological perspectives. Smythe illuminates the ebb and flow of researchers' engagement in *thinking*.

Nancy Johnston, in "Beyond the Methods Debate: Toward Embodied Ways of Knowing" (Chapter 7), explicates how the common subject/object split in research designs covers over the "doublesidedness" of human experience. Situating this study within multidisciplinary research, Johnston proposes new ways of thinking about research in the health and human sciences that enable holism and hope.

This volume, the fourth in the series *Interpretive Studies in Healthcare and the Human Sciences*, heralds a shift from competitive positions that debate the superiority of particular methods to one of thinking beyond methods (questioning) in ways that reveal new possibilities for research. Gathering the voices of scholars from across disciplines and around the world into converging conversations, this volume provides substantive paths to thinking in which researchers, students, and clinicians in healthcare and the human sciences can continue to inquire into complex human phenomena while keeping possibilities in play.

References

Baker, C., Norton, S., Young, P., & Ward, S. (1998). An exploration of methodological pluralism in nursing research. *Research in Nursing and Health 21,* 545–555.

Browne, A. J. (2000). The potential contributions of critical social theory to nursing science. *Canadian Journal of Nursing Research 32,* 35–55.

Diekelmann, J. (2004). *Hermeneutic phenomenology: An invitation from Martin Heidegger.* Unpublished manuscript. Victoria University, Wellington, New Zealand.

Diekelmann, J. (2005). The retrieval of method: The method of retrieval. In P. M. Ironside (Ed.), *Interpretive Studies in Healthcare and the Human Sciences: Vol. 4. Beyond Method: Converging Conversations of Philosophy, Methodology, and Epistemology*. Madison: University of Wisconsin Press.

Diekelmann, N. L., & Ironside, P. M. (1999). Hermeneutics. In J. Fitzpatrick (Ed.). *Nursing Research Digest*. New York: Springer.

Foss, C., & Ellefsen, B. (2002). The value of combining qualitative and quantitative approaches in nursing research by means of method triangulation. *Journal of Advanced Nursing 40*, 242–248.

Gadamer, H. G. (1986). In R. Bernasconi (Ed.), *The relevance of the beautiful and other essays*. (N. Walker, Trans.). New York: Cambridge University Press.

Gadamer, H. G. (1989). *Truth and method*. (Rev. ed.). (J. Weinsheimer & D. G. Marshall, Trans.) New York: Continuum. (Original work published 1960).

Gadamer, H. G. (1998). *Praise of theory*. (C. Dawson, Trans.). New Haven, CT: Yale University Press. (Original work published 1983).

Heidegger, M. (1962) *Being and time*. (J. Macquarrie & E. Robinson, Trans.). New York: Harper and Row. (Original work published 1927).

Heidegger, M. (1998). Introduction to *What is metaphysics?* (W. Kaufman & W. McNeill, Trans.). In W. McNeill (Ed.), *Pathmarks* (pp. 277–290). New York: Cambridge University Press. (Original work published 1967).

Honderich, T. (1995). *The Oxford companion to philosophy*. New York: Oxford University Press.

Krieger, D. (1979). *The therapeutic touch: How to use your hands to help or to heal*. Englewood Cliffs, NJ: Prentice-Hall.

Ironside, P. M. (2003). New pedagogies for teaching thinking: The lived experiences of students and teachers enacting Narrative Pedagogy. *Journal of Nursing Education 42*, 509–516.

Løvlie, L., Mortensen, K. P., & Nordenbo, S. E. (2003). *Educating humanity: Bildung in postmodernity*. Melbourne, Australia: Blackwell.

Morse, J. M. (1994). Designing funded qualitative research. In N. K. Denzin & Y. S. Lincoln (Eds.). *Handbook of qualitative research* (pp. 220–235). Thousand Oaks, CA: Sage.

Quinn, J. (1989). Therapeutic touch as energy exchange: Replication and extension. *Nursing Science Quarterly 2*(2), 79–87.

Sheehan, T. (2001). *Kehre* and *Ereignis:* A prolegomenon to introduction to metaphysics. In *A companion to Heidegger's introduction to metaphysics* (pp. 3–16, 263–274). New Haven, CT: Yale University Press.

Stevenson, C., & Beech, I. (2001). Paradigms lost, paradigms regained: Defending nursing against a single reading of postmodernism. *Nursing Philosophy, 2*, 143–150.

Beyond Method

1

The Retrieval of Method

The Method of Retrieval

JOHN DIEKELMANN

> A boundary is not that at which something stops but . . . is that from which something *begins its essential unfolding*.
>
> (Heidegger, 1954/1993a, p. 356)

Humans have always dealt with boundaries, whether self-imposed or forced, as the delimitations of political, economic, or social practices. Theologies and theoretical physics are claimed by boundaries as approachable via some ideal of perfection; God in the former, mathematics in the latter. Psychology and biology are in their own way, derivative of this kind of thinking. Psychology seeks to perfect the essential nature of the human mind, soul, and brain. The project of biology is to quantify organic functioning via a given conceptualization of evolution. The boundary is a limit that as mystery draws us by its very withdrawing.

Methodological procedures that turn on a sense of retrieval work to let possibilities *as* possibilities show themselves as they arrive into appearance. Retrieval as a proceeding (a non-algorithmic traversal) has the potential within it to also acknowledge that there is always a vital absencing that simply gives itself as absence. Methods that turn on the certainty of the closure of some pregiven totality cannot deal with the vitality inherent in absenting. This is the vitality of the *differ-ence* between presencing as always already presenting this or that and absencing as always already absenting this or that; vitality as a non-visible, non-calculable

3

phenomenon—nevertheless approachable via meditative, participatory, thinking practitioners.

In what follows, I will attempt to demonstrate that our dealing with the manifestness of what is present is given as our necessary "essential and therefore constant pointing toward what withdraws" (Heidegger, 1954/ 1968, p. 8–10; Sheehan, 2001b, p. 16–17). Total presence and any accompanying complete "knowledge" is a project that is striving to present the ideal. This is what is ownmost to what draws us to beyond the physical, that is, the metaphysical. Only as a questioning that turns on letting anything be its ownmost privation can there be a more inclusive seeing-of and listening-to what is present as phenomena. Interpretive thinking is an enactment of thinking that lets something be "as" it "orders" itself up. This is a possibility that can occur as dialogue that remains open to a "multiplicity of meanings" (Heidegger, 1954/1968, p. 71).

In this explication I will enlist Martin Heidegger as a guide. Taking his notions of thrownness, understanding, and language (1987/2001b) as a jumping off point, I will map out these phenomena onto Hans-Georg Gadamer's notions of historically effected consciousness, experience, and conversation. I will look at Jean-Luc Nancy's explication of meaning, figuration, and ex-position in order to suggest possibilities for methodical practices that release us *as a "we"* from the metaphysical notion that all time can be determined as "one unchanging present" (the *nunc stans*) (Heidegger, 1987/2001b, p. 179). I will not be using the "We" of the tradition's isolated ego conceptualizations. Instead I will explore the term "we" as a notion of be-ing-with-one-another joined with thinking as a co-being-in-the-world (Heidegger, 1987/2001b).

Lastly, I will offer an example from an everyday experience—that of an airport arrival/departure room. I will use this example to discuss the notions of absence and excess of meaning.

Where, When, and How We Find Ourselves

. . . science has developed such a power as could never have been met with on the earth before, and that consequently this power is ultimately to be spread over the entire globe.

(Heidegger, 1954/1977a, p. 156)

Method as it is known and practiced by contemporary techno-scientism is claimed by the necessity to seize the future and hold it fast (Gadamer, 1976/1981). For example, there is a belief that a model of the brain can be constructed such that its function can be somehow known once and for all. This necessary claim cannot be released, lest this letting-go jeopardize the certainty required to grasp the accessible. In science, in order for objects of study to be rigorously delimited, they must be accessible and graspable. But in order to grasp the accessible, the accessible *must* be graspable. The scientistic has ensnared itself in its own primitive tautology! The objects scientists study are determined by the frames scientists have placed around them. The assumption implicit in this framing is that this procedure captures the object itself and nothing more. The practices of including/excluding are central for empirical or statistical study. The dilemma of modern science is solved by itself for itself; nothing that is not presentified by some empirical or mathematicized means has significance and meaning via its ownmost complex of relationships and practices. Science cannot get around its own significance and meaning via its ownmost means and practices, because objects as "presences can appear, but never absolutely must appear" (Heidegger, 1954/1977a, p. 176). Scientistic thinking forgets or overlooks the fact that *all* knowledge is relative—it cannot avoid this specter.

As an alternative Heidegger (1977/2003) suggests "we need to learn to distinguish between *path* and *method*. In philosophy there are only paths; in the sciences, on the contrary, there are only methods, that is, modes of procedure" (p. 80). Interpretive thinking is a proceeding rather than a procedure. But this way of proceeding "is a path that leads away to come before. . . , and it lets that before which is led show itself" (p. 80).

The achievements of modern science have placed us into a world where human practices have led to radical polarities. On the one hand, the observation of microbes has led to a growing armament of antibiotics and advances in death control, which, on the other hand has produced a plethora of antibiotic-resistant, "super" infections and a growth in human population that has the potential to threaten the viability of the planet as a dwelling place.

Why does "method" need to be retrieved? After all, doesn't "the methodical" denote a rational/logical procedure by which the truth of some proposition or the quantification of some object can be achieved?

We find ourselves at a moment where the entire planet is affected by human activities. Heidegger (1943/1977c), writing on Nietzsche, contended: "Unexpectedly, and above all in a way unforeseen, man [sic] finds himself, from out of the [b]eing[1] of what is, set before the task of taking over domination of the earth" (p. 96).

Are we prepared/ready to deal with the issues at play in the dissolution of the putative human–nature dichotomy? The mystery that was the *Cosmocentrism* of the archaic Greek age is forgotten. *Theocentrisms* have lost their grip as a practice despite the fervor of religiosity that wells up from time to time; occurrences that are a reaction to the dominant subject-centered comportments inherent in the exercise of political power. The resulting anthropocentrism harbors the hidden dangers of:

- utopianism(s) as anesthetization *(Eliot's patient, etherized upon a table!)*
- technologism(s) as domination of all that is
- hypostasization of time
- valorizing as "unconditioned controllability" (Heidegger, 1989/1999, p. 311) : i.e., as the highest value

The modern tradition's play of the differences of humankind, as a product of Nature and/or God, has devolved into the will-to-will that "forces the calculation and arrangement of everything for itself as the basic forms of appearance, only, however, for the unconditionally predictable guarantee of itself" (Heidegger, 1954/1973b, p. 93, 99).

In this study I will attempt to pursue the signification "method" in terms of how it has unfolded from an historical use far different from that of today's. In order to get beyond the narrow contemporary usage of the term, I will trace method as method and subsequently offer possibilities for an opening that takes into account our "groundless groundedness" in historicality, dialogue, and always already exposure to meaning. Retrieval will be the pathway by which I will attempt a thinking that emanates from the self-unfolding of limit.

In *Zollikon Seminars* (1987/2001b), Heidegger notes the Greek root of the word method.

This word "method" is a composite from Greek μετα [*meta*] and οδος [*odos*]. 'Η όδος [*E odos*] means "way," while μετα [*meta*] means "from here to there," "toward something." (p. 101; see also Heidegger, 1982/1992b, p. 356)

Method is rooted in being on a way but not from a fixed point toward a predetermined end. Being on the way is a limit, not where something comes to an end, but where anything is enabled to reveal an ownmostness that is not necessarily rooted in human cognition but to which humans must necessarily relate. Limit is the "groundless ground" that advenes as interpreters peruse and listen to the becoming of unfolding. I will look at being-on-the-way as the "step back" later in this study.

The experience of limit as origin is an additional thread that I will attempt to weave through this exegesis in order to retrieve possibilities for "method." The Judeo-Christian tradition of the seventh to fifteenth centuries was typified by the efforts to combine faith and reason or logic. Method became a system of disputation wherein the existence of God was first and foremost the engine of speculative thought. The universe moved from a self-unfolding phenomenon to one that was created. But as Gadamer (1960/1990) works to demonstrate:

> The human word is used only as a counterpart to the theological problem of the Word, the verbum dei—i.e., the unity of God the Father and God the Son. But the important thing for us is precisely that the mystery of this unity is reflected in the phenomenon of language. (p. 419)

Renaissance humanists initiated a variety of attacks on

> the scholastics for trying to formulate necessary and universal propositions about God's existence and the structure of his creation. Such speculation, according to the humanists, is both illegitimate and useless: illegitimate because human reason cannot know the divine, and useless because even if we were to have contemplative knowledge, such abstractions would not help us direct our earthly civic affairs. (Kahn, 1997, p. 151)

With Renaissance humanists method became necessarily referred to reason as the logic of utility.

Method as way comes to a fork in its road: an idealism of persuasion versus a realism of apodictic certainty. In Europe, at least, the omniscience of the divine mind is superceded by the certainty thought to be possible via human cognition. Both paths held out promise: idealism included elements of Aristotelian prudence *(phronesis)* while realism held out the possibilities of access to fact-establishing laws. The idealist–realist (subject–object) split manifested itself in its views on language. Idealism adhered to an "expressive" view of language. This grew out of the belief that a "behind the scenes" cause, either as a transcendent psyche or deity, was responsible for language (Heidegger, 1987/2001b). Realisms eschewed speculation on causation because it called for judgment and use as a problematizing methodology. In terms of its side of the divide realism demanded for itself language that was representational in order to illustrate or solve problems (Kahn, 1997, p. 155). Procedures could not be divorced from conceptions of language.

At the dawn of the 16th century:

the Greek term *methodus* had no precise philosophical meaning, the humanists tended to identify it with the general pursuit and teaching of knowledge, that is, with the pragmatic arts of communication as both the means and ends of instruction. Method was technical only in the general sense that it involved the knowledge of the appropriate means to achieve a particular end. (Kahn, 1997, p. 157)

The sixteenth century saw the rise of mathematics as a method. For the practitioners, abstract epistemological principles would take precedence over the deliberations turning on the speculative (theological or metaphysical) or everyday (practical). Descartes argues that the true model of philosophical method would be mathematical (Kahn, 1997, p. 158). The mathematical moves from the Greek usage as that which can be learned and taught to the abstract relationships initiated by Newton in the seventeenth century (Heidegger, 1962/1967).

Realist methodologies purport to reduce phenomena to those that can be empirically verified and subjected to mathematically generated laws. The "thing-in-itself" could allegedly be determined by these methods. These must be repeatable at any time an experiment is performed. Idealist methodologies use speculative theories to determine the inner nature of the human subject (the idealization of phenomena). These theories derive their truth-value by elimination of competing possibilities. In the eighteenth century Kant, via the power of judgment in relation to sense experience, attempted to fuse the above threads into a cogent whole.

By the early twentieth century, theoretical comportment, in a way that was essential for it, was the necessary lawfulness of its progression. Theoretical comportment turns on its own necessitized necessity. Early in his career, Heidegger (1987/2000) explicated method as

. . . the *way* to the constitution of the context of states of affairs. In so far as the theoretical comportment is necessary, yet still a problem, it finds its lawful progression in method. (p. 177)

The theoretical attitude is comportment toward the maximum removal from any given situatedness; a science of explanation.

Theoretical comportment in so far as it is directed in a comprehensive way toward pure states of affairs in which every emotional relation is strictly disallowed, removes itself from life-experience. The theoretical world is not always there, but is accessible only in a constantly renewed divesting of the natural world. (p. 179)

Theory like method has its historical roots in Greek history. For the ancient Greeks θερία [*theoria*] was "the perceptual relation of man [*sic*] to [b]eing, a relation man does not produce but rather a relation into which [b]eing itself posits man" (Heidegger, 1982/1992b, pp. 147–148). On Heidegger's reading *theoria* was a clearing where humans were "delivered over to" as a gathering of meanings where concealing and revealing occur.

In *Truth and Method* (1960/1990), Gadamer retrieves the meaning of theory as *theoros;* "someone who takes part in a festival" (p. 124). *Theoria* was an active participation in things. More than this, Gadamer enacts a double retrieval by explicating *theoria* and the "theory" of modern science by relating this word to "verbal experience of the world" (p. 455). The participatory nature of the Greeks is different from that of modern science where theory and language are worked together to establish domination over the gathering of experiences and language in order to overcome their inherent tendency to resist quantification and control (p. 454–455).

Heidegger's "On the Essence and Concept of φύσις in Aristotle's *Physics B*, I (1939)" in *Pathmarks* (1967/1998b) is a discussion on the aspects of Greek language that facilitated, to some extent, the self-emergence of phenomena. The pre-Socratic thinkers for Heidegger let things be open as absence (privative presence) as they enacted a sense of preservation via the word (Sheehan, 1983). Heidegger's thinking of the essence of language, as we shall see, is pivotal in this explication of temporality.

The French philosopher Jean-Luc Nancy (1993/1997) elaborates on Heidegger and Gadamer by bringing out the circularity of the idealist/ realist dilemma:

the concept thinks and the intuition sees; the concept thinks what the intuition sees and the intuition sees what the concept thinks. *Signification is thus the very model of a structure or system that is closed upon itself* or better yet, *as closure upon itself* . . . the reality of man [*sic*] presents itself *right in* the ideality called "mankind" [*sic*] . . . the ideality of humans presents itself *right in* his sensible reality . . . (p. 23)

The circularity inherent in the subject-object paradigm is the limit from which it becomes visible. Any presentation of the unconditioned as the unconditioned is an idealization necessitated by the limit of conditioned-ness itself (p. 24). Humanism as anthropocentrism and certainty are inextricably intertwined as they assert themselves as "the complete system of the auto donation of meaning" (p. 25).

The danger of self-certainty, as Heidegger (1961/1973a) explicates it, is that self-certainty can obtain only as the will-to-will. One way or another we are self-interpreting (p. 48). Sheehan (1995a, 2001a) writes, we are "condemned to ontology" (p. 158, p. 12). We must deal with sense or meaning "amidst un-sense, non-sense, and no-longer sense" (Sheehan, 1978, p. 313). There is always already meaning in front of us as that which draws us into our future as an always already becoming.

For Nancy (1993/1997) meaning is understood as signifying an "as something." We assign presence, factuality, and sensibility to some mode that is intelligible. Reciprocally, assignment obtains as an assignment of intelligible determinations of some sensible mode that determines a particular materiality of the assigned itself (p. 22).

For many the subject-object paradigm has thus exhausted its intellectual possibilities as it swirls back and forth in its own self-circulation. Questions that arise might go something like this: Is the brain a computer analogue? Or, is the computer a brain analogue? How is "mind" defined? Located? Established? Nancy's explication explores this situatedness as an exhaustion of openings that point to any attempt to determine a *sovereign eternity of meaning*. The work of thought, or thinking, is thinking when its discipline and its rigor do not consist in mastering this sovereignty, but in attempting to move beyond it.

Enacting interpretive thinking is comportment (experience) such that we abide in an exposure to this sovereignty: our limit as "the West, history and philosophy." (Nancy, 1993/1997, p. 67) For Nancy this activity is not casual recreation "but, rather, a difficult, complex, and delicate set of decisions, acts, positions and gestures of thought and writing" (p. 67). As this practice, we are free for the weight of "what keeps signification—either willingly or reluctantly—oscillating dangerously on its limit"

(p. 67). Heidegger differentiates casual conversation from involved dialogue wherein the latter leads the participants in an asking after the problematic (Heidegger, 1954/1968).

The realist determination of object as object attempts to maintain certainty over issues of truth and falsity, but cannot deal with issues of good/bad. The idealist determination of the ultimate ideal loses itself in faith: either in God or some absolute ego-structure. Both approaches have made stunning contributions to human knowing. Realisms have gone beyond superstitions to demonstrate substantial facts. Idealisms have contributed to human self-knowledge by revealing a variety of the possible inner workings of human psyches. But, by locating all knowledge in the functioning of the human subject, they have overlooked or forgotten to look at the limit of the mysterious: being and time. For them, being is restricted to actual presences and time is necessarily frozen into an undifferentiated now.

In order to accept the interpretive method one must acknowledge one's finitude and historicity (historicality). Interpretive thinking turns on allowing that "historical knowledge of the past sets us before the totality of our human possibilities and therewith mediates us along with our future" (Gadamer, 1976/1981, p. 166). *Experience as interpretive phenomenology* is understandings that are transformative such that meanings and significances must be held open never to be completed.

For a group of thinkers the resulting subject-object split does not admit of closure. It is to three of these thinkers that I will now turn. They include Martin Heidegger, Hans-Georg Gadamer, and Jean-Luc Nancy. Heidegger is *the* pivotal thinker by which we are enabled to get beyond the subject-object paradigm of Greco-European metaphysics. Gadamer, a student of Heidegger, focuses his thinking on the play of direct human experience as given by historical situatedness vis-à-vis language as essential conversation and dialogue. Nancy extends Heidegger's project by working to extend the latter's exposition of the everyday. For him the world is and cannot be other than shared meanings.

Martin Heidegger: The Releasment of Time

Time is four-dimensional: The *first* dimension, which gathers everything, is *nearness*.

(Heidegger, 1967/1998a, p. 286)[2]

Heidegger's project was not existentialism. Nor was it the traditional sense of being (Sheehan, 1995a, pp. 157–158). Heidegger's project was to release time from the fetters imposed on it by modernist methodologies as they became articulated by their various realisms and idealisms. Heidegger's method, if we can label it as such, is the way-ness of a way. He has written that "A way *leads* through an area; it opens itself up and opens up the area. A way is therefore the same as the process of passage from something to something else. It is way as *being-on-the-way*" (Heidegger, 1967/1998b, p. 222).

Retrieval as being on the way has the character of movement. It consists, as Sheehan (1983) writes, "in letting possibility remain possibility, letting appearance appear by not directly appearing . . . a matter simply 'being-underway,' where the only operative authority is the ineluctable movement of disclosure" (p. 133). I propose that we release Richardson's terms of past, future, and present (Richardson, 1974, p. 612) into those that reflect Sheehan's notions of "letting into appearance" or "disclosing" (Sheehan, 1995a, pp. 161–172). In my judgment his translations, which grow out of the flux of movement, are closer to the fluidity that Heidegger worked to impart as the enactment of a rethinking of temporality.

Thereby, the temporalizing of retrieval can be thought of as the always already advening of three co-terminus moments: (a) the mediating "always already," (b) thought that lets the unsaid origin be revealed/concealed as "becoming," and (c) a "presence-to" that needs the unsaid to be brought into words. Human agency does not consist in being a passive receptor of phenomena, but is comportment that can deal with what self-shows as decisive. Heidegger wrote in *Being and Time* (1927/1962) that "retrieval does not re-actualize the past but responds to the already-possible" (pp. 437–438).

We belong to space and time as space-time where we are allowed presence to space as place, and as time is extended to us as if a gift. Time, as what is proper to temporality, is other than the undifferentiated now-points of a homogenized past, present and future. It advenes as the meaning of nearness as:

1. Keeping the past (as alreadiness) open by *denying* its advent as *the* present.
2. Preserving the openness of the approach coming from the future (as becoming) by *withholding* the present (as presence-to) in the approach.

3. The presencing out of presence-to, alreadiness and becoming—true time as the reaching out to each other of its ownmost constitutive moments. (Heidegger, 1968/1972, pp. 15–16)

In other words, authentic (proper) time will not allow itself to be brought to a stand.

Only homogenous, abstract time can be measurable. The proper temporality of openness dislocates the human as ultimate cause or agent from its traditionally determined central position in space and time. Dasein (as openness)[3] is a becoming absent (not as a past or a future) that brings it to how it is: finite. Proper or authentic temporality is not linear (Heidegger, 1989/1992a, p. 18E); it is how we all are always already brought together; brought near to each other (Heidegger, 1989/1992a, p. 21E; also see pp. 6E–11E for a point by point explication of Dasein as openness). In *The Concept of Time* (1989/1992a) Heidegger explicates Dasein's proper temporality. It is especially important to note the mistranslation of the German term *das Vorbei,* which is "the absence" not "the past" of Dasein as openness.[4]

Temporality for Heidegger is not restricted to the determinations of time as past, present and future. These mostly measurable moments have obviously had great utility. But temporality as nearness reveals us as "always on-the-way . . . stretched out towards full self-presence . . . but never arriving. We do not 'possess' our lack-in-being; it possesses us and defines our essence" (Sheehan, 2001b, p. 17). We overlook or forget our mortality if we insist on some variation of permanence.

Retrieval becomes the retrieval of possibility as possibility, not of what one has lost, but of what is always already yet to come, and is, thereby, at least for Heidegger, the acceptance of our finitude.

ONESELF	Retrieval 1 = freeing-up of one's own mortality or of culturally inherited possibilities—happens implicitly
ONE'S INHERITED POSSIBILITIES	Retrieval 2 = expressly knowing the historical provenance of the possibilities one frees up so that one can preserve them in radical possibility

Retrievals 1 & 2 are not a revival of what-is-as-having-been but are the imperative to live into one's becoming (Sheehan, 1995b, pp. 220–221).

Heidegger, Dasein as Openness and Being-in-the-World

Who are we? We remain cautious in our answer.
(Heidegger, 1968/1972, p. 12)

If it can be demonstrated that realisms and idealisms have reached an intellectual/cognitive dead end, what is left? Heidegger moves beyond the subject–object paradigm in order to get behind/beyond/prior to theological, psychological, biological, and/or idealized notions that attempt to freeze the nature of being human. His answer was *Dasein*. *Dasein* in German means existence. But Heidegger saw the need to get beyond existence as some fixed physical reality (realism) or eternal ideal (idealism). In his work Dasein as openness evolves as an open region where possibilities arrive and leave. Dasein as openness is Heidegger's retrieval of what it means to be human from the hypostasizing certainty claims of post-Cartesian thought.

Through the path of his thinking, Dasein as openness moves from center stage as the finite locus of occurrence to an integral part of what is.

In *Being and Time* (Heidegger, 1927/1962) being-*open* (*Da*-sein) means *being-*open (Da-*sein*). The 'Da' [of Da-sein] is determined here as "the open." This openness has the character of space [[as room]]. Spatiality [[roominess]] belongs to the clearing. (Heidegger, 1987/2001b, p. 225; also see Lovitt, 1977, p. xxxv n.2)

In the *Zollikon Seminars* (1987/2001b), Heidegger distills Dasein as openness down to three terms: Thrownness, Understanding, and Language. In turn each of these must take into account two interrelated phenomena: being and time. Being as what is ownmost to existing and temporality as nearness.

Thrownness and understanding mutually belong together in a correlation whose unity is determined through language. (p. 139)

Only on the basis of the belonging together of thrownness and understanding through language as saying is the human being able to be addressed by beings. (p. 139)

These phenomena are interpreted by Heidegger to be coterminous, that is they must advene together. They cannot be separated as quanta.

Thrownness

> Thrownness is neither a 'fact that is finished' nor a Fact that is settled.
>
> (Heidegger, 1927/1962, p. 223)

The open is here *already*. Thrownness includes mortality, situatedness, society, mutual interaction, things as available, presence–absence, building, and the capacity for thinking interpretively.

The "facticity" of Dasein as openness consists in its being handed over to its "can-be." Dahlstrom (2001) succinctly states that "facticity is not to be identified with the character of some brute fact ascertainable by perception observation and the like" (p. 298). Dasein as openness *has to be* and is able to be in some way.

Understanding

> All interpretation is grounded in understanding.
>
> (Heidegger, 1927/1962, p. 195)

Humans *must* take what is available as something. Understanding is already given as a capacity for utility, a surplus of meaning, and dwelling as possibility. Understanding for Heidegger is not primordially a cognitive representational process. It is the immediate givenness of the world one (Dasein) is thrown into (Heidegger, 1927/1962, pp. 182–195).

As thrownness "the [temporal] ecstatic [as not bound by the static] relationship [to the world] . . . is a basic structure of being human. What is founded in it, is that openness according to which the human being is always already addressed by beings other than himself [*sic*]. The human being could not live without this being addressed" (Heidegger, 1987/2001b). We are addressed by things other than us and *as* our own bodying forth. If we understand bodying forth in a more inclusive way, we are enabled to understand that openness as being-in-the-world is not completed in terms of mere sense perceptions.

In Heidegger's (1987/2001b) interpretation "*understanding* may be used only regarding an insight . . . [as] how something is connected with something else" (p. 186). He wants us to remember (retrieve) that "natural science according to its own means (method) cannot understand the link from seen object via perception as 'transformed' in the cerebral cortex" (p. 197). The "link" is the "as" of taking something as something.

There is no autonomous decontextualized relationship from object to subject. Any "understanding of being . . . belongs to being-in-the-world. . . . *Bodying forth* as such belongs to being-in-the-world" (p. 196).

Heidegger's (1987/2001b) analytic of openness was to understand comportment as an engagement of oneself that both sustains what beings are *as* presence-to, and one's comportment toward their being available *as* usefully understood (p. 198). The as-structure of interpretation is a kind of ongoing *circular circulation*. When any individuals say *as*, they "are always dealing with a predication of something about something" (p. 145). Heidegger's project was to explicate existence as an openness that is coterminous with a clearing. Openness as not opened by any agent and clearing as the necessary place of our comportment. He can then assert that "being open is only possible when the clearing has already happened to us, so that something can be present or absent. The being open 'to' lies in the manifestness of presence. There would be no relationship without it" (p. 145).

Language

The word—no thing, nothing that is, no being: but we have an understanding of things when the word for them is available. Then the thing "is."

(Heidegger, 1959/1971c, p. 87)

We should not forget that being is a question, not an ultimate cause, and that "manifestations of [b]eing to the human being does not mean, by any means, that [b]eing as such, or indeed its manifestness, is apprehended explicitly and thematically by the human being and by philosophical thought" (Heidegger, 1987/2001b, p. 121).

Humans *must* discourse. Humans are utilized to listen to the saying of the soundless. I am using "utilize" not in a theological or instrumental sense, but in the sense of the necessary reciprocity that obtains as any and all complexes of involvements that we find ourselves, as Dasein as openness, delivered over to. Silence, naming, recollective thinking, poesy, philosophical thinking, interpretive retrieval, and freedom-for all turn on discursive possibilities. Heidegger's work sought to broaden our relation to language. Language certainly is grammar, communication, utile, metaphorical, and so on. But he wants us to allow language to speak for itself. For him, naming and thing cannot be separated, as doctrinaire nominalisms would have it. This also means that any theoretical positions on how and why human language developed, while of interest, do not reach the heart of the matter.

What is at stake in language is how it is when it says "world": world as totality of significance involvements. Thus, for him "the usual meanings given-to-language are constrictions" that reveal themselves as a limit that can be looked on in what they self-conceal (Heidegger, 1987/2001b, p. 200). In an ontological sense, this concealing should not be looked on as a conscious scheme by some targeted elite force. Interpretive thought does not necessarily ignore repressive or exploitative political or economic phenomena but holds them open as they present themselves.

Everyday usage of language can be a phenomenon of "using-up"—a flattening. Heidegger (1959/1971c) struggled "to show possibilities that will allow us to become mindful of language and our relation to it" (p. 58). He worked to retrieve a hidden possibility; to prepare or enable the revealing of a transformative experience with language as a saying that gathers (p. 62). In uncovering the hidden "the reflective use of language cannot be guided by the common, usual understandings of meanings; rather, it must be guided by the hidden riches that language holds in store for us, so that these riches may summon us for the saying of language" (p. 91). Interpretive practices (ontologies) are always already an integral part of any saying. Language is more than saying or discursivity. It belongs to the play of time-space. It "gives us room and allows us to do something, gives us a possibility, that is, it gives what enables, means something else and something more than mere opportunity" (p. 93).

What does this "saying" of language mean for us? Humans are free for a range of possibilities. In general to say "means to show; to make appear, set free, that is, to offer and extend what we call World, lighting and concealing it" (Heidegger, 1959/1971c, p. 93). Humans can decide and choose whether they listen or do not listen.

As the play of openness, "the human being has something to say because saying, as letting-see, is a letting-see of something as such and such a being" (Heidegger, 1987/2001b, p. 90). Choice and decision are given by the fact that humans can never effect a completion in terms of a universal linguistic meaning but must always be ready for linguistic meaning that exceeds that which is given at any one place.

Heidegger wants us to let ourselves be involved with language in a richer way. For him a word is not an object relationship. Words disclose as they open up (Heidegger, 1987/2001b, p. 185). Language turns on the significance of an encountering where "every spoken word is already an answer" (Heidegger, 1959/1971f, p. 129). The saying of language does not exclude silence or what is not said. Thought interpretively, we come to the place where, "To speak means to say, which means to show and to let [something] be seen. It means to communicate and, correspondingly, to listen, to submit oneself to a claim addressed to oneself and to comply and respond to it" (Heidegger, 1987/2001b, p. 215).

Language needs humans to speak being. Being, as such, always already advenes as something humans must discourse about. So we see that "*language* is identical with the understanding of [b]eing, and without this one could not experience death as death, that is, as the uttermost possibility approaching Da-sein" as openness (Heidegger, 1987/2001b, p. 220).

Linguisticality exceeds finite mortals in that there is always an unsaid that cannot be specifically said—that is, mortality not as a death event, but mortality as an always already possibility. Gadamer writes that the necessary "'essence' of the word does not lie in being totally expressed, but rather in what is left unsaid, as we see especially in speechlessness and remaining silent" (Gadamer, 1967/1976a, p. 234). Our finitude turns on a phenomenon that does not and cannot admit of specificity.

Fundamentally, "the 'as' connotes discursiveness, not only as a human possibility but above all as a human necessity. We are 'condemned' to (or thrown into) relating to things mediately and discursively" (Sheehan, 1995a, p. 276). This obtains whether the things or others present to us are physically here or not here. Whether the "I" is here, or *as* a possible not, is not an issue of doubting one's existence or the existence of any external object. First and foremost there is involvement with the manifestness of entities we are thrown into.

Thrownness, understanding, and language are the moments where Heidegger's thought turns on the possibility of what it means to be properly (authentically) human. His earlier writings explicated this as "openness whereby sense-as-such is generated" (Sheehan, 1978, p. 313). This was specifically taken over as being-ahead-of-oneself-unto death. Later writings elaborated on this by discussing mortals as those who are apportioned openness and aheadness as possibility (p. 313). The latter is pursued by Heidegger in his writings that turn on the fourfold of earth, sky, mortals, and divinities.[5] Openness as a complex of ongoing meaning relationships is a response to "the summons of the fourfold" (Heidegger,

1954/1993a, pp. 351–363). The play of the above "moments" is, for him, one of their mutual belonging together as they reflect each other. To free these moments into their essence as "world" is an essential choice or decision to be made on how incessant practice and long experience of thinking is to be entered into (p. 362).

Retrieval turns on the possibility of any presence-to anything that is available as always already given by the absence of any determinable (by theory or scientific research) origin or by an equally undeterminable future, which can only be anticipated, which, in turn, can only be "concretized" as becoming. What is fundamentally proper to humanity is its finiteness as mortal being-in-the-world of infinite possibilities as given and as announced to us by the possibility of our very own absence. This announcement is other than mere irony, it is the call to which we must respond.

Insofar as we can use the term in the current technical sense, Heidegger's "method" *is* his enactment of thinking such that he is always already being-underway, drawn by *"the possibility whereby any given present moment understands how to be becoming"* (Heidegger, 1989/1992a, p. 20E; translation modified by Sheehan, 1999). Hermeneutical and other approaches to interpretive phenomenology turn on this "first principle." The discussion of "waiting" in "Conversation on a Country Path" (Heidegger, 1959/1966, pp. 67–69) is a later version of this thinking, where waiting is an enacting service to thinking. The caring explicated in *Being and Time* is transformed into an allowing of oneself to be possessed (claimed) by temporality.

Heidegger and Method

We must proceed on the "path toward" ourselves. But this is no longer the path toward a merely isolated, principally singular I.

(Heidegger, 1987/2001b, p. 110)

Becoming as the step back into our origin is a return to the elements of thrownness, understanding, and language that we are always already right at and cannot leave (Richardson, 1974). In section 7 of *Being and Time* (1927/1962), "The Phenomenological Method of Investigation," Heidegger writes that "The expression 'phenomenology' signifies a *methodological conception*" (pp. 49–63) characterized as the how of the philosophical research. Heidegger appropriates Husserl's slogan "To the things [matters] themselves." It should be taken into consideration that the operative word for both Husserl and Heidegger is "to." The term "matters" can be construed as either matters of concern to conceptualization or as matters that can be physically or theoretically determined via empirical determinations. Phenomena, either ontic, ontological, or mathematical can appear-as, disappear-as, be covered over-as, be forgotten-as, be absent-as, that is, the play of presence and absence as the self-giving of phenomena (Heidegger, 1927/1962). The play space of "letting something be seen . . . of the phenomenology of Dasein . . . is a *hermeneutic* . . . where it designates this business of interpreting" (pp. 58–62). Letting something be seen from itself is a conscious effort to get beyond the givens of some foreclosed present.

For Heidegger (1927/1962), then:

Ontology and phenomenology are not two distinct philosophical disciplines among others. These terms characterize philosophy itself with regard to its object and its way of treating that object. Philosophy is universal phenomenological ontology, and takes its departure from the hermeneutic of Dasein, which as an analytic of *existence,* has made fast the guiding-line for all philosophical inquiry at the point where it *arises* and to which it *returns.* (p. 62)

The hermeneutic of Dasein as openness was Heidegger's jumping off point from the guiding question of metaphysics, What is a being?; to his later thought revealed in his grounding question, What is the truth of be-ing (Heidegger, 1989/1999, p. 120)? How can we articulate, as demanded, by our fundamental discursiveness, the play of what comes to be seen, experienced, that which we are possessed by, but cannot possess? It can be claimed that there is a need for this to be effectuated whether we ignore it or not.

Later in his career, Heidegger drops the term method, unless it is to discuss its changed meaning. His project moves to thinking as a "step-back" (Heidegger, 1957/1969, pp. 49–74). The step back is not a return to some idealized epoch or ego-subject in order to effect an infinite repeatability but is a preparatory readiness to think in the face of what seems to be the most obvious or simple. A leap is required; one that accepts the possibility that results cannot be guaranteed.

The motto Heidegger chose for his collected works was *ways not works*. He did not articulate a method per se but, like his student Gadamer, thought that the methodologies as practiced by science were a symptom of the closures effected by the advent of "techno-scientism" (cf. the essays in *The Question Concerning Technology*). For him "all was way" (Heidegger, 1959/1971c, p. 92) and "following the movement of showing" (Heidegger, 1968/1972, p. 2).

I believe Heidegger is best read as he enacts a movement of showing, not as whether he is right or wrong. Heidegger enacts showing in his works when he begins with the most ordinary and obvious descriptions of phenomena. He proceeds to turn and return his readings to phenomena in order to give richer counter-resonances to their self-circulating. As I am on my way through this explication I will attempt to bring forth some circulations that have grown out of Heidegger's pioneering thinking.

Hans-Georg Gadamer: History, Experience, and Conversation

My paradigm of teaching and learning is the Socratic conversation, the question and answer between individuals who embody the pedagogical scene concretely in ever shifting and undefined ways, such that their respective identities may be thrown into doubt.

(Heidegger, 1945/2002, p. 41)

With these words, Heidegger positioned himself in a tradition that began with Plato's Socratic dialogues. Gadamer's project turns on working to come to mutual understandings via conversation and dialogue. If Heidegger's major project was to release thinking from the ossified dead end of the subject-object paradigm, Gadamer's work turned on the possibilities that are at play in "a reflection on what a human organization and shape of life is, can be." Philosophical hermeneutics "is not itself the art of understanding but only the philosophy of understanding" (Gadamer, 1997/1997, p. 52).

I will be using "interpretation" and "hermeneutics" interchangeably. In "A Dialogue on Language" (Heidegger, 1959/1971a, pp. 9–13, 29) Heidegger discussed his going beyond the use of the term hermeneutics.

It is my reading that this was an attempt by him to include a richer conception of dialogue in his work, especially to effect understandings with other traditions of thought. Any attempt to concretize the netherworld of human psychological phenomena or functioning is, for Gadamer, a practice that is the purview of disciplines other than philosophy.

Gadamer's (1967/1976d) elaboration of Heidegger's threefold description of Dasein as openness consists of historically effected consciousness (pp. 18–43), experience and conversation/dialogue. These are, in turn, the manifestations of a kind of participatory play, which "exists in and for those who play it, even if one is only participating as 'spectator'" (Gadamer, 1997/1997, p. 27). Play in Gadamer's writings is a back and forth involvement mutually belonging to the participants, be they individuals, texts or text analogues, productions, or things of nature other than humans. This conception of play is one without winners or losers but is not without rules. But these "rules" are of a different order from those established by grounding them in some transcendental consciousness. Like Heidegger, Gadamer works to pursue phenomena as they lay claim to us.

Gadamer's contribution to our being-on-the-way is the weaving of his thoughts of "play" and language with history, understanding, and speaking as conversation and dialogue. In his essay "Man [sic] and Language" (Gadamer, 1967/1976b, p. 64–68) he discusses three things that are peculiar to language as we are with it.

The first is that we are not consciously aware of grammatical structures when we are involved in everyday saying. The "real being" of language here is "what is said in it" as "it constitutes the common world in which we live" (p. 65). Grammatically incorrect double negatives, disagreement of verbs and nouns and group specific idioms (the figurative, the ambiguous, the metaphorical, the "mispronounced") are all readily understood by the participants of a given group. The *Chomskian hardwired grammar* is derivative of our historically effected meaning. We are first delivered over to meanings, not to abstract rules of grammar.

The second aspect of language for Gadamer is its "I-lessness" (p. 65). Language that speaks must be participatory. Its play is one-among-others. The ongoing movement of experience and understanding is always present.

The third is what Gadamer calls "the universality of language" (1967/1976b, p. 67). He brings up the example of translation in order to clarify his remarks. The task of translators must never be to copy what is said, but to place themselves in the meanings that belong to what is said in order to carry over what is said into the direction of their own saying. This endeavor has the possibility of avoiding a flattening of meaning that suppresses the range of meaning in the original saying.

For Gadamer then, the play of retrieval consists, in part, of acknowledging that "language is the real medium of human being" (Gadamer, 1967/1976b, p. 68). Gadamer admonishes us to see language as a realm that it alone fills out. Language is the realm of human beings with one another as common understandings and their continually replenished agreement/disagreements. Human existence depends on language games for everything we learn (Gadamer, 1967/1976b, p. 56). It is as necessary as the air we breathe.

One of the most misunderstood notions of Gadamer's writings is his notion of our being fundamentally "guided by preconceptions and anticipations in our talking in such a way that these continually remain hidden" (Gadamer, 1967/1976f, p. 92). The English translation of this notion is "prejudice," a word that has called out a misunderstanding that avers that Gadamer is in favor of arbitrary forms of discrimination. To my mind, the more important dialogue is effected when the examination of all preconceptions is a pivotal issue in *all* thinking.

For Gadamer, prejudice includes more than the generalized notion of unfounded discriminatory actions. It also includes those that pose as self-evident certainty. This can include ideology as well as any pretensions of being free of all prejudice. Philosophical hermeneutics as practiced by Gadamer makes the claim that its acknowledgment of its own possible prejudice is the first necessary step to the retrieval of any prejudice that is naively covered over. Open conversation/dialogue lets what is outside of a given point of view merge with it in order to generate a new one. For Gadamer the final product is not a synthesis, because the point of the other must be defended even in its stringent opposition. If there is a problem here, it is how an "unyielding repetitiousness characteristic of all dogmatism" (1967/1976f, p. 92) is to be overcome. Is there an aporia between what is revealed and what is enforced? Can any transcendental consciousness be determined once and for all?

To be nondiscursive is not an option for participatory humans (Dasein as openness). We are immersed in language as "the medium in which substantive understanding and agreement take place between two people" (Gadamer, 1960/1990, p. 384). David E. Linge, in his "Editor's

Introduction" to *Philosophical Hermeneutics* (1976) writes: "the 'thrownness' of Dasein is elaborated by Gadamer in his conception of the interpreter's inevitable involvement in effective history" (p. xlviii). Our history
is what self-effects; we *are* this history. For Gadamer (1967/1976e), it is
not possible for any interpretive method to be learned independently
from its application and consequences; its meaning.

Historically Effected Consciousness

> In living one always finds oneself already in a situation that is conditioned by
> effective history, . . . one can never by means of reflection place oneself in an
> externalized relation to one's situation.
>
> (Gadamer, 1994/2001, p. 46)

Consciousness here is not the central notion of the modern tradition,
that is, that human cognition is the determinant for everything that is.
For Gadamer, history gives in advance what objects we take as the most
worthy of inquiry. There is immediate experience; this is true. But humans forget that there is a possibility that this immediacy may conceal
more than it shows.

> [W]e are always already affected by history. It determines in advance both what
> seems to us worth inquiring about and what will appear as an object of investiga-
> tion, and we more or less forget half of what is really there—in fact, we miss the
> whole truth of the phenomenon—when we take its immediate appearance as the
> whole truth. (Gadamer, 1960/1990, p. 300)

The mission that claims techno-scienticism is to so objectify all forms of
experience such that any element of history that allows for thoughtful
experiences other than that of rationality and logic is excluded (p. 346).

In hermeneutic interpretation, time is not an unknown to be solved
for: "time is no longer primarily a gulf to be bridged because it separates;
it is actually the supportive ground of the course of events in which the
present is rooted" (Gadamer, 1960/1990, p. 297). What is proper to temporality is that human existing is more or less continuously made up of
multiple attachments (jointures) to multiple standpoints. There is no permanent horizon line (Gadamer, 1960/1990).

There is a mystery that dwells in a free openness, wherein we can
"learn by letting it say something to us" (Heidegger, 1968/1972, p. 66).
History is a mystery that "does not belong to us, we belong to it" (Gadamer,

1960/1990, p. 276). It is a self-revealing that arrives prior to any of our self-understandings. We comport ourselves as if the way of the family, society and state is self-evident. The focus on ourselves can be a distorting mirror. Any individual self-awareness of any individual "is only a flickering in the closed circuits of historical life" (p. 276). Thus Gadamer can claim that the presuppositions of individuals outweigh their judgments in the constitution of the historical reality of their existing.

Experience

> The truth of experience always implies an orientation toward new experience.
>
> (Gadamer, 1960/1990, p. 355)

In conversation, Gadamer mentions that he regards the chapter on experience to be the centerpiece of *Truth and Method* (1994/2001, p. 53). For Gadamer, experience turns on a richer conception of temporality. Proper experience is one that does not fulfill an expectation and can never be repeated exactly. It can only be retrieved as interpretation. All interpretive experience is linguistic, therefore, "the pure transcendental subjectivity of the ego is not really given as such but always given in the idealization of language; moreover, language is already present in any acquisition of experience" (Gadamer, 1960/1990, p. 348). Language is beyond/other than any idealizations. The form that the verbal takes and the content of tradition cannot be separated in interpretive experience (Gadamer, 1960/1990, p. 441). Experience is an essentially negating process, not describable as a string of continuous generation of idealized universals that give determinable results. Properly thought, experience takes place as typical when the generalizable is continually altered and thereby refuted (Gadamer, 1960/1990).

Experience always already arrives as (Gadamer, 1960/1990):

1. "an orientation toward new experience" (p. 355),
2. the genuine as the "experience of one own historicity" (p. 357),
3. co-terminus with understanding (p. 259). The origin of the openness that is being-in-the-world is not a "resigned ideal."

Gadamer's thinking of understanding manifests itself as:

1. "the original characteristic of the being of human life itself" (p. 259),
2. "the fusion of those horizons supposedly existing by themselves" (p. 306),

3. "always interpretation" (p. 307),
4. "the efficacy of history at work" (p. 456),
5. a moment that is constant from whole to part and back (p. 291),
6. essentially circular (p. 293),
7. not as a psychic transposition (p. 395).

As we experience and understand we do not recognize the power of effective history as it is integral to our understanding as such. In fundamentally Heideggerian terms, Gadamer explicates history as the always effectual. The questions we ask are founded by our self-finding. That is, we are always already within a situation, or better, we *are* a situation. Bringing the play of its relationships into a light can never be a finished task (Gadamer, 1960/1990, p. 301). Hopes and fears, for example, participate in what is nearest—we approach them as the alreadiness of their past influence. Our interpretive (hermeneutical) situation brings our prejudices with us. Our particular present as a presence-to something is a continuous arriving of necessities that we must test. Prejudices, presuppositions, and biases as horizons "of the present cannot be formed without the past" (Gadamer, 1960/1990, p. 306). These all draw into a future that is "finite becoming." A contribution that interpretive scholarship can make is to uncover what is currently covered over, but always with the presupposition that any interpretation can never be complete.

Horizons are necessarily "fused" or brought together, whether as conflict or harmony whereby the tension/compression interplay is an encountering experience. The historicality of a text or text analogue is mediated by a consciousness that is effected *as* history. Interpretive practices strive to bring-out, as a bringing-into-nearness, jointures as they come together and fly apart (Gadamer, 1960/1990, p. 306). One is called on to experience thinking in such a way that the self-bringing "about this fusion in a regulated way is the task of . . . historically effected consciousness" as a self-occurring (circular) occurrence (Gadamer, 1960/1990, p. 307). Perhaps this can be looked on as a series of concentric rings whose source fades into an absence that must be present as an origin and whose ownmost essence ever widens into an unknowable possibility of a "butterfly wing hypothesis."[6]

Learning a language exemplifies what is ownmost to experience. The experience of learning our first language is not a private experience. Learning a second language grows out of differentiating it from our first.

The experience of learning additional languages is akin to the interpretive process as they have their own meaning horizons and preset rules.

In this way, "to have learned a foreign language and to be able to understand it" is an exercise of capacity for understanding such that it "always means that what is said has a claim over one, and this is impossible if one's own 'worldview and language-view' is not also involved" (Gadamer, 1960/1990, p. 442). From out of this experience we can begin to see how our situatedness gives interpretations that continuously need adjustments in order to more adequately understand not only another language experience, but the ensemble of phenomena that we become thrown into.

We, each one of us, begin as co-undergoing a verbally constituted experience of the world. This occurs as what is meaningful and significant, not as a calculated product. Moral or ethical thought is able to recognize this. However "the methodological ideal or rational construction that dominates modern mathematically based natural science," is by nature removed from decisions of this kind (Gadamer, 1960/1990, p. 456). Thus because "language characterizes our human experience of the world in general," historically effected consciousness is essentially realized in language. World cannot be objectified in language. As well, any putative historical effect cannot be interpreted via hermeneutical consciousness (Gadamer, 1960/1990, p. 456). The effects of history can be the subject of interpretive practices, but can never be frozen in place and time.

The thinking of interpreters must deal with what words of a tradition reach them. Hermeneutic/interpretive practice releases control of words and their tradition to history in order to allow them to be listened to. "That to which we are to listen really encounters us and does so as if it addressed us and is concerned with us" (Gadamer, 1960/1990, p. 461). It is important here to note the use of the hermeneutic or interpretive "as" is not a representation of some mystical power, but generates ways in order to reveal how practices are listened to and seen.

Thus Gadamer writes that "If we stress . . . the fact of something's coming into language as what really occurs in the event of language, we are preparing a place for the hermeneutical experience" (1960/1990, p. 471).

Conversation and Dialogue

All life communities are speech communities,
and language is only language in conversation.

(Gadamer, 1994/2001, p. 152)

Every word causes the whole of the language to which it belongs to resonate and the whole worldview that underlies it to appear (Gadamer, 1960/1990). Every word is the eventuation of a moment. Every word carries with it the unsaid to which humans must relate to its summons with a response. Human speech cannot be considered imperfect if it is fluid and bound to context. Its logic is its power to bring meanings forth. The power of meaning is that it can never be exhausted by speech.

Interpretation cannot start from any other place than that of somebody who has a necessary connection to a tradition that is already a linguistic speaking out (Gadamer, 1960/1990). It is incumbent on the interpreter (as hermeneut) to discover the standpoint or horizon of the other via conversation and dialogue. This intelligibility does not necessarily entail agreement (Gadamer, 1960/1990). As one thinks historically, one arrives at an understanding of the meaning of what is already freed up as tradition (Sheehan, 1978).

The art of conversation "includes the art of having a conversation with oneself and fervently seeking an understanding of oneself" The art of thinking "means the art of seriously questioning what one really means when one thinks or says this or that. In doing so, one sets out on a journey, or better is already on the journey" (Gadamer, 1997/1997, pp. 33–34). Proper dialogue is involvement with one's traveling partners but not as an idealized, unattainable empathy. In "genuine dialogue something emerges that is contained in neither of the partners" (Gadamer, 1960/1990, p. 462); that is to say, what is ownmost to dialogue is revealed as revealing.

One of Gadamer's pivotal presuppositions is that there is "no transcendental principle of the self" (Gadamer, 1997/1997, p. 37). Therefore any self is inextricably part of the complexity that has been discussed as "world." Any putative reality beyond a given conception of "self" can become visible only via the medium of language (Gadamer, 1960/1990). Thus Gadamer emphasizes that *language is the universal medium in which understanding occurs. Understanding occurs in interpreting*" (Gadamer, 1960/1990, p. 389).

In terms of interpretive practices, language is more than a mere possession. In fact humans do not possess language at all; language possesses humans. Without language humans would not be in a world at all (Gadamer, 1960/1990). As being-in-the world, Dasein as openness is other than what can merely be determined by biological sciences, ego psychology, or theology. But as inclusive of these determinations, openness is coterminously determined and determining. To interpret this play "[w]e must be ready and willing to listen. Such readiness allows us to surmount the boundaries in which all customary views are confined, and to reach a more open territory" (Heidegger, 1954/1968, p. 13). The communities inherent in humans living a life are only possibilized as conversation and dialogue (Gadamer, 1994/2001).

Our whole experience of the world is made possible from *"language as a medium"* (Gadamer, 1960/1990, p. 457). This is especially true of thinking as hermeneutical/interpretive experience. All interpretations necessarily adapt themselves to the hermeneutical situation to which they belong. The hermeneutical situation turns on the truth of language as it occurs as tradition. In turn, "language has its true being only in dialogue, in *coming to an understanding*" (1960/1990, p. 446).

Understanding as fore-understanding comes first (Heidegger, 1927/1962, p. 191). In other words, we do not first deal with objects and/or subjects as mental constructs. We are always already actively engaged in purposes. The medium of language is what lets any object come into words: a mutual belonging of interpreters and language obtains (Gadamer, 1960/1990, p. 389). Letting come into words entails a hearing that engages us *as mortals* who are always already attuned (needed and employed) by the play of what determines us as mortals (Heidegger, 1957/1991).

I will proffer an example in order to bring what Heidegger, Gadamer, and Nancy are working to explicate via discussions of attunement into clearer focus. I once attended a musical performance where a Beethoven string quartet was performed by an ensemble playing matched Stradivarius instruments. An attunement obtained as the advent of a complex of instrument quality, interpretive performance skills, a magisterial composition, and the involved attention of the audience.

In this example, the elegance of the Stradivarius instruments needed us all as participants to enable (use) them in order for them to be what they already were. The musicians and the attendees did not sit around and weigh and measure or otherwise stare at the instruments and sheet music. The concert was not a linguistic experience as defined by parameters that turn on the operation of rules of vocalization and grammar. On the other hand it was, it could not have occurred without, the interpretive saying of language in all of its ontic and ontological ramifications and the attuned response of the attendees. We were enabled (claimed) by the necessary usage of the instruments *as* a revealing of their ownmost "need-to-be-used" in order for them to be what they already were. Conjointly, as present to this experience, all participants were the play of the nearness of what they already were. Thereby the context became itself, not as a tautology given by the rules of calculative logic, but as a revealing whose origin is concealed within itself.

Hermeneutic interpretation and understanding "need" and are "used" by each other to the extent that "understanding and interpretation are the same thing" (Gadamer, 1960/1990, p. 388). Subject and object as discrete originators of knowledge disappear as the reciprocating play of question and answer is enacted. The hermeneutic circle turns as "the questioner becomes the one who is questioned" (Gadamer, 1960/1990, p. 462). Interpreting is realized as the ongoing dialectic of question and answer.

Gadamer and Method

A word is always an answer.
(Gadamer, 1967/1976e, p. 151)

Echoes of Heidegger resound in Gadamer's work. He too articulates interpretive thinking in light of modern science as a rigid technoscienticism and "its effort to put knowledge into the hands of its anonymous society of investigators" (Gadamer, 1997/1997, p. 37). He writes that the methodological ideal of modern science "ensures that every one of its steps can be traced to the elements from which its knowledge is built up, while the teleological units of significance such as 'thing' or 'organic whole' lose their legitimacy" (Gadamer, 1960/1990, p. 459). In order to keep possibilities open, Gadamer stresses the need for continual questioning. For him questions do not presuppose any answer. He offers that "the essence of the *question* is to open up possibilities and keep them open" (p. 299). Interpretive questioning is always preparatory and requires readiness to listen. An interpreter (hermeneut) is "a person trying to understand a text and is prepared for it to tell him [*sic*] something" (p. 269).

How does one listen? There are a variety of aspects of which I will list a few (Gadamer, 1960/1990).

1. The understanding of something written is not a repetition of something past but the sharing of a present meaning (p. 392).
2. Hermeneutic work is based on a polarity of familiarity and strangeness. Here too there is a tension. It is in the play between the traditionary text's strangeness and familiarity to use, between being historically intended, distanciated object and belonging to a tradition. *The true locus of hermeneutics is this in-between* (p. 295).
3. The work of hermeneutics "is not to develop a procedure of understanding, but to clarify the conditions in which understanding takes place" (p. 295).
4. Certain "critical" methods in so far as they pretend to objectivity "are concerned to guarantee that . . . basic experiences can be repeated by anyone" (p. 347).
5. "An instrumentalist theory of signs which see words and concept as handy tools has missed the point of the hermeneutical phenomenon. . . . [C]oncepts are constantly in the process of being formed. . . . [U]nderstanding always includes an element of application and thus produces an ongoing process of concept formation. . . . [W]e must recognize that understanding is interwoven with concepts and reject any theory that does not accept the intimate unity of word and subject matter" (p. 403).

The above five aspects of listening attempt to correct previous assumptions about the nature of experience, tradition, and language. For the methodology of modern science, "experience is valid only if it is confirmed; hence its dignity depends on its being in principle repeatable" (Gadamer, 1960/1990, p. 347). Husserl's work can be read as attempting to take the idealized world of scientism into some original experience of the world. His work attempted to make perception per se, as directed toward some unspecified external physical appearance, the basis for experience as such (Gadamer, 1960/1990). Gadamer's task was to demonstrate that history was always at work prior to any perceptual uptake.

Wherever words are thought to be merely a sign function, any original joining of speaking and thinking is reduced to an instrumental relationship. Science is self-required to think language as a fixed set of relationships, which in turn is the manifestation of forgetting that the essence of living language continues. The scientific ideal of an unambiguous designation is an unattainable ideal (Gadamer, 1960/1990).

Instrumental relationships are part and parcel of being-in-the-world. But they fundamentally depend on contexts that shift historically and therefore cannot be considered final. Any ongoing "assimilation is no mere reproduction or repetition of the traditionary text; it is a new creation of understanding" (Gadamer, 1960/1990, p. 473). Creations of instrumental understandings are in play as history. For Gadamer as well as Heidegger, "it is . . . the game itself that plays" as the unfolding of our fundamental practices (Gadamer, 1960/1990, p. 490).

To be human is to understand, whether as an involvement with tools, in a tradition, or as an interpreter. Interpretive "understanding in the human sciences shares one fundamental condition with the life of tradition; it lets itself be *addressed* by tradition. . . . The objects that the human sciences investigate, just as for the contents of tradition, that what they are really about, can be experienced only when one is addressed by them" (Gadamer, 1960/1990, p. 282). As the ones who understand we are "always already drawn into an event through which meaning asserts itself" (p. 490). This manifests itself as play, which as a concept "unites event and understanding in their interplay, and also the language games of our world experience" (p. 557), which, as the one and the many, we are always already involved with. Articulated discourse is a step-by-step unfolding of the unity of the word. This unity is what we say to one another in conjunction with all that is said to us (Gadamer, 1960/1990). In this way we are enabled to listen to the one and the many, but not as result.

Jean-Luc Nancy: The Self-Announcement of Meaning

. . . wherever the One becomes a problem,
the problem of the Many is present as well.
(Gadamer, 1968/1980, p. 132)

I take the above words as Gadamer's pointing us from Socratic dialogue, via Heidegger to Nancy. The one and the many belong to and are used by "meaning as meaning" and is necessary as a counter-resonating of human "being-together." In "Sharing Voices" (1990), Nancy writes

meaning must be given in advance to the interpreter. . . . How could there be meaning without a meaning of meaning itself, preliminary to the meaning which can comprehend the semantic as well as the controlling meaning of the "meaning"? (p. 215)

Any method, be it scientific or interpretive, has to deal with the problem of the one and the many. Science attempts to isolate entities in order to describe and quantify them and their relationships to others of like kind. However, when research on humans obtains, it is impossible to study the autonomous, isolated individual owing to the fact that ironically there would be no one available to study this wholly unobtainable entity.

Research in the health and human sciences requires at least one person studying one other person so there are always at least two people. Sophisticated technology cannot be read by a comatose patient! Even if the patient is cogent, he or she must be instructed in the rules for reading the technology. This must necessarily be done by another individual, who in turn must be part of a given community. The autonomous isolated individual is techno-scientism's chimera. Every individual is simultaneously the group or community in which they reside. Is it possible to reduce an individual human being to a discrete entity determinable by the necessary repeatability of the scientific method?

Nancy (1996/2000) points out the problems inherent in any conceptualization of a single being, human or otherwise. "Such a being, which would be its own foundation, origin, and intimacy, would be incapable of *[b]eing* in every sense that this expression can have" (p. 12), thereby only obtaining as an unresolveable contradiction in terms: an aporia.

Appearing is a co-appearing such that the meaning of "together" can never come to some equilibrium point; it oscillates continually and without end. Together obtains as "either the 'together' of juxtaposition *partes extra partes,* isolated and unrelated parts, or the 'together' of gathering *totum intra totum,* a unified totality, where the relation surpasses itself in being pure" (Nancy, 1996/2000, p. 60). Both of these positions necessarily presuppose some kind of isolated particulars. How is one to establish a relationship to it (Nancy, 1996/2000)? If we listen we can hear limit as it is announcing itself as the impossibility of the possibility of a pure locale situated as some atemporal phenomenon.

Meaning

the co-appropriation of meaning and the real is precisely that by which existence always precedes itself, as itself, that is to say, insofar as it is without essence—insofar as it is the without-essence.

(Nancy, 1993/1997, p. 76)

There is always already meaning. To declare that there is no meaning is a powerfully meaningful assertion. We are thrown into the world.
Nancy (1996/2000) does not articulate this as an existence/essence dichotomy but as a gathering wherein meaning occurs in the sense that we
are the medium that allows for the mix of self-production and circulation.

The circulation that we are must occur as that which we are necessarily immersed in and cannot be released from via *any* means. Nancy's
(1996/2000) way of putting this is thus: "There is no meaning if meaning
is not shared. Pure unshared presence—presence to nothing, of nothing,
for nothing—is neither present nor absent" (p. 2). In his own way, Nancy
follows Heidegger's thought that "the nothing" must obtain as a privation
which, in turn, is the presence of an absence.

Presence and absence always already come to pass as something.
Heidegger's term for this is "the turning" (1949/1977b, p. 41; 1989/1999,
p. 129) wherein humans are grounded in terms of the play of presence
and absence, not in terms of themselves. Meaning's touch brings itself
into play as its own singularity, which in turn turns on bringing it (meaning) into play. The conjoining back and forth of every touch of meaning is
such that an undefinable mutuality arrives as both question and mystery
for humans (Nancy, 1996/2000, p. 6).

Meaning always already obtains as:

1. "the possibility of significations" (Nancy, 1993/1997, p. 59),
2. presentation, coming into presence (Nancy, 1993/1997, p. 59),
3. "the with" (Nancy, 1996/2000, p. 83),
4. "right at" existence (Nancy, 1996/2000, p. 10),
5. the disposition of the between (Nancy, 1996/2000, p. 27),
6. without provenance (Nancy, 1993/1997, p. 60),
7. a self-giving and self-abandoning (Nancy, 1982/1990, p. 244),
8. a setting of us in motion as a community (Nancy, 1993/1997, p. 61).

The notion of co-appearance is central to Nancy's thought. Implicitly
present in the work of Heidegger and Gadamer, Nancy (1996/2000) focuses on co-appearance in order to explicate the nature of being-with.
He writes that "co-appearance . . . must signify . . . that 'appearing' (coming into the world and being in the world, or existence as such) is strictly
inseparable, indiscernible from the *cum* or the *with*, which is not only its
place and its taking place, but also—and this is the same thing—its fundamental ontological structure" (p. 61). Given this position on his part,

Nancy must take into account some interpretation of the individual. Singularities as strangeness are concentrated in "sudden and headlong precipitation" (p. 8). Ontologically speaking, we must allow this precipitation in order for there to be someone at all. The someone must spring forth coterminously with "world" as an arrival that issues forth as "the coming of the 'always already' and the 'everywhere'" (p. 83). Each belongs to this proper origin, which then is a sharing of "originarity and originality" (p. 83). As *non-locatable locales*, origins are discrete points of spacing between *the us*, coterminus with the rest of the world: the world as the *"between all beings"* (p. 19).

Between does not represent a measurable space. The between is taken as a relationship such as one between friends or the between of birth and death. When we speak of proximity ontologically or interpretively it includes nearness as space—as well as intimate partners. Every possible origin is at once the necessary together of what it is for and via the singular plural being-for: "[b]eing-many-together is the originary situation; it is even what defines a 'situation' in general" (Nancy, 1996/2000, p. 41). Prior to any object or subject there is origin originating as the time-space between singular plurals. It is not a matter of defining "being" as a term, it is a matter of accepting that "[b]eing absolutely does not preexist; nothing preexists; only what exists exists" (Nancy, 1996/2000, p. 29).

The mystery of being is historical in that it continues to be a phenomenon around which, at least for Greco-European thought, there is a swirl of controversy. When Nancy (1996/2000) writes that "[b]eing is only simultaneous with itself . . . assumes movement, displacement, and deployment" (p. 38), he is not attempting to deify being, but to leave it to itself. If we leave being as a concept in order to arrive at some other origin as beginning, we must still realize that "[b]eing is *with;* it is *as* the *with* of [b]eing itself (the co-being of [b]eing), so that [b]eing does not identify itself *as such* (*as [b]eing of the being*) but shows itself, *gives itself, occurs, dis-posed itself* (made event history, and world) as its own singular plural *with*" (p. 38). The with is not added to what is, but is what enables any interpretable immanence or intrinsic condition to become self-presented at all (p. 62).

Any "with" essentially advenes from nowhere, but is already. The "with" is a becoming such that as a mark inscribed over the between it both spans it and underpins it at the same time. As a joining it constitutes the coming together or splitting apart (Nancy, 1996/2000, p. 62). I read this as Nancy's attempt to articulate the between as an invisible, unmeasurable phenomenon that abides, as the interval that humans must be. This obtains for both space and time as they are seen to always already become as a unity (p. 6).[7]

The open as cleft, rift, furrow, resists closure, but at the same time it is what is given to us. We are free for looking at this as curse or as gift. Meaning as opening-of or opening-to does not admit of imprisonment, finality, or enclosure (Nancy, 1993/1997, p. 65). Thus, Nancy writes, "at the point where we would expect 'something,' a substance or a procedure, a principle or an end, a signification, there is nothing but the manner, that turn of the other access, which conceals itself in the very gesture wherein it offers itself to us—and whose concealing *is* the turning itself" (1996/2000, p. 14).

What is to be retrieved is not meaning or significations per se; we have not lost or forgotten them. But for Nancy "the modern age has been the access to signification as will to produce signification, while the ancient age entered signification as the ordering of the world" (1993/1997, pp. 28–29). The centrality of producing significations is now located for better or worse in human cognition. Perhaps our task can evolve to one where retrieval as retrieval becomes one of working with the danger inherent in the finite essence of that which cannot be brought to a close.

Figuration

Who could weigh, and on what scales, the "materiality" of weighing, on the one hand, and the "immateriality" of thought on the other?

(Nancy, 1993/1997, p. 75)

Meaning needs to present itself in such and such a way that as inappropriable it includes the possibility of its own absence. Figuration needs a place to be presented, to become exposed as figuration. Nancy (1982/1990, 1993/1997) does not explicate figuration as a representation or as a standing for something other in an ordering whether by a divine power or cognition's representings. If one understands figuration as mere form, which it is, from certain given perspectives, this restricts this term to an unwarranted confinement. If figuration is heard in a musical sense, it articulates itself as syncopation and counterpoint, as brief melodic or rhythmic motifs. This analogy to music can be extended such that even if absent, the musical performance is still present in memory. It is still in front of us as a figure.

Independent figurations as meaning clusters (complexes) are heard simultaneously in their passage from presence to absence and vice versa. Figuration here can thereby be understood as the play of understandings-as. It is thus the circulation of the given and the taken, non-rule governed contrapuntal involvement of the available (Sheehan, 2001b) and our "always already becoming the moment of our mortality" (Sheehan, 1983, p. 306). It is the "right-at" that we must take part in. Figuration as a kind of experience "self-presents the disruptions of the exposed identity of meaning and the dispersion of meaning's meanings" (Nancy, 1993/1997, p. 83). There is incessant multiplication and twisting of figures that in turn reveal meanings as ephemeral yet concrete.

For Nancy, the grasping as grasping of a singular configuration/event completes its showing, yet "leaves it inappropriable, fragmentary, fractured, a fractal object of meaning" (1993/1997, p. 82). Whether we think from parts to whole or from whole to parts, similar conditions pertaining to meaning always obtain; they arc "woven into the opacity of meaning . . . and into its resistance to the breakthroughs of" (p. 83) humans as they themselves are placed into and as meaning as necessarily finite mortals.

I read figuration as the same as, but not identical to, "understanding-as" (Heidegger, 1927/1962, pp. 188–195). Figuration is another way of saying that fundamental human comportment always already occurs as figurations. The figurative is not the concretizing of an object in an absolute sense but it is the essence of human understanding that is sent by meaning to which we are necessarily (not as an option) exposed. We are delivered over to meaning that kaleidoscopically self-remixes. Coterminus with that, we are required by our finitude to be "right at" the meaning because we are exposed to (set out with) it in its infinity. Thus Nancy joins the struggle of the Greco-European philosophical tradition of the as-structure of human/world/history/nature (Sheehan, 2001b, p. 8–12).

Figuration is not the hypostatization of meaning via universal linguistic configuration; it is again releasement to the play of a between that is presented as absence. Figuration is the social, the political, the economic phenomena that humans are free for as they are enabled by them. Figuration as Heidegger's openness comports itself in all societal mixes. These know themselves to be made up of nonimmanent co-appearing. Fundamentally this is exposed as "knowing" through which collective comportment is revealed as a complex of practices (Nancy, 1996/2000, p. 69). In this revealing figuration becomes itself.

For many the unnerving "retreat of the political and the religious, or of the theologico-political, means the retreat of every space, form, or screen into which or onto which a figure of community could be projected" (Nancy, 1996/2000, p. 47). For Nancy (1996/2000), the self-presented retreat manifests itself in a pair of fundamental motifs: (1) the rigidity of rule or law governed realms, and (2) a withdrawal into a self that is intended to be nothing more than an impossibly isolated "I."

In terms of the first motif: "By experiencing an 'entry' into signification, the West experienced an exit from something that it could not signify, and consequently, the impossibility of signifying either its own advent or the establishment of the order of signification" (Nancy, 1993/1997, p. 28). The circle of the will-to-will must constantly renew itself by excluding anything that does not immediately present itself to any given individual's empirical experience

Our current state of affairs is certainly open to many interpretations. This "chiasma or circle worries us in our confused and anxiety-ridden awareness that society just 'turns around and around,' without substance, without foundation, without end" (Nancy, 1996/2000, p. 57). But is this anxiety-ridden awareness misplaced? It seems to me common knowledge that humans are social beings. The questioning that presents itself is one of being-with and together. If this is a valid question, it brings to the fore an anxiety about the sociality of humans. It is an injunction that we place upon ourselves, as that which we receive from a world that we have to be (Nancy, 1996/2000).

Nancy's (1996/2000) task is to retrieve the self-conception of our being-with. For him there is an irreducible strangeness that constitutes people as such. They are themselves as "primarily the exposing of the singularity according to which existence exists" (p. 9), not to be reduced to any primary substance or concept. People—they, us, I, you—are an exposition of singularity. As this singularity, the totality of beings is communicated with in the sense of experiencing "to" and "along with." Figuration obtains as "the spontaneous knowledge of society—its 'preontological comprehension' of itself" (p. 70), which, in its own turn, turns on nonepistemological knowledge about "being" itself. Social being revolves around, turns on itself, and no longer revolves around conceptions of Subject, Other or the Same (p. 57). The "from one to the other is the syncopated repetition of origins-of-the-world" (p. 6). Our togetherness is our essential singularity. We are contrapuntally assembled but not unified, united, or fused (p. 33).

Therefore, the world as significant is delivered over to understandings prior to any signifying. Our world does not need any constituted meaning in order for meaning to be presented as such (Nancy, 1993/1997). Meaning as interpreted thus "infinitely exceeds signification, and it neither has nor gives signification" (p. 63). This is neither lack of meaning, future as impossibility, nor a deadened deterministic fatalism. World as meaning has a sense of permanence to "*us* as exposed, to a space and to ourselves as a space, to a time and to ourselves as a time, to language, to ourselves" (p. 63). The advent of our signification exposes us to us as others and "to evil, to good, to choice, to decision, to choices and decisions, all as the event of our significations" (p. 63). For Nancy, thinking this "exposure-to" works to protect us and spare us from the trap that could ensnare us in the danger of thinking that a permanent signified presence can obtain.

After Heidegger, we can offer the thought that the world worlds. The world is always local. Its uniqueness as its unity and totality go to effect reticulated multiplicities, which in turn is not the production of a tangible result (Nancy, 1996/2000, p. 9). The world as it worlds is the always already. Moral or ethical conclusions are initially not determined as such: "our . . . disposition/co-appearance . . . is neither negative nor positive, but instead the mode of being-together or being-*with*" (p. 13). First and foremost for interpretive thought there is the play of the arrivings of phenomena as a giving of possibilities.

As mortals, finite humans, we always already begin to understand meaning as being-with-each-other-in-the world. Nancy writes, "this understanding is always already completed, full, whole and infinite. We understand ourselves infinitely—ourselves and the world—and nothing else" (1996/2000, p. 98). Being is always already thought interpretively (ontologically) as a shared question, as Heidegger asserts. Nancy adds that "we share understanding between us: between us all, simultaneously—all the dead and the living, and all beings" (p. 99).

The words of James Joyce come to mind for me here; his short story *The Dead* (1998) brings out the mystery of the western setting sun as an absencing that promises becoming. He presents the sea, which receives snow "softly falling into the dark mutinous Shannon waves," as that which never gives up its future of secrets. All we can hear is "the snow falling

faintly though the universe . . . upon all the living and the dead"
(pp. 203–204).

As a kind of createdness or advent existence is "the beginning and
end that *we* are. This is the thought that is most necessary for us to
think . . . that excess which is impossible to totalize" (Nancy, 1996/2000,
p. 17). Meaning is an excess of the sense of significances that pulls everything along such that there is an enabling that allows a freedom—the retrieval of possibility as possibility.

Ex-position

> . . . right at humanity, existence is exposed and exposing.
>
> (Nancy, 1996/2000, p. 17)

Humans are capable of being claimed by what is readily available. Yet
taking the readily available as a whole has the possibility of leaving other
"wholes" out. By taking ourselves as the standard we forget "world" not as
just the world of humanity, but world as "the nonhuman to which humanity is exposed and which humanity, in turn, exposes" (Nancy, 1996/2000,
p. 18). In addition, there is *always* the possibility of going astray as a fundamental human comportment. A possibility of being open for openness
is to see freedom as a letting-be (Heidegger, 1967/1998c, pp. 143–152).
We are free to be "exposed to the risk of no longer being able to understand or interpret ourselves—but also, that we are thereby exposed once
again to ourselves, and once again to one another, to our language, and
to our world" (Nancy, 1993/1997, p. 65). The ability to let ourselves be
openness such that questioning becomes a practice that does not close-
down-on as a given imposition, but lets the mystery of the whole arrive as
its own arrival is a possibility that openness allows for humans.

We learn from Nancy, "signification becomes empty precisely because it completes it subjective process; its only *meaning* is itself, in its in-
ertia, that is, at once its own desire, its own projection, its own representational distance, and its own representation of distance, insofar as this
distance constitutes its essential property; the ideality, transcendence or
future of meaning" (1993/1997, p. 44). There seems to be "an originary or
transcendental 'with' demanding with palpable urgency, to be disentan-
gled and articulated for itself. But one of the greatest difficulties of the
concept of the with is that there is no 'getting back to' or 'up to' this 'originary' or 'transcendental' position; the with is strictly contemporaneous

with existence, as it is with all thinking" (Nancy, 1996/2000, p. 41). The proper exposure to the origin is to reach it as mystery that is allowed to stand *as* mystery as opposed to a mere unknown that can be solved for. In this way we have not missed the origin. The origin is the whole, but it always already exceeds any whole that can be known.

Can the sense of wonder that was once ascribed to pre-Socratic Greece be retrieved as a contemporary sense of mystery? There is a resistance to mystery today that resides (dwells) as the faith that insists that science will conquer all unknowns. For Nancy, "to wonder today is nothing other than to wonder before this resistance and insistence of our strange community in meaning, in the exposure to meaning" (1993/1997, p. 66).

In his poem, *The Second Coming* (1983), William Butler Yeats wrote that: "The best lack all conviction, while the worst / Are full of passionate intensity." Perhaps somewhere between the to and fro of these extremes lies an answer. It is possible to participate in allowing the wonder of being-together to emerge. Others can no longer be established as an "It" of anthropological other, subjectivity, or psychology of cognition. For Nancy (1982/1990) "It no longer refers to subjectivity, indeed to the psychology of 'understanding.' It is, in the other of every dialogue, the one which makes it other. . . . It is this other of the other which never reappears as the same thing" (p. 246).

Echoing Heidegger, Nancy avers that we are part of and are constituted by the open as "the uncovered that puts us face to face. *There is only us,* that is, the thing out in the open, being without subjectivity, finite [mortals], and the unsignifiable provenance of meaning" (1993/1997, p. 66). Openness always already starts from what arrives (is given) as being (existence), which is itself-co-determined as being "with-one-another" (Nancy, 1996/2000, p. 32). The works of Heidegger and Gadamer resonate as Nancy describes language as "the exposition of the world-of-bodies as such" (p. 84). For Nancy, "language is the exposing of plural singularity. In it all of being is exposed as its meaning . . . the circulation of a meaning of the world that has no beginning, or end" (1996/2000, p. 84).

Being is never found at a location or as some determinable "in something." But the meaning of being resides in what is spoken. Thus "one 'speaks,' 'it speaks,' means '[b]eing is spoken'; it is meaning (but does not construct meaning). But 'one' or 'it' is never other than *we*" (Nancy, 1996/ 2000, p. 27). Language is an incorporeal exposition wherein all entities, relationships, theories, and so forth, are involved with human practices (p. 85).

Our existence as any interpretive practice is necessarily involved with language. Any ontology of what, how, or that something is "all that is and all that goes into making a word;" "a word is what it is only among all words. . . . As soon as a word is said, it is resaid" (Nancy, 1996/2000, p. 86). The interpreted context is always already on the move; not toward any resolution, but as movement itself. Dialogue is necessary, not to capture meaning, but to let involved partners near its movement. Dialogue as an offering can only offer "the with of meaning" (Nancy, 1996/2000, p. 87).

Nancy's (1996/2000) thought on language grows out of Heidegger's, when Nancy discusses the presentation of the point of view of significa-tion. Meaning gives in that one thing is presented by signification as an-other thing: essence, principle, origin, end, value. The task of interpreta-tion is to present the "as" as such (p. 88). Heidegger entered on this path when he wrote that we let "beings-be in a particular comportment that relates to them and thus discloses them," but this "conceals beings as a whole" (Heidegger, 1967/1998c, p. 148). For Heidegger, this is "errancy" not as an error but as an intrinsic possibility of openness (Sheehan, 1995a, pp. 160–161). We are called by thinking by Nancy to be right at "the moment when, and the move by which, the signifying will knows it-self as such, knows itself to be insignificant and by itself releases a new demand for 'meaning'" (1993/1997, p. 51). Openness on the other hand is necessary and must be ready to receive the releasement. For Heideg-ger, possibility in this releasement becomes the allowing of mystery as the concealing of what is concealed to hold sway as openness (1967/1998c, p. 148). For Nancy (1993/1997), thinking is what inscribes the limit of signification in language. Thinking is an enactment that allows language to obtain as the limit of signification.

Openness as limit is what ontology or interpretive practice lets the fig-urative be its ownmost, as an open inscription. As this occurs in "passing to the limit of signification, language registers the shock of the thing. The hollow or crack disjoins the signifying order. The inscription is the outline of this disjunction" (Nancy, 1993/1997, p. 70). Freedom becomes the "property" of the advening rather than the license of the human being. As the step back "one must think an anteriority of the origin according to some event that happens to it unexpectedly (even if that event originates within it)" (Nancy, 1996/2000, p. 39). The temporality of experience is such that the past is always in front of us (Heidegger, 1927/1962, p. 41) as always already openness and possibility.

Nancy and Method

. . . every presupposition of [b]eing must consist in its non presupposition.
(Nancy, 1996/2000, p. 56)

I have articulated how the letting-be of some matter or thing always already includes its possible concealed essence. Taking something as something is "the philosophical presupposition of the whole politico-philosophical order, which is always an ontological presupposition" (Nancy, 1996/2000, p. 37). Interpretations of presuppositions are essential to any way that works to explicate phenomena. Even takings-as can be taken-as! Any examining of "the subject of 'ontology' first of all entails the critical examination of the conditions of critique in general" (Nancy, 1996/2000, p. 55). Methodical procedure for Nancy entails thinking as questioning as it does for Heidegger and Gadamer. Thinking "needs to think in principle about how we are 'us' among us, that is how the consistency of our Being is in being-in-common, and how this consists precisely in the 'in' or in the 'between' of its spacing" (pp. 25–26).

If we sample questions from Nancy's writings we see also that the questioner is at issue. Nancy asserts and questions: "We will speak: Who is the 'we'? How are we with one another? What is at play in our communication" (1996/2000, p. 33)? Any "critique absolutely needs to rest on some principle other than that of the ontology of the Other and the Same; it needs an ontology of being-with-one-another, and this ontology must support both the sphere of 'nature,' and sphere of 'history,' 'as well as both the 'human' and the 'non human'" (p. 53) in order to remain a thinking that does not close down on possibilities. Contrary to some positions, philosophical thinking is charged with the task of "the thinking of being-with; because of this, it is also thinking-with as such" (p. 31). Thinking with is an extension of Heidegger's notion of being needing openness and openness claimed by being (Sheehan, 2001a, p. 14). We can also see that Gadamer's dialogue obtains as a thinking-with.

That there is "is" is a troublesome position to take. Certainly not something one would say if they wanted to get hired to perform a reimbursable

service! Be that as it may the "is" calls out to us all whether we be philosophers or participants in other walks of life. Are we enmeshed in an unbreakable circulatory system? We hear Nancy (1996/2000) calling to us,
exhorting us to come to grips with something we always already come to
grips with. He submits that:

Our task is to break the hard shell of this tautology. What is the being-with of
[b]eing? (p. 35)

How is the being-with of being? Is being a metaphor? Symbolic? To the
extent that metaphors and symbols are abstractions they are being as advent. "The sole criterion of symbolization is . . . the capacity for allowing
a certain play in and by the image-symbol, with the joining, the distancing, the opened interval that articulates it as *sym-bol* . . . so that the dimension, space, and nature of the 'with' are in play" (Nancy, 1996/2000,
p. 58). The significance of symbol and metaphor is the meaning that is always already in front of them; how they "take," how they are given, how
they arrive. Symbol and metaphor as phenomena are only approachable
via dialogue. Hence, "the essence of the dialogue is in the infinite altera-
tion of the other, and in that puts an end with out end to the end of the dialogue. At each time it is put to an end, the announcement is renewed"
(Nancy, 1982/1990, p. 246).

Interpretive practice is served by explicating symbols and metaphors
and their conjoined comportment as announcements-of. According to
Nancy (1982/1990), "the announcement is . . . the mode of the proper
presence of the other." Interpretation "is the announcement of finitude
by way of finitude: its division is infinite. This division is that of the dialogue" (p. 247), wherein, ala Gadamer, we as interpreting can be capable of arriving at a fusion of horizons. Nancy describes his project thus:

What I am trying to indicate by speaking of 'dis-position' is neither a simple position nor a juxtaposition. Instead, the *co* defines the unity and uniqueness of what
is, in general. (1996/2000, p. 39)

We can see traces in this project of Heidegger's thrownness and the
call that calls forth thinking (Heidegger, 1954/1968). In addition, for
Gadamer, a conversation *must* be with someone, some text or some tradition. For Nancy, dialogue only obtains as "exposing the 'with' as the category that still has no status or use, but from which we receive everything
that makes us think and everything that gives 'us' to thinking" (1996/2000,

p. 43). There is no political "with" as long as power as sovereignty "involves nothing more than an eager repression of the very question of being-in-common" (p. 43).

If political power seems mostly to be infused with practices of suppressing being-in-common, where are we to go? Respect for the ineffable, the mystery, the sacred, the essential finitude of openness is not enforceable. One of the problems, issues, criticisms, of interpretive methods is that they cannot admit of solutions. Insofar as these are well thought out, these criticisms must be part of any conversation. But interpretation as interpretation cannot be concreticized into a system. When this is enforced, interpretation ceases to be itself.

The future as becoming is presented by Nancy (1982/1990) as the divine. It is what gives itself and self-divides "in voice and in *hermeneia* [interpretation]" (p. 237). The divine gifts itself as the sharing of voices. The divine is a recognition that the temporalized openness that we are a non-separable part of is both to be respected as such and to be looked on as a gift to take to heart. To think "is not to reactivate the signs and significations that are in the process of being consumed in this exposure [to the limit]; it is rather to think the exposure itself" (Nancy, 1993/1997, p. 52). Thinking is a form of thanking by which we endeavor to reveal the sense of what is given, as ever an infinite giving which is not ours as finite beings to control (Heidegger, 1954/1968, pp. 138–147). Thinking stems from thoughts that are given, not from the opposite (Heidegger, 1954/1968). Thinking is to recall that:

We never come to thoughts. They come to us. (Heidegger, 1954/1971e, p. 4)

Thinking is what is given as our essential (ownmost) nature.

The Questioning of Method

The lasting element in thinking is the way.
(Heidegger, 1959/1971a, p. 13)

If there is a thread that self-weaves its way through the thinking of the interpretive thought of the three scholars that I have attempted to explicate, it is discursiveness. For Heidegger (1959/1971b), language speaks as not anything human, and "[w]e not only *speak* language, we speak *from out of it"* (Heidegger, 1959/1993b, p. 411), for Gadamer, "language speaks us" (1960/1990, p. 43), and for Nancy, "language says the world" (1996/2000, p. 3).

The genitive in the naming of this section (The Questioning of Method) is meant to be ambiguous, as are all the genitives in this exposition. Questioning is not the possession of method; method is not the possession of questioning. The ambiguous genitive is the play of verb and name; the play of action and naming. Openness as Dasein is what we are. Fundamental to this is the possibility of our own absence (or presence). Our proper temporality must include the possibility of the absenting or presenting of anything else. This is what "opens-up" human knowing (Sheehan, 2001a, p. 15).

There are thinkers who attempt to utilize empirical or scientific methods to quantify power, control, outcomes, and dominance practices. Interpretive methods at their best labor to explicate the specific problems inherent in the indiscriminant adherence to the ambiguous conceptualizations of power, dominance, and control. These terms are not unambiguous and finalizeable.

Methods as unquestionably practiced can be a polyglot. Methods as such are noncohering play between theory, which is unessentializable (i.e., the theory of theories of . . . *ad infinitum*), and objectification, which is, as a result of modern physics, unquantifiable. If this interpretation obtains, where does this leave us? To the will to will?

There is general consensus that coterminous with the rapid growth of its human population our home planet is warming, but there is a divide on what the cause is. Species are becoming extinct, but the very scienticism that enabled us to see this also avers that extinct species can be brought back to "life" via genetic reconstructions. The confrontations (I would not characterize these as debates!) that turn on abortion, gay and lesbian marriage, and patriotism, to name just a few, do not seem to be rooted in any attempt to understand the other.

Methods in the contemporary sense are fundamentally the assertion of hidden or forgotten values. Realisms assert their value as one of true versus false; idealisms must deal with good–bad distinctions. But in a complex of temporal, physiological, biological, ethnic, political, power, economic, social, and linguistic relationships what does a realism choose to measure? What does an idealist theory choose to exclude/include via its necessary progression of abstractions? What is decisive?

Interpretive practices are a way of keeping one's foot in the door that techno-scientism and some aspects of critical social theory consider closed. Heidegger's clearing *as* clearing is fundamentally kept open by it-self with no help from us. But without us, as mortals, there could be no clearing. Possibility as possibility means just that. No more, no less.

Arriving and Departing

[The] humble layer of our everyday experience contains another rudimen-tary ontological attestation: what we receive (rather than what we perceive) with singularities is the discreet passage of *other origins of the world.*

(Nancy, 1996/2000, pp. 8–9)

Let me submit a pedestrian example of the situatedness of airline travel as it reveals aspects of experience. Somewhere between arrivals and departures lies a complex place of alreadiness, presence-to, and be-coming. One does not arrive at an airport alone. One does not check in, verify his or her ticket, visa, and passport alone. And most certainly, one does not go through security alone. One is thrown into the trip, under-stands what is necessary, and must participate in various conversations in order to once again depart and arrive. And, of course, the ticket-buying public consists of mortals.

As an experiencing there can be interpretive multiplications or sub-tractions: there is always already being-with. There is a being-with the theory and objectness of the technological means, the necessity of being-with of others as they co-appear, the being-with of the plurality of singu-lar meanings, and the being-with of departures and arrivals. Every arrival is a departure from, and every departure is an arrival to. The world of "froms" is absent but still present. The coterminous world of "tos" is ab-sent but still present. This is the definition, if I may call it that, of priva-tion as Heidegger explicates it. There is always an excess of meaning that is delivered over to or gathered by the situation.

Air travel is a tradition we are thrown into as an historical meaning. We understand such travel as immediate experience and are required by our linguisticality to participate as a playing along within a given way which is an exposure as meaning event.

The arrivals/departures room is where there is no "metaphysical closure, full self-presence, and perfect self-coincidence" (Sheehan, 2001b, p. 17). The comings and goings cannot be measured according to any knowable standard—once a presence is seized upon, there is always already an olio of possible absences and impending presencings. We should not be surprised then if we discover via interpretive reflection that the room is open to interpretation and what we must be is open. For it and us to be open we belong to the room as it uses/enables us. The room needs us in order for it to be itself (Heidegger, 1954/1993a; Sheehan, 2001b).

Interpretive work is bound by the incompletability (finitude) of the infinite—it is a relation of counter-resonance (Heidegger, 1987/2000, p. 251); an "unbreakable reciprocity" (Sheehan, 2001b, p. 13). In interpretive work, dualisms such as history, nature, mind-body, true-false, and good-bad are not done away with (if they even could be!) but are allowed to stand in order to deal with the play of their belonging together, but not in order to arrive at some putative higher truth or ideal.

As an attempt to show a situation that presents an interpretation of the generation of the play of meaning, I am presenting an airport's arrivals and departures area as, "the *inter*lacing of strands whose extremities remain separate even at the center of the knot" (Nancy, 1996/2000, p. 5). I will submit snippets of a variety of conversations to illustrate that work to reveal that, "the world always appears [appears suddenly, emerges, wells up, surges forth] each time according to a decidedly local turn [of events]. Its unity, its uniqueness, and its totality consist in a combination of this reticulated multiplicity, which produces no result" (p. 9).

The area where this reticulated multiplicity occurs is not an abstract space, it is a locale that is a kind of magnet, a space in the sense of room. The German word *raum* is more akin to our word room. So space as room can be experienced as room-for, room-to, and simply as a place where and when dwelling occurs. Then the word *spielraum,* translated as "leeway" in *Being and Time* is more akin to roominess where the play of the open occurs. In "Building Dwelling Thinking" (1954/1993a), Heidegger writes that spaces are complexes of occurring and re-occurring significance/insignificance; not a pure manifold. A pure manifold cannot contain any excess of meaning and significance or by itself produce what it includes or excludes. I submit that thinking this abstractness is itself a veiled call for interpretive thinking.

The sense of "room" here includes the everyday play of outside and inside as well as the temporalizing of past, present, and future. Nancy's

(1996/2000) explication of Heidegger's work calls into question the brief treatment of the everyday in *Being and Time*. He asserts "Heidegger confuses the everyday with the undifferentiated, the anonymous, and the statistical. One cannot affirm that the meaning of Being must express itself starting from everydayness and then begin by neglecting the general differentiation of the everyday, its constantly renewed rupture, its intimate discord, its polymorphy and its polyphony, its relief and its variety" (p. 9).

Nancy's work retrieves the possibilities inherent in the everyday by thinking of its "obstinacy" and "domination" as another beginning. He takes Heidegger's thought that in this obstinacy and domination "there lie possibilities of my Dasein [as openness], and out of this leveling down the 'I am' is possible" (Heidegger, 1989/1992a, p. 9E). Significant for Nancy is his thought that "'people' are silhouettes that are both imprecise and singularized, faint outlines of voices, patterns of comportment, sketches of affects, not the anonymous chatter of the 'public domain'" (1996/2000, p. 7). Therefore, he adds: "from one singular to another, there is contiguity but not continuity" (p. 5). Thus we are together in a one to another as "the syncopated repetition of programs-of-the-world, which are each time one or the other" (p. 6).

Let us begin somewhere on the way. In common speech "the ordinary itself is originary . . . the exception is the rule" (Nancy, 1996/2000, p. 10). But in many instances what is common speech to a given group is taken as nonsensical or as jargon by another listener. But there can be no jargon either as some restricted terminology or idle chatter in interpretive thinking. All saying is a hinting.

We hear:

The child over there has never seen an airplane in an airport before; why is she waving good-bye? Because she knows what absence means and that her grandparents will always be present even if they never return. I get it. Absence is always a kind of presence. They are mutually codependent as possibility and cannot be any other way.

Departure (as well as arrival) times are more than an airline schedule. They are part of a complex of events. They are, however, concrete times that we can specify. Our own mortality, on the other hand, as always already nearness, is a phenomenon that leaves us incomplete. Thus it can be claimed that "meaning can only be right at existence" (Nancy, 1996/2000, p. 10), primarily as an unspecifiable, but concomitantly as the quotidian.

Everybody seems at home with their luggage. Yes, luggage only becomes manifest when it falls apart. To say the least!

We are always already using things in such and such a way. But they are also using us because we are involved with them in their availability.

We can also see that "this very humble layer of our everyday experience contains another rudimentary ontological attestation: what we receive (rather than what we perceive) with singularities is the discreet passage of *other origins of the world*" (Nancy, 1996/2000, p. 8–9). The arrivals and departures room is the locale of a variety of emotional states; better I should say it this way: there are attunements *as* their situatedness (their thrownness) obtains. These are, in turn, reciprocally given as their originations.

That group over there seems to be happy, but they all speak different languages. Their happiness is saying as showing. There is no scientifically determined univocity that can measure happiness and sadness. We know there is caring though. I agree.

In James Joyce's novel *Ulysses* (2002), he has Stephen Dedalus assert that God is a shout in the street (p. 34). From Nancy we hear that any "themes of 'wonder' and the 'marvel of Being' are suspect if they refer to an ecstatic mysticism that pretends to escape the world. The theme of scientific curiosity is no less suspect if it boils down to a collector's preoccupation with rarities" (1996/2000, p. 10). The rare and unusual as objects must necessarily reveal meaning. Does rarity entail the forever of species extinction or does the rare bring a higher price in the marketplace? Is the everyday the rare and unusual from an ontological perspective?

Those two people in hard hats are looking at something. What are they looking at? I heard one of them say that the architect Ludwig Mies van der Rohe thought that architecture begins when two bricks are put together carefully. Is that the sense of the two senses of articulation in *Being and Time*? The Greek philosophical sense of the discursive nature of synthesis-diairesis? Yes, it seems that jointures gather in one way or another.

We seem to have forgotten that things come together as well as they self-differentiate themselves. We must take part in an existence that we are necessarily estranged from. Nancy (1996/2000) offers that: "'Nature' is . . . 'strange,' and we exist there . . . [t]hen again, we say 'strange,' 'odd,' 'curious,' 'disconcerting' *about* all being" (pp. 9–10). Is there a need to let go of our attempt to subjugate all that is to our everpresent estrangement due to shifting human centered values?

From *Being and Time* we hear that we are that entity for whom our own existence is an issue for us. To speak of the strange is to hear what the strange says.

. . . did you hear him say that there was no such thing as power? Yes, I did, and I might add, that is about the strangest thing I have ever heard.

There is no "out there" independent of an observer, for how could we know if there is without observing it as such? On the other hand, "that which does not maintain its distance from the 'between' is only immanence collapsed in on itself and deprived of meaning" (Nancy, 1996/2000, p. 5). Therefore there is no "in-here" either because something or other has to put me (thrown me) into the, or better yet, *as* in-the-world.

Those people over there who are crying are not speaking but they are saying a lot. The way they body-forth is a showing of their conversation.

Conversation is always already a between, a meaning. There are no private conversations, even if one is thinking to oneself. One is always already *in* a world.

All of what you and I have happened to hear seems obvious. Why then, should we pay any attention to the taken-for-granted? Are we too nosy? Yes and no.

Situatedness obtains as a full complex and as surprise, and is sometimes shocking. There are also issues concerning personal privacy to be dealt with. On the one hand revealing (as best as possible) the taken for granted, as it self-reveals, always holds the possibility for being free-for an otherwise covered-over problematic. On the other hand, the taken for granted must always be allowed as the possibility of its invisibility. The taken for granted does not necessarily show up on a computer screen. Phenomena do not manifest themselves as a result of human willing, but occur as we deal with them. Perhaps, more significantly, a phenomenon may show up *as* a computer screen.

Aside from the fact that the room of arrival/departure is fictional; is my conversation selection scientific? Based on accepted statistical methods? It most certainly is not! But it is held out into the open such that I have attempted to submit it as a gathering, not as a closure. There are an infinity of interactions that could be selected and thereby interpreted. As such it is a sampling of what has come and by the absence of what is not in the conversational fragments. There is always already a not, but also the always already becoming as a presence-to.

As phenomena call out, any interpreter listens with interest. Which ones are selected are pregiven. Suitcases might not generate university research, but happiness and sadness could and indeed have. Unless one is a philosopher interested in equipment, suitcases disappear into the world of commerce and industry, or they obtain as a university engineering professor's world wherein he/she has become wealthy from a patent for designing more ergonomic luggage. Even the most trivial matters hold questions.

Conclusion

the one thing that matters is whether
. . . the dialogue . . . before us, be it written
or spoken or neither, remains constantly coming.
                                   (Heidegger, 1959/1971a, p. 52)

Heidegger, Gadamer, and Nancy are interrelated thinkers. Their work resonates with one another's insofar as each thinker attempts to move beyond a metaphysics that understands truth as only that which can be constituted empirically or epistemologically (Dahlstrom, 2001, pp. 17–29; Sheehan, 1983, pp. 297–303).

Heidegger enables us to be free for proper temporality as the claim absence has on presence. Presence-to needs a receptor and a place to advene. Gadamer explicates this place as the necessity and universality of hermeneutic dialogue. Nancy's project is to generate respect for the singular that is determined by the plural due to the fact that they are mutually determined by each other and they are needed by each other.

If, for Heidegger, silence speaks out of the unspoken (Heidegger, 1927/1962, pp. 208, 342–343; Heidegger, 1959/1971f, p. 120) of the nothing, for Gadamer every word reveals questions, and for Nancy we are exposed to the nothing as immediate singular plural co-appearance-to (1996/2000, pp. 67–71), then method must turn on being methodically nonmethodological; as a being free for waiting (Heidegger, 1959/1966, pp. 67–90; Heidegger, 1985/2001a, pp. 138–139).

There is no imperative for conversation/dialogue but there is necessity for acknowledgment for the place of the singular plural: Dasein as openness. Dasein as openness is the always already present-to becoming the moment of its mortality.

How does something get from nothing to here? Physics has its big bang theory and the Judeo-Christian tradition has its creation story. But prior to the big bang or the creation of the universe there was what? The past and the future remain unfinished (and unfinishable) projects. We are only free for living out our incompleteness.

The retrieval of method is a retrieval of what it means to release temporality forward into its origin. Decisive for any retrieval are interpretations that work to explicate involvements that we are always already in the midst of as the enduring whiling of Dasein as openness. There is no ideal communicative activity, no pure transcendental ego, and no abstract particular that can be established once and for all. There is only listening and responding.

Notes

1. The words [b]eing, being and beings that are part of this paper indicate the is-ness (being) of what is (beings) or entities; things that are. See Sheehan (2001b, pp. 8–10).

2. The fourth dimension of time as nearness shows up not only in the above marginal note but also in Heidegger's *The Concept of Time* (1989/1999, p. 22E) "Conversation on a Country Path About Thinking" (1959/1966, pp. 88–90), and *Time and Being* (1968/1972, pp. 15–16). In addition, I refer the reader to pages 101–108 of "The Nature of Language" (1959/1971c), where Heidegger works to demonstrate how time and space cannot be reduced to some given "universal-theoretical formula."

3. I am choosing to leave the term Dasein unitalicized and referred to as "Dasein as openness." The literal translation of the word is "existence, being here or being there." I am following the position of Heidegger that some terms are untranslatable (cf. 1957/1969, p. 37; 1982/1992b, p. 99). Others have translated it as existence (Sheehan, 1979, p. 78). Sheehan moved to openness in his later works (2001a, p. 8), there-being (Richardson, 1974), being-here (Dahlstrom, 2001), and openness-for-[*being*] (Lovitt, 1977). Leaving this pivotal term undefined is not a promissory note, contra Sheehan (2001b), but my attempt to let the term become its own way of self-showing.

4. See Sheehan (1979, p. 80) and Sheehan (1995b, p. 219).

5. An exhaustive explication of the complexities of the fourfold cannot be pursued here. Readers are encouraged to consult related materials in Heidegger's *Basic Writings*, *On the Way to Language*, and *Poetry, Language, Thought.*

6. The butterfly wing hypothesis is where the beat of a butterfly's wings can start a

chain reaction that affects the history of the entire planet. It is based on computer driven models where a minute initial difference in "input" can lead to a massive difference in "output." The hubris of techno-scienticism?

7. This harks back to the cleft (cleavage) articulated in *Contributions to Philosophy* (Heidegger, 1989/1999), the rift of *Origin of the Work of Art* (1960/1971, p. 63), and the furrows of *What is Called Thinking* (1954/1968, pp. 190–193).

References

Dahlstrom, D. O. (2001). *Heidegger's concept of truth*. New York: Cambridge University Press.

Gadamer, H-G. (1976a). Heidegger and the language of metaphysics (D. E. Linge, Trans.). In D. E. Linge (Ed.), *Philosophical hermeneutics* (pp. 229–240). Berkeley: University of California Press. (Original work published 1967).

Gadamer, H-G. (1976b). Man and language (D. E. Linge, Trans.). In D. E. Linge (Ed.), *Philosophical hermeneutics* (pp. 59–68). Berkeley: University of California Press. (Original work published 1967).

Gadamer, H-G. (1976c). On the problem of self-understanding (D. E. Linge, Trans). In D. E. Linge (Ed.), *Philosophical hermeneutics* (pp.44–58). Berkeley: University of California Press. (Original work published 1967).

Gadamer, H-G. (1976d). On the scope and function of hermeneutical Reflection (D. E. Linge, Trans.). In D. E. Linge (Ed.), *Philosophical hermeneutics* (pp. 18–43). Berkeley: University of California Press. (Original work published 1967).

Gadamer, H-G. (1976e). The phenomenological movement (D. E. Linge, Trans.). In D. E. Linge (Ed.), *Philosophical hermeneutics* (pp. 130–181). Berkeley: University of California Press. (Original work published 1967).

Gadamer, H-G. (1976f). Semantics and hermeneutics (D. E. Linge, Trans.). In D. E. Linge (Ed.), *Philosophical hermeneutics* (pp. 82–94). Berkeley: University of California Press. (Original work published 1967).

Gadamer, H-G. (1980). Plato's unwritten dialectic (P. C. Smith, Trans.). In *Dialogue and dialectic: Eight hermeneutical studies on Plato.* (pp. 124–155). New Haven, CT: Yale University Press. (Original work published 1968).

Gadamer, H-G. (1981). Philosophy or theory of science? (F. G. Lawrence, Trans.). In *Reason in the age of science* (pp. 151–169). Cambridge, MA: MIT Press. (Original work published 1976).

Gadamer, H-G. (1990). *Truth and method.* (2nd rev. ed.). (J. Weinsheimer & D. G. Marshall, Trans.). New York: Crossroad Publishing Company. (Original work published 1960).

Gadamer, H-G. (1997). Reflections on my philosophical journey (R. E. Palmer, Trans.). In L. E. Hahn (Ed.), *The philosophy of H-G Gadamer* (pp. 3–63). Chicago: Open Court. (Original work published 1997).

Gadamer, H-G. (2001). *Gadamer in conversation: Reflections and commentary* (R. Palmer, Trans. & Ed.). New Haven, CT: Yale University Press. (Original work published 1994).

Heidegger, M. (1962). *Being and time* (J. Macquarrie & E. Robinson, Trans.). New York: Harper & Row. (Original work published 1927).

Heidegger, M. (1966). Conversation on a country path about thinking. In M. Heidegger,

Discourse on thinking (pp.58–90). (J. M. Anderson & E. H. Freund, Trans.). New York: Harper & Row. (Original work published 1959).

Heidegger, M. (1967). *What is a thing?* (W. B. Barton, Jr. & V. Deutsch, Trans.). Chicago: Henry Regenery Co. (Original work published 1962).

Heidegger, M. (1968). *What is called thinking* (F. D. Wieck & J. G. Gray, Trans.). New York: Harper & Row. (Original work published 1954).

Heidegger, M. (1969). *Identity and difference* (J. Stanbaugh, Trans.). New York: Harper & Row. (Original work published 1957).

Heidegger, M. (1971a). A dialogue on language (P. Hertz, Trans.). In *On the way to language* (pp. 1–54). New York: Harper & Row. (Original work published 1959).

Heidegger, M. (1971b). Language (A. Hofstadter, Trans.). In *Poetry language thought* (pp. 187–210). New York: Harper & Row. (Original work published 1959).

Heidegger, M. (1971c). The nature of language (P. Hertz, Trans.). In *On the way to language* (pp. 57–108). New York: Harper & Row. (Original work published 1959).

Heidegger, M. (1971d). Origin of the work of art (A. Hofstadter, Trans.). In *Poetry language thought* (pp.15–87). New York: Harper & Row. (Original work published 1960).

Heidegger, M. (1971e). The thinker as poet (A. Hofstadter, Trans.). In *Poetry language thought* (pp. 1–14). New York: Harper & Row. (Original work published 1954).

Heidegger, M. (1971f). The way to language (P. Hertz, Trans.). *On the way to language* (pp. 111–136). New York: Harper & Row. (Original work published 1959).

Heidegger, M. (1972). Time and being (J. Stambaugh, Trans.). In *On time and being* (pp. 1–24). New York: Harper & Row. (Original work published 1968).

Heidegger, M. (1973a). Metaphysics as history of being (J. Stambaugh, Trans.). In *The end of philosophy* (pp. 1–54). New York: Harper & Row. (Original work published 1961).

Heidegger, M. (1973b). Overcoming metaphysics (J. Stambaugh, Trans.). In *The end of philosophy* (pp. 84–110). New York: Harper & Row. (Original work published 1954).

Heidegger, M. (1977a). Science and reflection (W. Lovitt, Trans.). In W. Lovitt (Ed.), *Question concerning technology and other essays* (pp. 155–182). New York: Harper & Row. (Original work published 1954).

Heidegger, M. (1977b). The turning (W. Lovitt, Trans.). In W. Lovitt (Ed.), *Question concerning technology and other essays* (pp. 36–49). New York: Harper & Row. (Original work published 1949).

Heidegger, M. (1977c). The word of Nietzsche: God is dead (W. Lovitt, Trans.). In W. Lovitt (Ed.), *Question concerning technology and other essays* (pp. 53–112). New York: Harper & Row. (Original work published 1943).

Heidegger, M. (1991). *The principle of reason* (R. Lilly, Trans.). Bloomington: Indiana University Press. (Original work published 1957).

Heidegger, M. (1992a). *The concept of time* (W. McNeill, Trans.). Oxford, UK: Blackwell. (Original work published 1989).

Heidegger, M. (1992b). *Parmenides* (A. Schurer & R. Rojcewicz, Trans.). Bloomington: Indiana University Press. (Original work published 1982).

Heidegger, M. (1993a). Building dwelling thinking (A. Hofstadter, Trans.). In D. F. Krell (Ed.), *Basic writings* (pp. 343–363). New York: Harper & Row. (Original work published 1954).

Heidegger, M. (1993b). The way to language (D. F. Krell, Trans.). In D. F. Krell (Ed.), *Basic writings* (pp. 397–426). New York: Harper Collins. (Original work published 1959).

Heidegger, M. (1998a). Introduction to *what is metaphysics?* (W. Kaufman & W. McNeill,

Trans.). In W. McNeill (Ed.), *Pathmarks* (pp. 277–290). New York: Cambridge University Press. (Original work published 1967).

Heidegger, M. (1998b). On the essence and concept of φύσις in Aristotle's *Physics* B, I (*1939*) (T. Sheehan, Trans.). In W. McNeill (Ed.), *Pathmarks* (pp. 183–230). New York: Cambridge University Press. (Original work published 1967).

Heidegger, M. (1998c). On the essence of truth (1930) (J. Sallis, Trans.). In W. McNeill (Ed.), *Pathmarks* (pp. 136–182). New York: Cambridge University Press. (Original work published 1967).

Heidegger, M. (1999). *Contributions to philosophy (From enowning)*. (P. Emad & K. Maly, Trans.). Bloomington: Indiana University Press. (Original work published 1989).

Heidegger, M. (2000). *Towards the definition of philosophy* (T. Sadler, Trans.). New York: Continuum. (Original work published 1987).

Heidegger, M. (2001a). *Phenomenological interpretations of Aristotle* (R. Rojcewicz, Trans.). Bloomington: Indiana University Press. (Original work published 1985).

Heidegger, M. (2001b). *Zollikon seminars* (F. Mays & R. Askay, Trans.). Evanston: Northwestern University Press. (Original work published 1987).

Heidegger, M. (2002). Heidegger on the art of teaching (V. Allen & A. D. Axiotis, Trans.). In *Heidegger, education and modernity* (pp. 27–45). Lanhan, MD: Rowman and Littlefield. (Original work published 1945).

Heidegger, M. (2003). Seminar in Zähringen, 1973 (A. Mitchell & F. Raffoul, Trans.). In *Four seminars* (pp. 64–81). Bloomington: Indiana University Press. (Original work published 1977).

Joyce, J. (1998). The dead. In *The Dubliners* (pp. 159–204). New York: Vintage International.

Joyce, J. (2002). *Ulysses*. New York: Random House.

Kahn, V. (1997). Humanism and the resistance to theory. In W. Jost & M. Hyde (Eds.), *Rhetoric and hermeneutics in our time* (pp. 149–170). New Haven: Yale University Press.

Linge, D. E. (Ed.). (1976). Editor's introduction. In *Philosophical hermeneutics* (pp. xi–lviii). Berkeley: University of California Press.

Lovitt, W. (1977). Translator's introduction to *Question concerning technology and other essays*. In W. Lovitt (Ed.), *Question concerning technology and other essays* (pp. xiii–xxxix). New York: Harper & Row.

Nancy, J-L. (1990). Sharing voices. In G. L. Ormiston & A. D. Schrift (Eds.), *Transforming the hermeneutic context: From Nietzsche to Nancy* (pp. 211–260). New York: State University of New York Press. (Original work published 1982).

Nancy, J-L. (1997). *The gravity of thought* (F. Raffoul & G. Recco, Trans.). Atlantic Highlands, NJ: Humanities Press. (Original work published 1993).

Nancy, J-L. (2000) *Being singular plural* (R. D. Richardson & A. E. O'Byrne, Trans.). Stanford, CA: Stanford University Press. (Original work published 1996).

Richardson, W. J. (1974). *Heidegger: Through phenomenology to thought*. The Hague: Martinus Nijoff.

Sheehan, T. (1978). Getting to the topic: The new edition of *Wegmarken*. In J. Sallis (Ed.), *Radical phenomenology: Essays in honor of Martin Heidegger* (pp. 299–316). Atlantic Highlands, NJ: Humanities Press.

Sheehan, T. (1979). The original form of *Sein und Zeit: Heideggers Der Begriff der Zeit, 1924. Journal of British Society for Phenomenology 10*, 78–83.

Sheehan, T. (1983). Heidegger's philosophy of mind. In *Contemporary philosophy: A new survey* (pp. 287–318). Boston: Martinus Nijhoff Publishers.

Sheehan, T. (1995a). *Das Gewesen:* Remembering the Fordham years. In B. E. Babich (Ed.), *From phenomenology to thought, errancy, and desire* (pp. 157–177). Boston: Kluwer Academic Publishers.

Sheehan, T. (1995b). Heidegger's new aspect: On *In-Sein, Zeitlichkeit* and the genesis of *"Being and Time." Research in Phenomenology* 25, 207–225.

Sheehan, T. (1999). Heidegger, M. *The concept of time.* (Thomas Sheehan, Protocol translation for University of Wisconsin–Madison School of Nursing Institute for Heideggerian Hermeneutical Studies).

Sheehan, T. (2001a). *Kehre* and *Ereignis:* A prolegomenon to introduction to metaphysics. In *A companion to Heidegger's introduction to metaphysics* (pp. 3–16, 263–274). New Haven, CT: Yale University Press.

Sheehan, T. (2001b). A paradigm shift in Heidegger research. *Continental Philosophy Review* 32(2), 1–20.

Yeats, W. B. (1983). *The poems.* New York: Macmillan.

2

Representing

Interpretive Scholarship's Consummate Challenge

KATHRYN HOPKINS KAVANAGH

The give and take of interpretive inquiry prompts new understandings of the meaningful experiences and multiple realities of peoples' lives. The question is, then, what to *do* with those—the *how* and practices of representing. This chapter deliberates the challenges of interpreting and representing (not to be confused with statistical representativeness in sampling), which is by definition political (Goldberg, 1998; Ross, 1999), and argues that a critical praxis informed by and echoing the realities of multicultural society is essential to socially responsible scholarship (James, Hockey, & Dawson, 1997).

Researchers are more than instruments through which voices and experiences are interpreted. How we study phenomena influences what we find. Researchers elicit and interpret experiences and realities of others and represent both those and their interpretations through language. Understandings are unabashedly filtered through our own interpretations, which are influenced by our own histories and biographies. Many stories that deserve to be told are those of peoples whose worldviews and lives may differ greatly from those of the inquirer. The scholarly product—written, oral, or in combination with other forms (for instance, metaphorical visual representations, drama, or poetry)—is the inquirer's responsibility. That responsibility extends well beyond formalized ethical concerns (informed consent, confidentiality).

Denzin and Lincoln refer to representing as "the most open-ended of the controversies surrounding phenomenological research today" (2000, pp. 184–185). Communication and meaning involve layers of interpretation of complex symbolic capital as we grapple with issues of reflexivity, incorporation of voices, meanings of "otherness," patterns of thinking, ideologies of categorization and hierarchy, and creation of identities (Susser, 2001b). Diverse ways of representing (multi–voiced, collaborative, negotiated, empowering [James, Hockey, & Dawson, 1997]) are language-dependent. Indeed "reality happens within language" (Gadamer, 1976, p. 35). While interpreting and representing become more complex when language and cultural orientations differ, the fact is that we live in a culturally complex society. We need to move beyond methods to make explicit these aspects of scholarship.

Language and Thinking

And I wonder at the words. *What are they?*
(Momaday, 1993, p. 217)

Issues around language are important in interpretive scholarship because languages and peoples relate to one another in complicated ways (Burling, 1970; Goodenough, 1971; Leininger, 2002). People adopt the values and perspectives of their social groups so that those come to shape their views of the world, what matters and what does not, and what they attend to and what they ignore (Dewey, 1916; Kincheloe & McLaren, 2000). It is through language that beliefs and preferences are, as Foucault (1994) put it, signified and represented. Much of that is through words. Speech and writing, the former having existed since the dawn of humanity and the latter for at least six thousand years (Kottak, 2003), so dominate human interaction that other means of communication are often devalued. Western cultures traditionally privilege the spoken over the written and the written over nonverbal communication (Derrida, 1978).

In the larger scheme of things, oral traditions dwarf written literature in size and diversity (Foley, 2001). In some ways, the precedents of oral traditions are more congruent with the goals of interpretive inquiry than are those of the alphabetic ways that we have learned to depend upon and privilege. Language in indigenous oral cultures is experienced as a property of the sensuous life-world (Abram, 1996). Spoken words, being attributed with animistic power, are viewed as real presences that make

the coherence of human language inseparable from that of the surrounding ecology and the sentient terrain. In such traditions, language refutes
western tendencies toward anthropocentrism (the belief that humankind
is the central fact of the universe) and reinforces the idea that words are
to avoid extremes and are not to be wasted (Abram, 1996).

Exactly what humans have to work with in terms of language is neither fully nor clearly understood. Whereas some linguists, such as Chomsky (1957), believe that the human brain dictates that all languages share
a set of deeply structured elements, others, such as Sapir (1931) and
Whorf (1956), theorize that different languages lead their speakers to
think about things in different ways. For example, because gender exists
as a feature of English grammar ("her heart attack," "his sed rates") and
we use a system of noun gender and adjective agreement, we are likely to
pay more attention to gender than are speakers of the many languages
that do not genderize what or whom they are talking about (Kottak,
2003). In sum, according to the Sapir-Whorf hypothesis, the language we
use shapes our thinking. Thus we have trouble conceptualizing anything
for which we do not have words at the ready.

In "The Nature of Language," Heidegger (1971) dwells on the final
line of Stefan George's poem, "The Word": "Where word breaks off no
thing may be" (Heidegger, 1971, p. 62). Heidegger speaks of *logos* as simultaneous Being and Saying. There is nothing where the word is lack-
ing. "Only the word makes a thing appear as the thing it is, and thus lets it
be present" (Heidegger, 1971, p. 65). That the "being of language" is the
"language of Being" (Heidegger, 1971, p. 94) clarifies the essential relationship between interpretive inquiry and language. According to Heidegger (1971), dictionaries have "plenty of terms, and not a single word"
(p. 86), for such compendia cannot use those terms as words. In short,
collecting and storing is not *Saying*. The transformative power of language is in speaking. Language is literally and figuratively the "tongue"
(lingua) of human saying (Heidegger, 1971, p. 114).

Whether reflecting innate or cultural patterns, the constellation of
language and tradition is interwoven with patterns of thinking. There is no
universal viewpoint, source of knowledge, or method of communicating
that qualifies the storyteller or interpretive scholar. Western languages
and societies are partial to binary opposition (white/black, male/female),
with the primary terms being privileged and designated as norms of
cultural meaning (white/non-white, male/non-male) (McLaren, 1998).

Society and language (not nature) compose binaries in which power always occupies both sides (Ross, 1999).

To Spinoza, kinds and individuals were infinite in profusion and expression, with each striving for power and resisting neutrality through innate ranked statuses. Ranking from high to low implied that the lower ranks existed for the sake of the higher in a world marked by proximity, fear, and power without intimacy (Spinoza, 1988). Kindredness emerges from links among humans and other kinds—genders, races, animals, plants, machines, nationalities, and other repetitions of mastery. In these epistemic orderings, the secondary terms exist only in relation to the first (Stam & Shohat, 1998). That conceptual framework strongly influences the categories we use.

The ways of interpretation are intertwined with the histories of concepts, for example, nature, the soul, the social, and the body (Riley, 1988; Warnke, 2002). For Aristotle, the essence of women was rooted in their imperfection as misbegotten males, a theme that grew to encompass feminine identity. In the nineteenth century, the opposition between body and soul was replaced with that between natural and social. For women this meant being different from men not so much in body and soul as in role—being suited to nurturing and domestic life (Warnke, 2002). Such is the hegemonic power of linguistic and conceptual meaning to incline understanding (through interaction between our self-understanding and our ideals) in certain directions (Taylor, 1998; Warnke, 2002).

Genderized western languages dualistically collude with hierarchically stratified views of the world and its inhabitants to polarize and rank the categories we use (Césaire, 1972; Hernández, 1997; Kavanagh, 2003). We struggle to discern inbetweenness and continuities in a world systematically and discretely (even concretely) dichotomized into *either-or* (black *or* white, masculine *or* feminine, us *or* them, right *or* wrong, even *or* odd, Democrat *or* Republican) a world in which it seems anomalous to think of phenomena as continuous (both good *and* evil, for instance, or light *and* dark, educated *and* ignorant, Christian *and* non-Christian).

More monistic peoples experience less conflict between categories (Feng, 1937/1983; Nisbett, 2003). They might, for example, comfortably affiliate with both Christian and indigenous animistic religions as they would utilize both conventional biomedicine for curing and shamanism for healing. "[T]he pueblo *kiva*-priest who attends Catholic mass and then officiates over the arrival of the *Kachinas* in the pueblo plaza sees no contradiction in these diverse activities" (Hunt, 2002, p. 224), despite professing the *Kachinas* to be deities. In the western world, attempts to refute or avoid dualism have generally failed (Lovejoy, 1930/1996). Our language and its usage, couched in the value of efficient rationality, encourage us to interpret such flexibility as contradictory.

In addition to comparing, polarizing, and accentuating opposition, competition, and difference with our naming and categorizing words, western languages convey strong sociolinguistic inclinations toward deduction, logic, and chronology—in other words, order (Foucault, 1994). Such rational standards obfuscate wholes, dialectics, and relationships. To be understood, science-based and arithmetically inclined worldviews plead for reduction to the simplest forms. Relative to English, eastern languages and those of many indigenous cultures around the world demand *fuller* understanding. Words or their parts usually have multiple meanings so context is required to understand them (Nisbett, 2003). Action is undertaken in concert with others or as the consequence of the self operating in a field of forces (Nisbett, 2003). Each word is seen in terms of relationships. While studying Navajo, I translated written passages only to be informed by the Navajo teacher that my efforts could not be accurately evaluated because the printed Navajo textbook did not (*could* not) provide enough of the context for a fluent Navajo speaker to know which words were truly appropriate. To persons grounded in contextualized thinking, the stripping away of situatedness that is associated with writing is highly problematic (Cooper, 1998; House, 2002).

Indo-European languages, including English, emphasize nouns that lend themselves to categorization. Nearly any property of an object can be objectified by adding the suffix "ness" ("thrownness," "situatedness") or its equivalent. English is a highly subject-prominent language and the language is agentic. That is, the person, place, or thing does the acting. "The nurse used her stethoscope to listen for a heartbeat." The world is seen in terms of static groups: nurses (versus other people), stethoscopes (versus other things), and heartbeats (versus things symbolized by no heartbeat or irregular heartbeats). Even as children learning language, westerners have their attention directed toward objects and the categories to which they belong.

Not all languages emphasize the words that lend themselves to taxonomic classifications. Children of Asian cultures have their attention directed toward relationships (Nisbett, 2003). The traditional Chinese world, as an example, consists of continuities so it is the part–whole dichotomy that matters. In an ancient Chinese encyclopedia called the *Celestial Emporium of Benevolent Knowledge,* animals are classified as "those that belong to the emperor, embalmed ones, those that are trained, suckling pigs, mermaids, fabulous ones, stray dogs, those that are included in this classification, those that tremble as if they were mad, those drawn with a very fine camel's hair brush, others, those that have just broken a flower vase, and those that resemble flies at a distance" (Nisbett, 2003, p. 137; paraphrased in Foucault, 1994). Obviously, class membership was not contingent upon shared attributes. Instead, classes formed around the ways items were thought to influence one another through resonance, as in the Chinese system of Five Processes in which the categories spring, east, wood, wind, and green all influence one another, and a change in wind (or any other category) affects all of the others (Nisbett, 2003). In the life-world of this philosophy, there is no concern about relationship between a member of the class and the class as a whole because classifying or limiting knowledge fractures the greater knowledge. That is, a part–whole representation does not presume that objects in a category share properties, so one cannot induce that if one mammal has a liver, all mammals do.

In contrast, the Greeks, for whom the world was composed of objects so individual–class relations seemed natural, assumed that all things in a category have the same properties. Hence one can induce from a single case: one mammal has a liver so all mammals do. Reflecting our deep cultural roots, westerners tend to categorize objects more than easterners, and we discern or learn new categories by applying rules about properties to specific cases. Relationships are, in the West, more often viewed as fulfilling than defining (Taylor, 1998). Since peoples in the East tend to organize the world in terms of every fact in its potential relation to every other fact (by thematic relationship rather than by taxonomic category), in selecting whether the chicken or the grass should be grouped with the cow, the grass wins every time.

Eastern societies distrust decontextualization and resist ideas based on underlying abstract propositions alone (Nisbett, 2003). While western societies reward reductionism and tend to disparage wordy contextualization, a language like Navajo (with its Athabaskan roots in Asia) is dominated not by nouns but by verbs to emphasize the world in motion— "talking the land," telling stories, and explicating innate interrelationships

(Cajete, 2000; Cooper, 1998; Goossen, 1995). Motion is so intrinsic to the Navajo worldview that there are nearly thirty verbs just for handing something to someone else (Young & Morgan, 1995).

In Heideggerian terms, for the Navajo something does not first exist and then move, but is constituted by its movements—its falling and thrownness, happening or historizing (Heidegger, 1967). That is, it is contextualized by its situatedness—the experience-founded interpretations and assertions about the world that Husserl called "horizon" (Gadamer, 1976; Husserl, 1994). So highly contextualized is the simple occurrence of transferring an object from one person to another that the very act is shaped semantically by the relationship between myriad properties of the action and those of the entity being handed over, in addition to other aspects of the situation. In the English language, in contrast, words are not seen as dependent upon context to be understood. They stand on their own. Words can speak to us with the power of the metaphysical, but it is often hermeneutical practice to attend to them etymologically (Kincheloe & McLaren, 2000) while neglecting the "horizon" from which they come.

In the ongoing process of meaning-making and interpreting, there are no simple relationships between linguistic form and cultural traits, although the form and structure of discourse figure strongly in interpretation and identity (Urciuoli, 2001). Generally in Native American cosmologies, everything has the possibility of intimate knowing relationships, for everything is both sentient and interrelated in the unified world (Deloria & Wildcat, 2001). Language both reflects that holism and becomes metaphysical. While the landscape is chanted, talked, and prayed, language animates and connects the breath of the person with that of others and of the world (Cajete, 2000). Language is culture and culture is lived. Language is Being. Words are the power that results in moving. Native American storytellers compare words with items in medicine bundles— "each piece, not just the most symbolically powerful pieces, is whole in itself and is essential to the whole. . . . Stories can cure or kill" (Bataille, 2001, p. 224). The Navajo, for instance, do not speak of death or dying, for words have the power to result in events occurring.

Written or spoken, words and languages are not *things* with neatly matching categories or types (Urciuoli, 2001). They are not rooted in a world that gives them meaning so much as they are thought itself (Foucault, 1994). Words have both linguistic and conceptual meanings.

For that reason, direct translations of words are seldom adequate for communicating authentic meanings of lived experiences. Stories are legion of embarrassing consequences of imperfect understanding of other languages. Consider how the slogan "Come alive with Pepsi" was translated in Asia as a promise that "Pepsi brings your dead ancestors back from the grave," or the American Dairy Association's "Got milk?" was translated in Mexico as "Are you lactating?" (Ferraro, 2001). Snickers aside, implications for corporations who lose credibility through muddled messages model those for the researcher who fails to *understand*. Assuming simple equivalence of word meanings within or between vocabularies is as perilous as assuming that literate persons or societies are superior to those that are not (Cooper, 1998).

In addition to the complexity of words and the structure of language, we must concern ourselves with the reality that writing always involves some alienation or distancing from spoken words and experience. Writing words inherently influences their meaning and interpretation. Paper transformed into written documents (paper money, licenses, court subpoenas) means something other than "paper" and takes on the status and power of the institutions it represents.

Interpretive inquiry is not only dependent on language but typically uses *written* texts. Hermeneutics designates that text interpretation, whether naïve or reflective, says (ontologically speaking) *we are* (Crusius, 1991). But "[t]he real question is not in what way being can be understood but in what way understanding is being" (Gadamer, 1976, p. 49). Emphases on method may foster dependence on words and underestimation of their value and authority by way of prescribed form.[1] While philosophical hermeneutics argues that understanding is an essential condition of being human and that understanding *is* interpretation (Gadamer, 1976; Schwandt, 2000), it is our task to come to grips with the vagaries of that humanness in interpreting and representing—in which language and writing play major roles.

Humans dwell in possibility. "Living a life is being in a world of possibility possibilizing; being open to possibilities and [to] how language speaks is a way to increase understanding of being human" (Diekelmann, 2003). So it is that "[o]ral traditions work like language, only more so" (Foley, 2001, p. vii). Language functions to express (which was the primary use of language in ancient cultures) or to communicate (which is the primary focus of language in contemporary, westernized cultures) (Cooper, 1998). Scholars who study indigenous oral communities have concluded that it is difficult for literates to experience the world, and in particular the natural world, in a way that approximates the intensity and vividness of the discourse that oral peoples have with the world around them (Abram, 1996).

The animistic perception of a natural phenomenon (such as a shadow shifting across a boulder) as a meaningful gesture, or entering into conversation with clouds or owls, reflects an inherently participatory disclosure of surroundings not as inert but as expressive entities, powers, and potencies. "Inanimate" rivers spoke to tribal ancestors much as "inert" letters on a page speak to us. In our distancing from the land, we no longer experience the enveloping earth as expressive and alive—despite Heidegger's early interest in the fourfold (earth, world, gods, and humans) later seen in reference (and opposition) to technology (Inwood, 1999). Yet in our anthropocentric alphabetic world, we take it for granted that writing "speaks," which is a form of animism (Abram, 1996), and the fourfold is mirrored in our ideas about relationships and differences. In efforts to get something into words, on the screen or into print, we may be lured into attending more closely to the words than to what they are representing. It is only fair to ask whether we have replaced the metaphysical world of our ancestors with a linguistic one rendered physical by writing language—and what the trade-offs are.

Silence is as much a part of language as are words. What is not said speaks loudly and is storied. In indigenous ethics, it is usual for language to be accompanied by lengthy silences so that partner, thought, will be fostered (Abram, 1996). With silence so potent, important words are preceded by silence until the interpersonal atmosphere and climate for communication is clear and harmonious (Cooper, 1998). Nonverbal techniques are important in interviewing and storytelling (Fontana & Frey, 2000; Hall, 1973). The Lakota are fond of claiming, for instance, that two of them can be back to back with neither saying a word while they hold an entire conversation. Proxemic communication uses interpersonal space to communicate attitudes while kinesic communication includes body movements or postures. Paralinguistics communicate through variations in volume, tone, pitch, and quality of voice, while chronemics reflect patterned pacing and length of silences in conversation (Fontana & Frey, 2000). Despite being essential for accurate representation, these aspects of language, like silence, tend to be neglected in, or even completely absented from, text-based interpretation.

To early humans, language was sacred and creative. It included communication with animals and divinities and extended to such phenomena as visions and dreams (Hunt, 2002). Communication was perceived as release of a stored power; speaking, singing, shouting, gesturing, staring, and other expressions allowed potential energy to become kinetic energy, a psychodynamic power closely associated with thought or consciousness (Cooper, 1998). As such, language is powerful; it could restore peace, harmonize a "patient" with his total environment, reenact creation, or change the air from being negative to positive (Witherspoon, 1977). The moral rules and printing tools imposed upon language and its use by colonialism concentrated on external communication, while indigenous expression relied more upon internal transmission (intuition, silent communication, memorized myth, internalized power) (Cooper, 1998) in which language is both spiritual and substantial, and in which, if in doubt, one remains silent.

Human languages allow displacement (speaking of things or events that are not present) and productivity (generation of new expressions through combining old ones) (Ember & Ember, 2002). Prioritizing words over silence and print over listening can leave interpretation on thin ice. To Heidegger, "speaking is at the same time also listening" (1971, p. 123). We speak by way of language (the sounded word and nonverbal forms) because we listen to it and appropriate (come to own) it. "Language is the house of Being because language, as Saying, is the mode of Appropriation" (Heidegger, 1971, p. 135). Meanings and stories are born of these capabilities. But there are great linguistic divergences, often among even closely related groups (such as generations) for we are, through language, endlessly (re)symbolizing (re)articulating (re)allegorizing, and (re)metaphorizing who we are and how we live in the world (Willett, 1998).

If there is a typical interpretive scholar, most likely he or she is from an English-speaking westernized society, highly dependent upon spoken and written words, and more a participant than a critical student of language and culture. The point is that we bear a responsibility to examine and reveal to ourselves and others how it is we construct and *say* our world, for how we do so cannot help but be reflected in our words, interpreting and representing. Being is as normally transparent to us as language, yet both Being and beings exist in concealment and hiddenness.

Meanings

Meanings are embedded in symbolism (which ranges from personal to universal) and in patterned styles of usage. In addition to communicating, speech (in all of its verbal and nonverbal forms) is manipulated to express feelings and evoke them in others, for instance, to insult or flatter, to construct images, and to generate moods. But we do not all think or express ourselves in similar ways. In communicating, North Americans (being highly individuated) characteristically overestimate their distinctiveness, while the Japanese do not even have a traditional concept of "a lively discussion" because such activity threatens the ideal of group harmony (Nisbett, 2003).

Linguistically, words are merely terms—as Heidegger saw them in the dictionary. It is in *showing* that something comes to light (Heidegger, 1971). In communicative speech, meaning is always associated with indicative relation (Husserl, 1994). Conceptual meanings denote more than words, as "caring nurse" expresses something that differs from the words "registered nurse." "Discourse," which in ordinary language connotes a formal expression of ideas, values or opinions, in Foucault's sense denotes vocabulary empowered to support certain forms of social dominance in specific contexts (Kohl, 1992; Warnke, 2002). Words reveal more than they communicate. "She was a real 'Nurse Ratchet'"; "he is an angel of mercy." To everyone everywhere, it is meaning that matters. Snowmobiles, "iron dogs" in Netsilik Eskimo, denote a significant advantage over live dog teams because they eat only when they work (Oswalt, 2002).

Meanings in translation, transcription, and interpretation reveal connections among text, author, and reader (Derrida, 1976; Ellis & Bochner, 2000). There is a strong impetus to attend to the cultural and situational significance of spoken and written accounts and to the nature of discourse in their production and reproduction—that is, how it is that the world is embodied and represented in speech and writing (Atkinson, 1994). Of course, there is no single or simple way to do that. Foucault, for example, advocated exploration of the use of words in terms of power and knowledge in dialectical practices that regulate what is considered reasonable and true (Foucault, 1972, 1973, 1980). For Derrida, words have meanings only in relation to their differences in a system of language (Derrida, 1978), thus meanings are constantly deferred by their contingency upon other words and are revealed only through intricate deconstruction. Both are radical departures from notions of the "natural world" as "out there" and empirically distinct from perception or interception (Schutz, 1962, 1964, 1967).

Human life is fundamentally dialogical. Language is essential to self-definition and the essential message of hermeneutics is that to be human is to mean, and only through the multifaceted nature of human meaning can we hope to understand people (Josselson, 1995). Locally shared meanings and interpretations are used to compose lives and, writ large, societies and cultures (Gubrium & Holstein, 1995). Today, in our multi-cultural and postmodern world, it is our challenge as interpretive scholars to make explicit and undermine the dualistic and hierarchical values that shape much of linguistic meaning in western cultures. It is through interpretation that the double binds of social and political forces in the production of meaning and value are exposed (Willett, 1998). Some of the most effective ways to throw open interpretive space is with multiple perspectives (e.g., feminist, critical, marginalized, boundary-crossing) that unsettle meanings and make them vague with contingency. But even then, efficient western decontextualization results in different ways of interpreting than those traditionally shaped by eastern integration and centering on relationships (Nisbett, 2003). The contrast suggests fundamentally different assumptions about the world, as well as variations in skills necessary for discerning and attending to relationships in complex environments. The implications for interpreting and representing are myriad.

Contextualizing and Worldview

For several years I co-taught a series of graduate qualitative research courses with a phenomenologist. Our conversations recurrently came down to this:

COLLEAGUE: It does not matter that the participant is Israeli and I am not.

KHK: It does matter. We need to know as much as possible about him—his culture, how he thinks, his language, his view of the world—who he is.

COLLEAGUE: If it matters to his story, he will tell me how being Israeli matters.

KHK: How can you interpret meaning in an Israeli man's story without exploring what it means to him to be an Israeli man? How does he know that it is safe to bring it up?

COLLEAGUE: He is Israeli. That does not mean his story is Israeli.
   Context is barely relevant.
KHK: His story is an Israeli man's story. His background is crucial to
   understanding how his story is situated and he in it.

And around we went. The goal here is to neither dismiss nor reify context
but to remind scholars of the importance that differences (implicit and
explicit) may have in meaning, telling, interpreting, and representing. In
inquiry, foregrounding makes it possible to understand concrete and social realities as constitutively meaningful in interpretation (Gubrium &
Holstein, 2000). Heidegger (1969) spoke of *Weltanschauung*, view of life
or worldview, as relating to the world in ways that contrasted with science
and philosophy. He questioned the relationship of worldview to *Dasein*
(Heidegger, 1969). While confronting the interplay of meaning and context is akin to opening Pandora's box (James, Hockey, & Dawson, 1997;
Mishler, 1979), ignoring it may be as spurious as positivist notions of objective independence between phenomenon and researcher. Heidegger's
conviction that worldview (relative to philosophy) narrows and constricts
real experience (Inwood, 1999) is precisely *why* the interpretive inquirer
needs to attend to it in both reflexive and interpretive work.

   "[N]ever-ending reflectiveness on our forehaving—preunderstanding in the sense of meaning-orientations implicit in our practices—is a
significant part of the hermeneutical task" (Crusius, 1991, p. 27). There is
no privileged access to understanding and meaning-making. Only in
interpreting the intersubjective world with sensitivity and skill can we
safeguard diverse realities from misrepresentation. Meanings may be
what we make of them, but as interpretive researchers we must ask how
it is that we interpret. How much knowledge and understanding of the
sociocultural constellation in which experiential phenomena occur is
necessary to keep our interpretations from reflecting our own stories and
worlds—that is, our own constellations?

Narrative and Story

   Interpretive inquiry thrives on narrative. We access peoples' lives and
worlds through their descriptions and stories, so the best narratives are
those that are individuated (though still social), are experiential, and disclose personal transformation (Bateson, 2000). Story is the medium that
allows the past and those who lived it to take hold of the imagination

so that the listener may confront what is considered sacred, eternal, and timeless (Miller, 2001)—what matters. Narrative approaches claim openness to whatever realities are brought to them as conversations and interviews generate plausible accounts (Silverman, 2000). Personal narratives evolve from humans communicating with other humans and their worlds—from being inside those exchanges with all of the negotiations, accommodations and integrations of good story. This means gathering the compelling and the mundane, apparitions of culture and its disrupting gaps of nothingness—the "cultures of no culture" (Taylor, 2003)—to represent complex understandings of experience and living.

Narrative and storytelling, like other uses of language, are culturally patterned. The organization of text affects its meaning. Oral societies retain and refine memories with mnemonic means, rather than through written storage systems (Cooper, 1998). Native American storytellers, for example, often speak in forms of measured verse (Basso, 1988). Their myths and stories (used to provide drama, educate, resolve issues, experience the artistry of storytelling, evoke mystery, connect generations, experience catharsis, and heal) are affected by print and electronic media. When presented as prose, as they typically were by Europeans and Euro-Americans, those transformed Native American stories led to inaccurate representations (as well as distorted translations) of the peoples whose stories they told.

Time is another phenomenon that is attended to differently among nonliterate peoples. Personal narratives matter in part *because* they fracture the boundaries of clearly framed representing and breach separations between the researcher and the researched (Ellis & Bochner, 2000). A storied life keeps the past alive with all of the incompleteness and tentativeness of real-life circumstances. To commodify that story for the convenience of the reading market begs questions about ownership and exploitation. "Narrative is both about living and part of it" (Ellis & Bochner, 2000, p. 746). As such, it deserves realistic as well as evocative representing (Richardson, 2000).

In representing, storytelling reveals meanings that used to be referred to as "insider views," but are now viewed more inclusively (and optimistically in terms of shared meanings) as intersubjective. These teach us how meanings and significance are and are not revisable in relation to present-day contingencies (Ellis & Bochner, 2000). In health care, illness narratives (Kleinman, 1988) and clinical narratives (Diekelmann, 2002;

Good, 1998; Miller & Crabtree, 2000) tell stories and create space for multiple realities that move toward listening and questioning. Stories make actions explainable and challenge assumptions and stereotypes. They form and shape. In reference to a figure in his childhood, master storyteller Momaday claims, "I am created in the old man's story" (1993, p. 219). Collective stories resist conventional cultural narratives by supplying alternatives (Silverman, 2000) and allowing people to be empowered through speaking (Madriz, 2000).

My name is Rigoberta Menchú. I am twenty three years old. This is my testimony. I didn't learn it from a book and I didn't learn it alone. I'd like to stress that it's not only *my* life, it's also the testimony of my people. . . . My personal experience is the reality of a whole people. (Menchú, 1984, p. 1)[2]

Stories may be formulated or fluid and free-flowing, being told until "[t]here are no more words to the story" (Mather & Morrow, 1994, p. 200). They are both open to change and susceptible to it. The hard part is recognizing the line between those. Hermeneutics takes dialogue as its mode of inquiry from Plato, and circular, dialectical understanding as permanently tensive and concealing from Hegel (Crusius, 1991; Ross, 1999). There are no subjects, only participants, in dialogue and in the intersubjectivity of genuine dialogue (whether between persons or between text and the interpretive inquirer), "something different comes to be" (Gadamer, 1976, p. 58) in a "fusion of horizons" (Gadamer, 1989, p. 273–274) that both reveals and conceals "beyond the spontaneous, unscrutinized projections of preunderstanding" (Crusius, 1991, p. 38).

"Who has not looked at the computer screen, read a paragraph he or she has written, and then chosen to alter it?" (Richardson, 2000). Stories are like writing: telling them reveals new questions, meanings, interpretations—possibilities. Creative conversation is shaped by feelings—ours as inquirers *and* those of participants, often shared. We gather stories, theirs and ours. Different approaches to inquiry elicit different stories. We make choices about portraying stories, representing people and interpretations. Perhaps we leave some parts out, find special appeal in others, and reinforce or dispel dominant representations through our choices. We are repository, archivist, analyst, interpreter. These roles of representational praxis are not to be taken lightly.

The vagaries of language aside, in examining the "hows" and "whats" of storytelling, it is no more possible for us to be *fully* aware of our contributing and intercepting biases (that is, those coming from our own experiences and who we are) than it is for those who share the stories with us to fully disclose their personal meanings. We are analogous to the oral epic singer, but with the challenge of doing a culture-straddling balancing act facilitated by being both insider and outsider, performer and investigator, sorter and keeper, collector and teller. Often the best we can do is collaborate, but at the same time, collaborations can multiply the natural mutability of realities (Foley & Moss, 2001). Our scholarship is made valuable and vulnerable by our very uniqueness.

Labeling and Naming

The thing is not known until it is named.
(Merleau-Ponty, 1962, p. 177)

What do we do when we begin to "see" and understand a phenomenon? We wrap it with words, possess it through description, label and name it categorically (as a theme, perhaps). This is an important process. From our earliest days, names populate our world. "Creation says to the child: Believe in this tree, for it has a name" (Momaday, 1993, p. 215). The power of naming and labeling came to the forefront in the 1960s when labeling theory presented meaningful links between social etiology and social pathology. Drawing on social interactionism, it was noted that social reactions to people or their actions, and the labels applied (for example, "juvenile delinquents") powerfully affected their interpretations of themselves and their expectable behavior (Becker, 1963; Goffman, 1961, 1963; Rose, 1962).

In recent decades the impact of labeling and stigmatizing has been so absorbed by western societies as to be taken nearly for granted (Albrecht, Fitzpatrick, & Scrimshaw, 2000). For example, the World Health Organization was sufficiently convinced of the importance of the perspective to introduce a now widely-accepted revised classification of handicap as directly related to the social problems stemming from labeling or the fear of being labeled (WHO, 1980; Wood, 1975). Health care professionals and lay populations were sensitized to the meaning and power inherent in affiliation between clinical interaction and specific people and places. For example, by virtue of diagnostic recognition and acknowledgement by credible practitioners in powerful places (such as medical centers, hence, the pun "edifice complex" [Torrey, 1984]), patients might share their gravest concerns and feel free to progress toward being cured or even healed. Naming a health condition, whether by divination or physical examination, gives the named phenomenon a culturally recognizable form and imposes order on a previously chaotic set of experiences. This release from the tyranny of singularity (Ross, 1999) through provision of a set of expectations and a basis for acting, has all of the power that knowing the name "Rumpelstiltskin" did in the German fairy tale collected by the Brothers Grimm (Torrey, 1984). For better or for worse, naming, labeling—recognizing kind and classifying—becomes a form of culture-oriented domination (Ross, 1999). Heuristically, a name is both liberating through identity and limiting through its "referential bondage" (Tschaepe, 2003, p. 68).

Naming has its downside when social and historical conditions lead to stigmatizing. Leprosy was not stigmatized in Hawaii, for example, until its incidence increased concurrently with the arrival of Chinese immigrants working the burgeoning plantations. From that time the Chinese were stigmatized in part because they were blamed for having brought leprosy to the islands (despite its being already there), and leprosy was stigmatized because it was identified with the Chinese—transforming a relatively unknown and unimportant disease into a morally threatening sickness and social conflict (Waxler, 1981). Conditions such as epilepsy, AIDS, pelvic inflammatory disease, and cirrhosis of the liver still carry powerful negative meanings embedded with moral connotations (Freund, McGuire, & Podhurst, 2003). In mental health, labeling remains wrought with discrediting and tainting stigma. "The stigma can be worse than the illness. . . . Stigma is about disrespect: it hurts, punishes, and diminishes people" (Anti-Stigma Project, 1998).

Reframing language ("crazy," "lunatic," "deficient," "wacko," "loony tune," or "psycho" into "mentally ill" or "psychiatrically disabled," for instance, or "handicapped person" into "person with a disability") has merits and limits ("normal" into "nondisabled person"). The boundaries are vague, for naming and labeling are meaning-creating undertakings and rarely neutral. Reflecting the perspectives from which they come, they point and push in certain directions. The power to name (even against one's will) is an expression of control, for to name a being both expresses power over and conjures up powers latent in that being (Dixon,

2002). While names have the power to cast people, places, and things in favorable or unfavorable light, the ability to name oneself is an act of liberation from semantic bondage. Aboriginal peoples everywhere assert that a name is sacred and must be treated as such (Somé, 2000). Many groups today are reasserting their own names for themselves (Lakota rather than Sioux, Lenni Lenape rather than Delaware, Diné rather than Navajo, and numerous others) in place of labels that were arbitrarily or even pejoratively applied to them during colonial times (Dixon, 2002).

A common scenario in traditional research involves the use of pseudonyms to safeguard anonymity of persons and locations. Since the Enlightenment, notions of self, uniqueness of personhood, and private domain have been sacrosanct. Codes of ethics insist on confidentiality, and the greatest risk in inquiry is the disclosure of private knowledge (Punch, 1994; Reiss, 1979). At the same time, "there is no consensus or unanimity on what is public and private" (Christians, 2000, p. 140; Punch, 1994, p. 94).

This brings up a number of heuristic issues for interpretive scholarship. How does the inquirer foreground participants' voices and identities, that is, who *they* are and what *they* are saying, in ways that are safe, acceptable, respectful, *and* confidential (Evers & Toelken, 1994)? Along with identities, aliases can mirror external frames of reference and function as a way of distorting perspective. What are the ethical issues involved in altering identities, and how far can such changes go without compromising credibility and interpretation? The guidelines are not without contradiction. However, it is notable that ethical guidelines tend toward "majoritarian ends" (Christians, 2000, p. 138). Along with informed consent, avoidance of deception, and privacy and confidentiality, accuracy is a primary consideration, which precludes "[f]abrications, fraudulent materials, omissions, and contrivances" as unethical (Christians, 2000, p.140).

Herein lurks the contradiction. For Merleau-Ponty, the name of a thing resides "on the same footing as its colour and form" (1962, p. 178). To be accurate, it can be argued that names of participants should reflect their social statuses. At the same time, it is also sometimes claimed that social identities should reveal themselves only when directly pertinent to the study. In the first situation, for example, if participants "Bill" and "Sue" of an interpretive study are ethnically Chinese, their names might be altered to imply their heritage as a way of communicating the actual diversity that exists within the study's participants—that is, to attest to the reality that persons of Asian extraction are participating in the research. Interpretive inquiry by those ascribing to the second scenario, on the other hand, would not include that identification because ethnic identity would be considered pertinent *only* if the participants indicated that it was.

While the former scenario assumes that it is preferable to imply equitable opportunities for participation in the study, it also implies that "Wen" and "Ming" differ somehow from other (presumably more western and "white") participants and that the difference may be significant. Despite making a positive statement for equality, this does not move toward assimilationist or "majoritarian" ends. By contrast, the latter representation, that is, leaving ethnicity unstated, ignores differences that may well be significant either to Bill and Sue or to interpretation by the researcher in a racist society. It is also possible that the majority status of an interpretive inquirer obviates recognition of the import of ethnicity, that is, that he or she does not recognize the deeper meanings and experiences of ethnic or racial status (or other social status or labeled situation) that is outside of his or her own experience.

This essentially no-win state of affairs clearly echoes the United States's perennial ambivalence toward difference and its history of both punishing and celebrating it. With a multiculturalism that is not fully theorized (Willett, 1998), the dialectics of recognition, communication, self-naming, and articulation are debated. Representing is struggled over in a confusion of politics, "correctness," and multicultural possibilities for self-expression (Goldberg, 1998; Taylor, 1998). These are interwoven by past and present realities to the extent that the challenge becomes one of encountering the past as the future inasmuch as it continually reintroduces otherness (alterity) within the present (Bhabha, 1990). The following dialogue from the comic strip *The Boondocks* illuminates the general dis-ease of the situation—the thin line between not enough and too much when it comes to [nomitive] recognition and labeling.

"I'm tellin' you, Huey—just by giving the characters in a movie really *black* names, it'll seem like a totally different flick."

"I think I'll start with a romantic comedy. There just aren't enough good black romantic comedies."

"*When Lamont met Boqueisha*—a screenplay by Michael Caesar."

"Oh, boy." (McGruder, 2001, 7/26)

These issues of identity are of increasing concern in light of new regulations regarding access to data collected in funded studies and for researchers who work in sensitive areas (such as reproductive health, genetics, or sexual orientation, among numerous others) (Olesen, 2000). There are also concerns for protection of those participants whose identities are difficult to conceal due to their unique positions in society and who must be cautioned that their confidentially cannot be assured (Chambers, 2000).

From a purely practical standpoint, two strategies reveal themselves for consideration in the pros and cons of representing identity. One is the value of autonomy, which in "the logic of social science inquiry" revolves around that ethic of democratic life (Christians, 2000, p. 139). People have the right to label themselves as they see fit. Such self-determination has led to practices such as encouraging participants to choose their own "identities" (names and descriptors) in studies, with some inevitably retaining their real names and others not. Researchers' written assurances that identities are protected or pseudonyms provided disguise authentic as well as artificial names and characterizations.

A second stratagem is presented in the acculturated or hybridized names used by individuals who wish to communicate their biculturalism. Examples, among many others, include such Asian American authors as Maxine Hong Kingston (*The Woman Warrior* [1977]; *Chinamen* [1980]), Gus Lee (*China Boy* [1992]; *Honor and Duty* [1994]), and Amy Tan (*The Joy Luck Club* [1989]; *The Kitchen God's Wife* [1992]). But, however recognizable and memorable, this heuristic ploy in no way alleviates the deeper issues of discerning, identifying, and labeling.

Classifying, Ranking, and Stereotyping

It is part of daily living to work at making sense out of the world. People typically organize that world from within the tradition of value orientations of a given society (Kottak, 2003). We generally do our decoding, judging, assessing, evaluating, choice-making, and systematizing to our advantage or to that of things or relationships that matter to us. With preunderstandings rooted in immersion in generally social and specifically cultural and personal experiences, we are predisposed to see things in certain ways, that is with knowing gained from what Heidegger called "forehaving" (Crusius, 1991). Comparisons are made, situations interpreted, commonalities and differences recognized and dealt with in patterned ways. The product of perspective is otherness or difference, which is usually tailored by self-perceived superiority (Wernitznig, 2003). By definition, difference is exclusionary—a mark of delineation to cut off from that for which there is an *a priori* understanding of *likeness* (Goldberg, 1998; Heidegger, 1981; Inwood, 1999). Thus others are judged to be different (in essence, strange to the self) and characteristically defined and labeled in ways that solicit agreement or commonality (kindredness) in standing (Ross, 1999).

Discerning difference always results from history, culture, power, or ideology of groups and must be understood in terms of the specificity of its production (McLaren, 1998). The contrast to difference is heterogeneity, the *logos* or neutral totality of infinite kinds—but this is interrupted by essentialism (belief in real essences of things to be defined by science and philosophy) and identity politics (Ross, 1999). Despite claims of some postmodern stances, there is no denying history or potential real break with the past; whatever possibilities there are for understanding and interpreting reside in our own forehaving (Crusius, 1991). Language is a major constituent of that—but not the only source of orienting influence.

Classificatory schemes and stable orders are rational, but meanings can congeal and be reified, making them monolithic and static in ways that being is not. Changes in thinking have led to demanding resistance to domination (as the link between kinds in terms of hierarchy) and to moving beyond ranking (Ross, 1999). While labeling and categorizing are increasingly considered ethical issues, old patterns of organizing the world are persistent and polarity and ranking haunt western thinking. Other descriptive associations (such as those based on idealized or imagined resemblance or relationship) are not always sought or considered (Foucault, 1994). In sum, relationships have many possibilities and interpretations. Kind might be found in function rather than form, for example, bringing together such disparate entities as tuning forks, microprocessors, pendulum clocks, the human pulse, sundials, water clocks, hourglasses, marked wax candles, the sun, leaves that turn colors with the season, and tree rings (Rosenberg, 1993).

Hermeneutics aims to hold open alternative possibilities for ways of showing (Crusius, 1991). Whether those of our own or others, it is difficult to recognize taken-for-granted patterns used to organize the worlds we or others live in. Gadamer calls those familiar assumptions and expectations that provide the initial orientation to what we are trying to understand "prejudices" (Gadamer, 1989; Warnke, 2002). Because even perception (seeing, hearing) is shaped by such prejudicial preunderstandings, continuous reflection upon these meaning-shaping orientations is a significant part of the hermeneutical task (Crusius, 1991).

Part of hermeneutic reflexivity involves recognizing and confronting prejudice in the form of stereotypes. Those most significant to and embedded in society involve class (relative economic resources), ethnicity, race, and gender—or a confounding of several or all of those concepts. Ideas about inequality are typically intertwined with socially interpreted and constructed meanings that are justified with culturally exaggerated differences, for instance, between genders, between immigrants and the native-born, and between indigenous peoples and descendents of colonists (Susser, 2001a). Ranking is typically superimposed upon such categories, albeit viewed naively as natural and innate.

Patterns of thinking and language conspire in many (and often complex) ways with those of bias and prejudice. From the days of the first European settlers, heterogeneity in the U.S.A. influenced delineation of class, racial, national, cultural, and gender categories that are closely related to the historical development of capitalism (Patterson, 2001; Susser, 2001a). At the same time, the word "ethnic" (which is derived from *ethnos* in reference to those tribes or nations beyond the Greek city-states and, as such, is inherently marginalizing) came into use as an alienating characteristic of *other* people. Although *ethnic* is a term so common in North America today that it lacks interpretive precision (Tuleja, 1997), the concepts of class and ethnicity have been conflated in such a way that the American "underclass," for example, is often characterized by public media and politics in terms of lack of family values and presence of criminal activity. This is further complicated by projection of a bifurcated prejudice toward opposing images, such as the successful assimilated minority and the "gangster/welfare mother" (Baker, 2001).

Not all prejudicial reinvention is pejorative, although it is almost always unappreciated. It is common practice, for example to "occidentalize," a pattern by which eastern cultures are interpreted from western values and norms, or to exoticize, which involves the conjuring up of mysterious, unchanging exotic peoples and ways. There are other techniques, intended and unintended, that marginalize through Othering and stereo-typing. The salient fact is that misrepresenting reduces people to impen-etrable differences and distances (sometimes even from themselves) and imposes identities that are not theirs. And misrepresenting occurs with remarkable ease if care is not taken to avoid stereotyping and other tools of misinterpreting.

Categorizing and Classifying Race

For all of our enlightenment and knowing, the tangle of race contin-ues with ominous regularity to entrap western scholarship into either contributing to it (often unwittingly) or trying to ignore it, which, since race and other categories of difference have real impact on real lives, brings into question issues of authenticity and credibility in inquiry. Interpretive scholars have an opportunity and a responsibility to help correct the morass of confusion common around "race" in society today—although that requires coming to grips with issues that many people find uncomfortable.

Platonic notions of ideal types held that the physical and material world derived from pure ideals. These ideals were unchanging except for their devolution from the pure form. Since humans could be assessed in terms of ideal types (that is, ideal male and female types, or ideal soldiers, nurses, teachers, or servants), this provided, in union with the Christian concept of a great chain of being (Lovejoy, 1996), a foundation for the idea of race. Thus the great chain became a ladder with white Europeans occupying the top rungs. Everyone else (based on characteristics such as color or creed) was further down, somewhere between Europeans and the nonhuman primates, with each rung and each race having a fixed place relative to God (Goodman, 2001).

The problem with ideal types, and the lack of reflectiveness that fosters them, is that they simply do not hold up. But with science and politics popularizing the theory of racialism (that is, of a fixed number of distinct human types), "race" was accepted as natural and real—as is gen-erally the case with ideas that are useful to the classes with control of leg-islation and information. For more than two centuries, an ensemble of sciences and their adjutants secured fixed taxonomies and stable racial-historical and gender identities that could be and were complied into a "natural" sociology of hierarchy that retains a haunting presence

(Robinson, 1998). Today, despite a century of scientific evidence that human "races" are social figments, "race" remains encoded in all our lives with political, intellectual and emotional meanings (Thompson & Tyagi, 1996). Self-depreciation, one of the most potent instruments of oppression (Taylor, 1998), is still widely exploited.

Notions of biological race embodied beliefs that the human species is divisible into a small and discrete number of fixed and old categories, that behavior is at least in part explainable by racial classification, and that races are hierarchically arranged (Goodman, 2001). That humans manifested the idealized discrete categories in neither their biological nor behavioral characteristics did not prevent natural historians from tinkering with the classificatory schemes until race explained (as it did for Linnaeus) such phenomena as customs, psychological attributes, and systems of government (Goodman, 2001).

Race is a typological and non-evolutionary concept that should have been replaced a century ago, given the dominance of evolutionary theory and biology and an abundance of evidence that division points between races were purely arbitrary since human variation is a continuous trait (Goodman, 2001). Prior to the idea of race, "us" and "them" distinctions were common, but they were not correlated with biology (Goodman, 2001). Yet today "[w]e are blacks or whites in a way that a sixteenth-century Xhosa could not be" (Warnke, 2002, p. 316). It is claimed that in "the micropolitics of racial cross-traffic" (Frankenberg, 1996, p. 15), "before America no one was white" (Kaye/Kantrowitz, 1996, p. 121).

Although common racial distinctions correspond to neither genes nor internal properties (but are rooted in the economic and social history of Atlantic trade and African slavery), racial thought spawned traditions of meaning leading to full-blown racial hierarchies (Warnke, 2002). The paradigm is tenacious, although the categories shift with time and circumstances—often arbitrarily. For instance, some groups, such as Jews, Irish, and Southern Europeans, were "whitened" with acceptance over time and became "ethnic" groups rather than "races" (Lesage, Ferber, Storrs, & Wong, 2002; Sacks, 1994). Class ascendance also contributes to whitening. Economic power partially "whitens" Asian immigrant capitalists allowing them access to privileged occupations and residential spaces, while others continue to be racialized (Goode, 1998; Ong, 1996). Yet, despite—or perhaps because of—its slipperiness, instead of disappearing, human "race" has been reified by constant use, conflated with human variation, seldom seriously questioned or challenged, and continues to be politically manipulated (Barkan, 1992).

Kinds and Identities

"Race" is only one way in which essentialism produces hierarchies that authorize exclusion (in the name of essence and kinds) and domination of *other* kinds (such as genders, classes, educational levels) (Ross, 1999). Whereas essentialism alludes to classifying singular individuals into kinds by their fundamental nature (types), the politics of identity today speak more often of those who classify themselves by their kind ("we" women, Jews, scholars, Onondaga, surgical nurses) to claim allegiance and seek alliances and community (Ross, 1999). This search for commonality may be, at times, much like Don Quixote's quest for similitude, thus transforming flocks, serving girls, and inns into armies, ladies, and castles (Foucault, 1994).

A ready-at-hand example of how kinds and identities entangle themselves involves Native American Indians and the deceptively simplistic query: *Who is an Indian?* Politically correct labeling (which now generally eschews issues and labels involving race) cites ethnicity as an easy answer. Either "Native American" or "American Indian" is technically correct as a category, although individuals often have strong preferences for one or the other (or against either) term. Traditionally there was no pan-Indian overarching concept; members of tribes or bands identified themselves by the indigenous names for those social groupings. Today, many Native Americans do not have tribal knowledge or connections but share a pan-Indian identity (Lobo, 2001; Straus & Valentino, 2001). Thus ethnicity is, at best, an imprecise term. Even putting confusion between Indians in the Americas and peoples in India completely aside, does ethnicity mean culture or ancestry? In reality, the boundaries are constantly renegotiated and redefined through social interaction (Gonzales, 2001) and personal interpretation (Warnke, 2002).

Political correctness aside, another way of dealing with the question *Who is an Indian?* might employ race (Straus & Valentino, 2001). During the nineteenth century, when biology spawned and nurtured the concept of race, blood was believed to be the carrier of physical and behavioral characteristics (Gonzales, 2001; Tapper, 1999). Existing concepts of race led to legal creation of racial categories in the U.S.A. and their application in regulations governing immigration, citizenship, entitlements, and the census (Merry, 2001). As if race were not mystifying enough, its nomenclature has increased in complexity with the government adding more categories and subcategories of "race" (some of them ethnic, i.e., cultural, rather than racial, i.e., biological) for the 2000 census, thus providing sixty-three possible combinations to use to characterize racial identity (Lesage, Ferber, Storrs, & Wong, 2002). But racial identity is always ambiguous and arbitrary. Even on the colonial frontier, race was mutable; the same individual might be white or black in one circumstance, Indian in another (Patterson, 2001). *Who is an Indian?* indeed.

If ethnicity and race will not serve to define "Indianness," how about genetics? The problem is that four migration periods of Asian-derived peoples moving into the New World resulted in morphologically distinct craniofacial and genetic patterns still discernible today (Brace & Nelson, 2001). These were not minor variants of the same people but correspond to distinct mitochondrial DNA haplotype lineages (Wallace & Torroni, 1992). In western societies it is common for "Asians" to be glossed as a homogeneous "Mongoloid" category and "American Indians, Native Americans, and Alaskan Natives" as a homogenous lot either Asian or separate enough to be AmerIndian. In reality, each of these superchunking categories includes many greatly varied subcategories. Given the heterogeneity among peoples who crossed the Bering land bridge and their descendants, and despite stereotypes of long, straight, black hair, dark eyes, and brown skin, physical characteristics, whether phenotypic or genotypic, do not answer the question *Who is an Indian?* (Gonzales, 2001).

Another way to go at the issue of identity is with socially constructed categories, such as "minority" (Straus & Valentino, 2001), which implies relative powerlessness. But such imposed tags are politically imprecise at best, and often unappealing and pejorative. One might also explore tribal identity, but that always ranged widely in meaning and usage, and continues to do so today. In its simplest forms, tribal identity might mean enrollment in a recognized tribe or documented blood quantum (a persistent federal designator that implies that the higher the percentage of "Indian" blood, the more "Indian" one is) (Gonzales, 2001; Pickering, 2000). Many people who identify as Native Americans or American Indians today fit only one or neither of those criteria. Authority repudiates neutrality even while professing to institute it (Ross, 1999).

Residence on an Indian reservation or preserve might also be considered a viable indicator, but more than half of all American Indians live in cities and there are now second- or third-generation urban Indians (Gonzales, 2001). Cultural markers, such as living "traditionally" (versus being non-traditional or assimilated into the mainstream or dominant society) or ability to speak a tribal language or to demonstrate use of Indian colloquialisms rules out a huge proportion of "Indians" after centuries of cultural oppression. And identity based on participation in practices associated with American Indian community or spirituality—powwow dancing, drumming, "sweating," burning cedar, vision quests, and so on—does nothing to clarify differences between "wannabes," pretenders, and "authentic Indians" (Gonzales, 2001).

In sum, there is no universally acceptable way to answer the question "Who is an Indian?" Kinds are always plural (Ross, 1999). Everyday stereotypes and ideologies are locally created and enacted. Most non-Indians, for instance, conceive of "real" Indians as the aboriginals that they *imagine* they once were, not the peoples they really were or are now (Berkhofer, 1979). And, in binary fashion, the past European image of Native Americans oscillated between the noble and the bloodthirsty savage (Dippie, 1982). Despite the inadequacy of any defining classificatory scheme, and despite efforts to eradicate the people (through ethnocide, genocide, or rendering them invisible and labeling them "vanished" [Dippie, 1982]), there are several million "Indians" in the United States and many more throughout the hemisphere.

Essentialism and categorization inflict individuals within their kinds with ethical-political obligation (Ross, 1999). Whereas identity is generally conceived as a bond (the affinity and affiliation of associates so identified) that holds the collective together (Goldberg, 1998), it can also be experienced as a form of bondage by insistence on an essential character, for instance, or requirements of ethnic or other group solidarity. There are also phenomena, whether social or personal (such as the effects of trauma or disability), that can be more powerful than racial or ethnic identities (Frank, 2000; Kess-Gardner, 2002; Thompson & Tyagi, 1996). As interpretive scholars, we must have a sense of the possibilities and be open to new ones before we ask *"What is the meaning and experience of being an Indian/woman/nurse/whatever and whoever you are?"*—or we will not know to inquire. Who we are *matters.*

Categories as Fabricated Horizons

Ethnic identity and its political implications are dialogic and potentially always changing. The reification of categories and the influence of those on interpretations of identity and difference is problematic. At the same time, the fluidity of categories is striking, whether they are social constructions or personal interpretations, indigenous or imposed. Native American identities traditionally involved local (tribal or band) affiliation and individual identity. For years the U.S. government supported Pan-Indianism (basically a blending of American Indian tribal cultures) as a replacement for tribalism and a step toward assimilation (blending into mainstream European American society), despite evidence of continuity of many of the separate groups (Lobo, 2001; Oswalt, 2002). Then the government's Bureau of Indian Affairs reversed its approach by advocating acknowledgement and recognition of indigenous groupings (Dippie, 1982; Leacock & Lurie, 1988; Lobo, 2001; Oswalt, 2002). Although pan-ethnic identity efforts following the 1960s civil rights movements often included groupings of culturally and historically dissimilar peoples, when opportunities arose to reify the categories (for instance, to qualify for resources or political representation), old identities and social constructions had new saliency for collective boundaries (Espiritu, 1992). Tribal and band identities reemerged.

Generally, seeing (i.e., what is noticed and attended to) is permeated by the language and categories at hand. Despite the social tenacity of "race," some categories that held fast in the sciences are changing in response to the expansion of genetic knowledge (Olson, 2002). Phenotypic differences (i.e., those that are physically apparent) lose significance when genetic evidence collapses categories (Gore, 2003). For example, it is increasingly recognized that congenital abnormalities and genetic diseases (such as Tay-Sachs disease, cystic fibrosis, and sickle cell disease) that occur more frequently in some populations than others involve explanations of population structures and gene flow that are far more complex than either genetics or notions of "race" account for (Mwaria, 2001). This is not to say, however, that new fabrications could not replace the old ones.

The limitations of available language and familiar mindsets continue to complicate life, as is the case when the term "biracialism" is used to represent peoples in Polynesia, the Caribbean, and many other places

who have been "multiracial"—if "racial" is at all a useful descriptor—
for centuries (Hall, 1996). Categories fluctuate with paradigmatic domination and political expediency, as is the case with the medicalization of
deviance as medical systems redefine normality, abnormality, identity
(Santiago-Irizarry, 2001), and moral issues under medical genre. In this
movement, what was thought of as badness is transformed into sickness,
as has occurred with alcoholism, homosexuality, promiscuity, drug addic-
tion, arson, suicide, child abuse, civil disobedience, and many other phenomena now subsumed under the spreading biomedical umbrella (Conrad & Schneider, 1992).

Challenging the Lists: Contested Categories, Borders, and Trouble Spots

Identities, as interpreted and negotiated constructions, are highly
susceptible to change. Categories shift. Individual subjectivities form,
reform, and transform as people grow, mature, and negotiate their
way through diverse, expanding networks of relationships in differently
situated (usually local but ever more globalized) spaces (Goode, 2001;
Warnke, 2002). Challenging essentialism, categorization, and labeling to
see and experience these intersubjectivities requires recognizing cate-
gorical boundaries and traversing borders. Such figurative delineations
might be linguistic, epistemological, ideological, geographical, cultural,
economic, political, or otherwise constructed of idiosyncratic or social
interpretation.

Borders demarcate otherness and stipulate the manner in which otherness is maintained and reproduced (for instance, as a medical or ethnic
struggle). It is at the margins that colonized and decolonized spaces form,
often as the consequence of boundary processes rather than individual
identity. Border cultures, where normative structures and codes collide
with alternatives, are anticentering places where living crosses the lines
of linguistic, cultural, and conceptual realities. In theory, despite—or
perhaps because of—the disruption inherent in such liminal situations,
there are opportunities in border regions to live multidimensionally
(McLaren, 1998). Identities that dispense with traditional boundaries
cannot be subsumed under either dialectical or analytic logic (Hicks,

1992; McLaren, 1998). There is new agency involved that is outside of the usual Euro-American, Cartesian, and other familiar discourses. On the other hand, modernist concerns about liberation from oppression remain relevant to a borderless interactive universalism that dismisses the identities of rationality (Benhabib, 1992; McLaren, 1998).

The Politics of Recognition

Recognizing meanings of *otherness* and *sameness* become urgent because of their links with personal identity and the potential for damage with misrecognition (as when society mirrors a confining or demeaning picture of the self) (Taylor, 1998). As an indispensable part of recognition, "whiteness" is being (and has been for more than a decade) explored as a culture—for without addressing white ethnicity there can be no critical evaluation of the construction of *the other* (McLaren, 1998; Wallace, 1991). "Whiteness" is traditionally and mythically heralded as neutral, despite arbitrariness (as noted above in the extension of "whiteness" to formerly racialized groups or individuals).[3]

Race has been used to commodify "blackness," "whiteness," difference, *other*, or strangeness (Bateson, 2000) to its own ends. Manipulating *others* without recognizing and interpreting "Otherness" as a tool of exploitation reflects and perpetuates the prevailing social texts in the politics of signification (that is, in which social norms are established and altered) (McLaren, 1998; West, 1990). Privilege is something that white people often deny they exploit or even have, despite the simple fact that being white implies having choices about when to focus on race—a luxury that people of color do not have (Lesage, Ferber, Storrs, & Wong, 2002).

Having reached its lowest level of acceptance in a century, "race," as applied to humans, is now being characterized as a "perishing paradigm" (Lieberman, Kirk, & Littlefield, 2003). This is not because bias and prejudice have disappeared but in large part because "race" as a human attribute goes against the growing bodies of knowledge in genetics and biology. Even those who continue to use the concept seriously doubt its utility since it fails to connote the extensive store of variation that characterizes modern peoples (Lieberman, Kirk, & Littlefield, 2003). The race concept, being biologically unrealistic, is really valueless in practice. *Nonetheless,* "race" still has very real social meanings that lead to suffering and injustice (Cartmill & Brown, 2003).

Shifting Paradigms: From Race to Multiculturalism

Immigration during the nineteenth and twentieth centuries was assumed to be the beginning of assimilative processes that would obliterate cultural distinctions (Nash, 2001). The gatekeepers of society—educators, employers, legislators, industrialists, and religious and labor organizations—embraced an Anglicized model of cultural assimilation as the path to progress (Lamphere, 1992). Then the civil rights and countercultural movements of the 1960s marked a shift from the prevailing assimilative standard of monoculturalism to a new ideal of inclusiveness and integration. This prompted deconstructing and reconstructing sociocultural boundaries around a supposedly neutral set of common (yet hardly universal) economic and legal values. The expanded margins alleviated intergroup tension and conflict and generally improved ethnoracial relations, but they left a hyphenated ethnicity (with labels such as "African-American" or "Asian-American") that implied being ethnic in private and American in public. Overall, revisions were still grounded in difference from the monocultural "norm" (Goldberg, 1998).

The struggle to emancipate ourselves from biased beliefs about the nature of society is ongoing. The morally unacceptable impact of those beliefs on people has led to an unruly mix of political identities. Among many others, these include nationalistic, ethnic, feminist, religious, occupational, and myriad other orientations—many being highly individuated and personal affiliations (Rosenberg, 1993). There is an increasing recognition of community as sets or networks of relationships that bond people together and, therefore, function as both a medium for establishing identity and as a locus for expression (Lobo, 2001).

Coexistence of multiple and often conflicting interpretations, meanings, implications, and problems of category frame current debates around multiculturalism. Somewhat simplistically, multiculturalism generally implies communities characterized by opportunities (public space without barriers) for enriching interaction and growth in preferred ways, at self-appointed paces, and amid reflections of those distinguishable identities (Giroux, 1998). Ongoing critique of multiculturalism is inherently political in the sense that redefinition of public values to make them more open to transformation must, in practice, deal with issues around plurality and the distribution of power (Goldberg, 1998). The theoretical, philosophical, pedagogical, and political presuppositions of multiculturalism require the same critical examination as any other societal ideals to avoid being nothing more than a "tug of war over who gets to create public culture" (Kessler-Harris, 1992, p. 310; McLaren, 1998). In classic Heideggerian terms, the multicultural ideal is Being as a groundlessness within which beings reveal themselves in ways that serve to frame meaning and identity (Crusius, 1991). To date, multiculturalism, not being fully theorized (Willett, 1998), remains expressed in a continuum of types.

Conservative multiculturalism, being fundamentally a compromise of monocultural views, hints at historically imperialist and colonial attitudes of Europe and North America (McLaren, 1998). From such a stance, for instance, African Americans might be recognized and patronized as entertainers and athletes who are descendants of slaves. In contrast, liberal multiculturalism is a perspective based on notions of intellectual sameness among peoples—a cognitive equivalence that allows equitable competition in capitalist society (McLaren, 1998). However, this view often collapses into an ethnocentric and oppressively universalistic humanism with norms that strongly reflect Anglo-American cultural politics and ideas about community (McLaren, 1998). Both conservative and liberal multiculturalisms feed what Momaday refers to as a "morality of pity" (1997, p. 69).

So-called left-liberal multiculturalism, on the other hand, may emphasize equality to the point of smothering important cultural differences that are responsible for variations in behaviors, values, attitudes, cognitive styles, and social practices. Rather than stanch differences around race, class, gender, and sexuality, for example, the left-liberal approach may encourage "otherness" to the point of exoticizing it with cultural authenticity (McLaren, 1998).

In sum, multiculturalism without a transformative political agenda may be just another accommodation to the existing larger social order. What is more, the notion of sharing cultures and practices is not automatically prized. Many members of indigenous groups, for instance, believe that use of traditional forms of ceremony and healing by people from outside the group is disrespectful. Respectful use is inherently associated with, and to be accompanied by, unbroken strands of traditional knowing (Cruden, 1995). If the trappings of ceremony lack reference points in the community (or if form is merely imitative), they may be viewed as patronizing or even dangerous (Cruden, 1995; Deloria, 1993,

1997). Neoshamanistic endeavors by non-Natives, as an example, are often interpreted as self-authorizations for appropriating Indian culture in neo-imperialistic ways. In addition to issues around property rights, interpreting and representing, such activities may be associated with making "Natives *re*vanish," in part because they typically avoid critical, problematic, and controversial issues faced by indigenous peoples today (Wernitznig, 2003, p. x).

Neither good will nor theory can do what requires institutions, societal commitment, and unbiased media to recharacterize changing public order and realign what is now often understood as merely insurgent, reactionary, dominant, or marginal (Taylor, 1998). We do not yet know how to effectively bring together multiple cultures (that is, culture in the broad sense of sets of values and behavioral norms) without threatening to compromise the identities composing those cultures. However, discomfort generated by this state of affairs does not justify failing to attend to it.

To move beyond these limitations, a critical multiculturalism is required from the perspective of a resistant, poststructuralist approach to representing in the construction of meaning and identity (McLaren, 1998). Since "prejudice against prejudice is also a prejudice against tradition" (Crusius, 1991, p. 34), the trend toward revised politics of identity and more fully realized multiculturalism—albeit still open and problematic—suggest that no one will be at home everywhere and, at the same time, in that homelessness, that every one will have many homes (Caws, 1998). It may be like the proverbial cup being half full or half empty, but it connotes shifts in paradigms and perspectives that are unsettling. Meanwhile, attempts to speak a new language are complicated by the need to make it comprehensible to those whose terms of reference may still be, at least in part, rooted in the old. Those are stories that interpretive scholarship can help tell.

The PC Spin

The emergence of various contemporary multiculturalisms is understood in relation to the twentieth century's dominance of monoculturalism—an ideology that went largely unchallenged (by the dominant, anyway) for a long time. The belief that imposing ideas, views, or identities on others is not acceptable has led to inventive new social contrivances under the banner of political correctness (PC). It is socially unacceptable to lock others (through stereotyping or criticism, for instance) into images not of their own making, but there are ways to communicate that the links between culture, politics, and identity remain contested, ambiguous (Taylor, 1998), and hierarchical. For many the shift is one from intolerance to tolerance tinged with pity (Momaday, 1997), rather than to an appreciation of diversity. It all goes back to interpreting and representing.

It is increasingly acknowledged that single-stranded explanations tell, at best, only a partial story: unemployment is never only about money, HIV is not only about sex (Wallman, 1997). Ethical practice requires representing capabilities in tandem with limitations to include both the experience of the issue and the options made sensible and available by the situation (Wallman, 1997). It is in learning to live with the realities (both capabilities and limitations) of complex circumstances (such as professional practice or culturally diverse society) that prompts both political correctness *and* an appreciation for deeper understandings and interpretations.

In the guise of "political correctness," the practice of using culture or ethnicity as a surrogate for race has encouraged denial and blurring of racial politics and widespread failure to understand how racial categories emerge and persist (Baker, 2001; Goode, 2001; Hallam & Street, 2000). Culture, seen as a neutral, safe, or even a "good" concept, has in large part replaced discussion of race, but as race is hidden, the two (culture and race) are confounded (Dominguez, 1995). Perhaps even more important than culture becoming the polite proxy for race in discourse, the worldview fosters romantic idealism of a multicultural and colorblind society. Despite being completely impossible (given the deep roots that "race" has in American culture), the colorblind approach would simplify societal reality by eliminating such responses to discrimination as affirmative action, majority-minority electoral districting, and school desegregation (Baker, 2001). In light of the old truism that not being part of the answer implies being part of the problem, to deny racism, either personally or professionally, in a society founded on racist ideologies and practices (and certainly not purged of those) is in effect condoning it.

"Blind" is the critical descriptor for the eye that chooses not to note discrepancies in health care (for instance, that black babies in the United States are three times more likely than non-black babies to be born without prenatal care and twice as likely to die within their first year) and a

litany of discrepancies in employment and wage statistics, prison sentenc-
ing patterns, and other social indices that manifest an incipient race-
influenced class formation process (Baker, 2001; Boone, 1989; Brooks,
1992; Feagin & McKinney, 2003; Tapper, 1999). Racism, particularly in
relation to economics, has profound implications for health status and
health care access (Mwaria, 2001; Singer, 2001). If scholars in the human
and health-related sciences have social responsibilities (and it is difficult
to argue that they do not), fully recognizing and representing the realities
of persistent racism are surely among those.

Representing: Who and How?

The crucial challenge is representing alterity while neither objectifying it (Bowman, 1997) nor distorting its meaning. A critical examination
of hermeneutic praxis is indicated. Reflexivity, like contemplation, is by
its nature potentially self-alienating. One has only to consider biomedical
health care's role in imperialism for an intimidating example (e.g.,
Brown, 1979). Self reflection alone is necessary but not sufficient for significant transformation. It must be accompanied by a language of criticism that serves as an antidote to the atheoretical use of "personal experience" in advancing claims for emancipatory action (McLaren, 1998).

Whether individual or collective, it is reflexivity that can reveal meanings, or undisclosed assumptions (Cooper, 1998; Hirshberg & Hirshberg,
1998). While Gadamerian hermeneutics calls for continuous reexamina-
tion and revision of understanding, there is an accompanying need in
interpretive work for increased emphasis on situatedness and contextualization as part of reflexivity. Just as the "faceless researcher," like the
myth of neutrality, works against disclosure of meaningful understandings and multiple realities, failing to explore possibilities reinforces the
power of the discourses from ideological traditions that still occupy contexts of social privilege (McLaren, 1998). There is a need in interpretive
scholarship for moving beyond method and "sharedness of meanings"
(Fontana & Frey, 2000, p. 660) to developing a sensitive and persuasive
praxis for intersubjective, embodied, and ethical representing of personal
and social experience (Simpson, 1997) that encompasses sharedness of
more and deeper meanings.

Textualization and Voice

Interpretive scholars work with texts, and the quandary of textualization is that there is no possibility of neutrality—for a text is as much an artifact of convention and contrivance as is any other cultural product (Atkinson, 1994). Text is always part of a tradition, a thing with a history. "In whose voice do we write?" (Fine et al., 2000). Who and what does even dialogic and dialectic text actually represent? Critical perspectives advocate a self-conscious awareness of reflexivity with special reference to the work of language and texts—their transcription, edition, analysis, and interpretation. Neo-Kantian approaches to interpretation are justifiably criticized for their "belief that the text can be examined as a 'thing' innocently out-there, without situation, and that their interpretation could proceed without understanding the 'hermeneutics of facticity'" (Mehta, 1976, p. 18).

Scholarly textualization and interpretation involve numerous ethical issues around representing, to include (among others) property rights, preserving diversity and multiplicity, avoiding excesses, and finding and foregrounding authentic voice. Who determines which representations of domestic, interpersonal or intimate relationships are to be considered appropriate, acceptable, adequate, or accurate (Simpson, 1997)? Interpretive strategies use writing to bring together horizons, context, or situatedness for understanding, and an empathic stance toward life experiences to uncover the dialogic nature of the self (that is, within the self and in dialogue with the world) (Josselson, 1995). Text (often altered with distancing, writing, and the horizons of its interpreters) may reflect incipient prejudgments, expectations, and foremeanings (Orr, 1991). Questions arise about who owns (versus appropriates) the text or the accumulated knowledge upon which it is based. Whose reality is represented after changes and interpretation? "When I cannot make sense of it, my explanation changes" (Warnke, 2002) does not necessarily imply movement in accordance with the reality experienced by the originator. Indeed, when a worldview is challenged, people are generally more likely to reconstrue the situation or the facts than they are to modify the worldview (Mack, 2003). For those who get to choose when to attend to such issues as race, ethnicity, or gender, there is tendency to put those aside.

We routinely transcribe, edit, and translate before and while interpreting (Foley, 2001). This reflects an orientation to a print-focused and text-shaped culture, but the practice can be crippling in the case of oral traditions and in situations in which we stand to lose far more than the spoken word (Foley, 2001). By its nature, transcription involves reduction. Written texts (far more than speech, which is accompanied by interpretive-delimiting acts such as gesturing, tone and pitch of voice, stress, and other contextual features) are vulnerable to being misunderstood due to a "kind of self-alienation through being written down" (Gadamer, 1989, p. 354–55). In textualizing, the scholar extracts an acceptable but inert composition that may forever eliminate parts of the meaning that voice, background, movement, facial expressions, and general interactive context provided. In essence, the experience of a phenomenon or event is taken out of context and edited into a written translation. Translations between languages risk additional potential distortion and distancing. Thus interpretation—the transformation back to original *situated meaning in speaking*—is the *real* hermeneutical challenge (Orr, 1991).

Concerted attempts to take textualized work back to the people who originated it at some earlier time are not always successful and are seldom emphasized in final scholarship. Ongoing negotiated collaboration (which may need to be plural, multifaceted, cross-cultural, and multisite to reveal the multiplication of realities or expectations of even a few participants) can become prohibitive in light of time and money crunches. Some scholars unfairly control for such complexities by leaving the more conspicuously diverse people or situations out of their studies or by screening out sensitive (racial, gender, multicultural) issues. In sum, deep-level engagements with language can be readily compromised by other agenda. It takes commitment to minimize the risk of constructing texts resembling "an outsider-centered, bookish medium" (Foley, 2001, p. viii) that fails to fully convey the realities pledged to them.

There are additional concerns with interpretive text because the reader cannot avoid interpreting while reading. That in itself is problematic because "the understanding of something written is not a reproduction of something that is past, but the sharing of a present meaning" (Gadamer, 1989, p. 354). Gadamer's response to these problems is insistence on questioning, conversation, and revision, going beyond taxonomies and classifications to almost inexhaustible complexity (Palmer, 1969), horizons, deeper meanings, and understandings. These are not parameters laid down for convenience, but they reiterate the conviction that "[a]ny project worth doing must take account of the cultural constellation" surrounding each narrative and story (Foley, 2001, p. viii).

Hedging and Hegemony

Informed discussion of scholarly interpreting and representing requires examination of hegemony (influences that control but may appear neutral or natural). Given the part that history plays in interpretation, and that of interpretation in history, exploring the legacy of the colonial gaze in research is vital. Worldwide colonialism, a potent and often persuasive reality between the eighteenth and twentieth centuries, included the promotion of literacy in European languages. Missionary schools, government agencies, and international aid programs assumed that reading and writing constituted a substantial, unquestionable, and self-evident benefit (Knack, 2002). It was assumed that benefits would accrue to people who acquired those skills, deemed as they were to be measures of civilization and progress. Bias and literacy joined forces to increase complexity and sophistication (often where these already existed in forms unrecognized or unappreciated by outsiders) in hegemonic creation of national identities, citizenship, gender divisions, sexual orientation, race (whiteness and non-whiteness), and changing notions of class consciousness that resulted, in large part, in making the poor invisible, scapegoating the racially defined poor, and collapsing "class" into the broader (but less antagonistic) category of socioeconomic status. The foundations of traditional knowing and "truth" were shattered for all involved.

Symbolic Capital and Power: Needing the Big Picture

The politics of representing link questions of access and cultural production to what people actually do with the perspectives they use within historically specific public spaces (Giroux, 1998). New flavors of democratization have unsettled the confidence of modernist ideologues and forced hegemonic powers descended from colonialism to loosen their grip on non-western cultures. With science, research, and phenomenology growing up in the wake of (actually intertwined with) colonialism, postcolonialism, and some forms of neocolonialism and postmodernism, exploring the influence of cultural hegemony on interpretive scholarship is essential to an informed critique of representing in inquiry. Grounded in the hermeneutic tradition, postmodern critique, and the reality of no extant pristine model for interpretation, critical research looks closely at textual claims to authority and the inadequacies of thin descriptions of decontextualized facts—that is, the stripping out of history and culture (Kincheloe & McLaren, 2000). But the lives of both the scholar and those studied are still being influenced by those historical, social and economic realities left behind when the earth-mover of overt colonialism driven by *"Homo hierarchicus"* (Quigley, 1997) moved on.

A dominant society conquers a subordinate one and labels the defeated group culturally and biologically inferior. The same is true of countless other aspects of life and preference, many of them abstract and subtle. The psychological function of slurs is to dehumanize and shape ideas about (and conduct toward) the object of the slur (Montaño, 1997). The "invention of tradition" (involving, for instance, women, nurses, and other subaltern groups) within modern states functions much the same way—to sustain "novel, symbolic, generally normative behaviors that served to establish continuity with a suitable historical past" (Tuleja, 1997, p. 1).

Colonial Americans rapidly provided themselves with a usable past: history, legends, symbols, paintings, sculpture, monuments, shrines, holy days and holidays, ballads, patriotic songs, heroes, and villains (Tuleja, 1997). Postcolonial management of such symbolic capital is designed to bring homogeneity and continuity. There is little wonder that revisionist histories are needed to sort out the myths and practices rooted in such stories as those of conquests, colonial exploitation, patriarchal assumptions, labor migration, and slavery (Susser, 2001a). In the interdependence of creativity and tradition, knowledge and other products of human agency are manipulated to create private heritages, micro-identities, and "invention"—one of the meanings of which is "to show oneself" (Tuleja, 1997).

Transformative epochs are *experienced*. As they are lived, stories are generated that deserve telling. Those stories represent lives and times. Enter the interpretive inquirer, who is as much a product as a student of some part of this ongoing (but increasingly globalized and privatized) era and who has a history and biography both unique and shared. It is that history and biography (the sociological imagination [Mills, 1959]) that informs how he or she sees the world—who and what is cited, remembered, ignored, forgotten (Susser, 2001a). But it is at best a world of contested realities, histories, and views (Eurocentrism, Afrocentrism), any of which can be naturalized as commonsense and become endemic in thought and education (Stam & Shohat, 1998).

The rhetoric of egalitarianism laid the groundwork for political roles and ways of participating in the public sphere. Multiculturalism, antiracism, antisexism, women's rights, and political correctness are all associated with the inequalities that exist between communities, in power relations, and in the social strata and cultural hierarchies that crystallized in the United States (Patterson, 2001). A large part of this involves issues around intellectual property rights, misrepresentation, and appropriation—that is, intellectual sovereignty (Bataille, 2001). The interpretive researcher works with manipulated knowledge as both a product and tool of social inquiry. The ethic of inclusion involves issues around justice, fairness, truth, beauty, and values. Self-representation through gendered, ethnocized (identitied) narrative expressions provide texts in which differences are recognized and understood not as fixed, romanticized, or essentiallized notions of history and experience but as metaphors for flow and indeterminacy (Giroux, 1998).

The Challenge in Interpretive Study

The ethical political obligation of our time is toward individuals with multiple and heterogeneous identities (Ross, 1999). While focusing on misery, poverty, and crises leads to objectification of populations (Susser, 2001a), emphasis of subjectivity may be seen as repressive and distorting and has been replaced by transformative ideas about intersubjectivity and empowerment. Meanwhile, narratives burdened by longstanding stereotypes, stripped of historical inequalities, or communicating neutered characterizations suggest distortion in interpreting and representing.

The most debilitating labeling is not that secondary to blatant discrimination against individuals but that which becomes "naturalized" and institutionalized as neutral and innocuous. With more assimilated people of color and even governments unable or unwilling to explicate the contradictory processes that both challenge and articulate the cultural politics of racism (Baker, 2001; Merry, 2001) and the other "centrisms" still afoot, ways are needed to identify salient, systematic bias and discrimination—or the disparities persist unrevealed. The challenge is to take up issues of difference in ways that do not replay the monocultural essentialism of the "centrisms" (sexism, racism, ageism, medicocentrism, and so on) (McLaren, 1998). This implies profound changes in education of health professionals and reorientation toward sensitivity and knowledge about alternative paradigms for understanding health in context, and in particular those ways of knowing that extend beyond biological health to an indivisible mind, body, and spirit.

Interpretive scholarship is learning how to denaturalize commonsense cultural categories to make explicit ways in which global, national, regional, and local institutions shape formation, maintenance, and shifts in categories and hierarchies of difference (Goode, 2001). Essentialist views of cultures as primordial with dynamic processes are being replaced by notions of power-shaping boundaries within which cultural ideas and practices occur (Barth, 1969; Hannerz, 1992). Conversations are changing. Critical pedagogies are extending to recognize more subtle dominations; for example, by media, which produce a "multitude of objectified cultural others" (Foley & Moss, 2001, p. 357).

The interpretive scholar must understand what happens at both the textual and institutional levels to appreciate the influence of such images on political and economic interests. In our texts we are obliged to recognize and interpret discourses around consumption and production of images, whether we are representing privileged ideological positions of social status or location, or counter-hegemonic images and messages of marginalized others. Historical "backlash" and "romanticization" of groups must be discerned, as well as the struggles of the stigmatized to produce their own self-valorizing cultural images. These are aesthetic and political expressions (Foley & Moss, 2001) that deserve to be made explicit.

In sum, we need to learn nonreductionist views of the social order and to see society as an irreducible indeterminacy. Interpretive inquiry must move beyond naïve issues of methodology to concerns about how reflexive intersubjective consciousness will lead to new border narratives and sites of possibility and enablement (McLaren, 1998). Representing dissenting voices of stigmatized others ("strangers") in oral and written texts, and recognizing how we own and use language, are parts of the ongoing de-objectification process. Narrow dichotomous ways of thinking about each other (black vs. white, gay vs. straight, native-born vs. immigrant) call for contextualization to personalize gray areas and broaden views. Bringing stigmatizing discourses closer to everyday experience to see how cultural misrepresentations occur, and personalizing these issues, heightens ideological consciousness and makes images easier to recognize and change (Foley & Moss, 2001). We cannot assume that those of us who are from "marginalized" identity groups (nurses, women) are not complicit in producing unrealistic images.

It is not that we should give up communicating experiences of poverty or oppression, or the imposition of identities (of "patient for life," for instance, or other "imperfections of representation" [Susser, 2001a, p. 245]), but that we need to find ways for interpreting to include the humanity and resilience of those hidden from view and to ask how we can fight against the misery we see (Susser, 2001b). Presenting counterstories is not enough. Shifting from objectifying to intersubjective methodologies requires transformation in representing. Critical hermeneutics fosters willingness to recognize and integrate perspectives—to recognize, acknowledge, and represent in evocative ways, for instance, how powerful symbolic categories (such as family, religion, race, gender, and sexuality) both generate caring and communal solidarity and serve to maintain inequalities.

There are examples (albeit not as many as one would hope) that illustrate inclusively transforming perspectives on representing. An outstanding example is provided by Frank (2000), who, in presenting the autobiography of a woman who was born without limbs, astutely critiques (from both the individual's and the social scientist's perspectives) the implications of both medical and educational intervention. Other examples among the most helpful resources in the literature are in the first volume of the same book series in which this chapter appears (Diekelmann, 2002). Fletcher, Silva, and Sorrell (2002), for instance, valiantly critique use of the concept *quality of life* and demonstrate the need for new ways of representing the experiences of people who cannot share their realities verbally with others or whose identified impairments imply to others that their lives lack quality. From the stance of teaching and learning, excellent sources include Chávez and O'Donnell (1998), who present the costs of non-engagement in multicultural contexts, and such texts as those edited by Willet (1998) and Goldberg (1998), which present multiple views on multiculturalism (and its theory) from micro, middle, and macro perspectives. Additionally, the medical anthropological literature is replete with examples of inclusive inquiry with emphasis on representing. The journals *Medical Anthropology Quarterly* and its European counterpart *Medical Anthropology* are highly recommended. Similarly, many ethnographic (e.g., Ho, 2003) and ethnohistorical works (e.g.,

M'Closkey, 2002; Richardson, 2003) are strong additional starting places for understanding implications of their representing experiences.

Overall, it is the level and quality of theoretical critique and reflectivity that determines real value. To be useful, today's inquiry is relational, compelling and inclusive of crises of legitimation and vocality. It questions the rights of others (such as medical personnel or scientists) to appropriate experience, action, traditions, and representations. Often this requires testing or challenging available literature by going to the source. When preparing courses about Native American cultures and healing traditions, for example, I contact (preferably by visiting) tribal organizations and colleges to collect the materials used by specific indigenous peoples to represent themselves. In my experience, attempting to understand culture and history from the inside has been warmly welcomed. With students, however, I continue to qualify my use of the materials by pointing out that my interpretation is one of an outsider, as well as biased toward inclusivity. On a far grander scale, the Smithsonian Institution's evolving National Museum of the American Indian, which represents some 1,500 cultural entities throughout the hemisphere, actively elicits from indigenous groups how it is that they want to be represented. Think how different that perspective is from former depictions, which were often based on stereotype and popularity.

Most interpretive scholarship involves writing. To be memorable, narrative has recognizable characters, well-described scenes that are historically and otherwise situated, and identifiable cultural & social issues (including injustices). To communicate productively, writing is political, ethical, and savvy. As such, interpretive inquiry contributes valuable and vulnerable scholarship. Perhaps the best to be hoped for in its literary craftsmanship is a form of coherence in which methodologies, principles, and values exist explicitly and uneasily (but creatively and effectively) alongside each other (Goldberg, 1998). There is no full separation of ideology and politics from methodology, but there is responsible recognition in representing.

It is the goal of interpretive inquiry to articulate a politics of hope. Identities are shaped by traditions of interpretation rather than those of power, and by self-understanding rather than construction (Gadamer, 1989). Now how do we integrate that with moving "from recognizing that history affects us or that discourses of power construct us to the possibility that we can consider our effective history or identities critically"

(Warnke, 2002, p. 317)? We must develop the imagination to acknowledge the textual construction of reality (Atkinson, 1994). The inquirer's identitied self is portrayed in ethical relationships with nature and humanity through direct and indirect, symbolic and rhetorical means. Convergence of interpretive inquiry with critical multiculturalism allows use of the capacity of culture (for self-creation of diverse human ways of living, however individualized in ideological variation) and empowerment of self-definition, production, and assertion of identities.

Interaction across cultures when indigenous views are not fully understood and well represented is dangerous (Kumar, 1979). Given the diversity of society, however, failing to cross cultural boundaries is unrealistic and perhaps unconscionable. The issue of representing becomes one of the "substantial rightness" of interpreting individuals as raced, ethnic, or gendered identities when acknowledging someone as black or white, male or female, adds little to understanding (Warnke, 2002). But in representing realities, we *must* reveal how people have suffered or flourished under those identities. If we do not acknowledge them, or at least, from a Foucaultian perspective, represent how the social identities we and others have result from power that cannot be evaded (Warnke, 2002), we fail in the task of revealing and representing experienced realities.

Categories and interpretations of identity must be challenged, but they are still more than inconsistent incoherencies in defining who we are. Transformative multiculturalists aim to establish, in the margins of hegemonic systems, alternative sources of meaning and moral authority. That requires decentering practices that work with the cognizance of oppressed identities and occluded differences in ways that the narratives of modernity were not aware (Willett, 1998). It is up to us to find practices that better reflect meaningful differences and commonalities in hermeneutical realities, and in interpreting and representing those. We are all ethnic. We live multiculturally. We are all strangers (Bateson, 2000). Who if not us?

Notes

1. The reader is advised to see Janesick (2000, pp. 390–391), for a frank discussion of "methodolatry."

2. Arias (2001) is recommended for discussion of the controversy that has arisen around Menchú's work.

3. As the adoptive mother of a child whose birth "race" was officially changed by the state of Ohio in the early 1970s from "black" to "white" to match mine (thus legally labeling

an individual who appears "black" as "white"), I have long been interested in the problematic nature of the untheorized use of both "race" and whiteness. The practice of changing race upon adoption, for example, was "explained" to me by social workers and court personnel as a "favor." Whatever the incentive, such misguided naturalizing or normalizing masks institutional discrimination in the sense that the relabeled individual, no longer legally a "minority" despite remaining a person of color, is then disqualified for Affirmative Action and other integrative efforts. See Fine et al. (1997) for a thorough discussion of whiteness.

References

Abram, D. (1996). *The spell of the sensuous: Perception and language in a more-than-human world*. New York: Vintage Books/Random House.

Albrecht, G. L., Fitzpatrick, R., & Scrimshaw, S. C. (Eds.). (2000). *The handbook of social studies in health and medicine*. London: Sage.

The Anti-Stigma Project. (1998). Flyer. Baltimore, MD.

Arias, A. (Ed.). (2001). *The Rigoberta Menchú controversy*. Minneapolis: University of Minnesota Press.

Atkinson, P. (1994). *The ethnographic imagination: Textual constructions of reality*. London: Routledge.

Baker, L. D. (2001). The color-blind bind (pp. 103–119). In I. Susser & T. C. Patterson (Eds.), *Cultural diversity in the United States*. Malden, MA: Blackwell.

Barkan, E. (1992). *The retreat of scientific racism*. New York: Cambridge University Press.

Barth, F. (Ed.). (1969). *Ethnic groups and boundaries*. Boston: Little Brown.

Basso, K. (1988). A review of "Native American discourses: Poetics and rhetoric," *American Ethnologist* 15, 805–810.

Bataille, G. (Ed.). (2001). *Native American representations: First encounters, distorted images, and literary appropriations*. Lincoln: University of Nebraska Press.

Bateson, M. C. (2000). *Full circles, overlapping lives: Culture and generation in transition*. New York: Ballantine Books.

Becker, H. S. (1963). *Outsiders: Studies in the sociology of deviance*. London: Free Press.

Berkhofer, R. F., Jr. (1979). *The white-man's Indian: Images of the American Indian from Columbus to the present*. New York: Vintage Books.

Bhabha, H. K. (Ed.). (1990). *Nation and narration*. London: Routledge.

Boone, M. S. (1989). *Capital crime: Black infant mortality in America*. Newbury Park, CA: Sage.

Bowman, G. (1997). Identifying versus identifying with "the Other": Reflections on the siting of the subject in anthropological discourse (pp. 34–50). In A. James, J. Hockey, & A. Dawson (Eds.), *After writing culture: Epistemology and praxis in contemporary anthropology*. London: Routledge.

Brace, C. L., & Nelson, A. R. (2001). The peoplings of the Americas: Anglo stereotypes and Native American realities (pp. 46–56). In I. Susser and T. C. Patterson (Eds.), *Cultural diversity in the United States*. Malden, MA: Blackwell.

Brooks, R. L. (1992). *Rethinking the American race problem*. Berkeley: University of California Press.

Brown, E. R. (1979). *Rockefeller medicine men: Medicine and capitalism in America*. Berkeley: University of California Press.

Burling, R. (1970). *Man's many voices: Language in its cultural context*. New York: Holt, Rinehart & Winston.

Cajete, G. (2000). *Native science: Natural laws of interdependence*. Santa Fe, NM: Clear Light Publishers.

Cartmill, M., & Brown, K. (2003). Surveying the race concept: A reply to Lieberman, Kirk and Littlefield. *American Anthropologist 105*(1), 114–115.

Caws, P. (1998). Identity: Cultural, transcultural, and multicultural (pp. 372–387). In D. T. Goldberg (Ed.), *Multiculturalism: A critical reader*. Oxford: Blackwell.

Césaire, A. (1972). *Discourse on colonialism* (J. Pinkham, Trans.). New York: Monthly Review Press.

Chambers, E. (2000). Applied ethnography (pp. 851–869). In N. K. Denzin & Y. S. Lincoln (Eds.), *Handbook of qualitative research* (2nd Ed.). Thousand Oaks, CA: Sage.

Chávez, C., & O'Donnell, J. (1998). *Speaking the unpleasant: The politics of (non)engagement in the multicultural educational terrain*. Albany: State University of New York Press.

Chomsky, N. (1957). *Syntactic structures*. The Hague: Mouton.

Christians, C. G. (2000). Ethics and politics in qualitative research (pp. 133–155). In N. K. Denzin & Y. S. Lincoln (Eds.), *Handbook of qualitative research* (2nd Ed.). Thousand Oaks, CA: Sage.

Conrad, P., & Schnieder, J. W. (1992). *Deviance and medicalization: From badness to sickness*. Philadelphia: Temple University Press.

Cooper, T. W. (1998). *A time before deception: Truth in communication, culture, and ethics*. Santa Fe, NM: Clear Light Publishers.

Cruden, L. (1995). *Coyote's council fire: Contemporary shamans on race, gender, and community*. Rochester, VT: Destiny Books.

Crusius, T. W. (1991). *A teacher's introduction to philosophical hermeneutics*. Urbana, IL: National Council of Teachers of English.

Deloria, V., Jr. (1993). *God is red: A native view of religion*. Golden, CO: Fulcrum Publishing.

Deloria, V., Jr. (1997). *Red earth, white lies: Native Americans and the myth of scientific fact*. Golden, CO: Fulcrum Publishing.

Deloria, V., Jr., & Wildcat, D. R. (2001). *Power and place: Indian education in America*. Golden, CO: Fulcrum Resources.

Denzin, N. K., & Lincoln, Y. S. (2000). The discipline and practice of qualitative research (pp. 1–28). In N. K. Denzin & Y. S. Lincoln (Eds.), *Handbook of qualitative research* (2nd Ed.). Thousand Oaks, CA: Sage.

Derrida, J. (1916). *Democracy and freedom*. New York: The Free Press.

Derrida, J. (1976). *On grammatology* (G. C. Spivak, Trans.). Baltimore: Johns Hopkins University Press.

Derrida, J. (1978). *Writing and difference*. London: Routledge & Kegan Paul.

Diekelmann, N. (2003). *Personal communication*. Advanced Institute for Heideggerian Hermeneutic Phenomenology, University of Wisconsin–Madison.

Diekelmann, N. (Ed.). (2002). *First do no harm: Power, oppression, and violence in healthcare*. Madison: University of Wisconsin Press.

Dippie, B. W. (1982). *The vanishing American: White attitudes and U.S. Indian policy*. Lawrence: University Press of Kansas.

Dixon, H. (2002). A Saponi by any other name is still a Siouan. *American Indian Culture and Research Journal 26*(3), 65–84.

Dominguez, V. (1995). Multiculturalisms and baggage of "race." *Identities 1*(4), 297–426.

Ellis, C., & Bochner, A. P. (2000). Autoethnography, personal narrative, reflexivity:

Researcher as subject (pp. 733–768). In N. K. Denzin & Y. S. Lincoln (Eds.), *Handbook of qualitative research* (2nd Ed.). Thousand Oaks, CA: Sage.

Ember, C. R., & Ember, M. (2002). *Cultural anthropology* (10th Ed.). Upper Saddle River, NJ: Prentice Hall.

Espiritu, Y. L. (1992). *Asian American panethnicity: Bridging institutions and identity.* Philadelphia: Temple University Press.

Evers, L., & Toelken, B. (1994). Collaboration in the translation and interpretation of Native American oral traditions (pp. 1–14). In L. Evers & B. Toelken (Eds.), *Native American oral traditions*. Logan: Utah State University Press.

Feagin, J. R., & McKinney, K. D. (2003). *The many costs of racism*. Lanham, MD: Rowman & Littlefield.

Feng, Y.-L. (1983 [1937]). *A history of Chinese philosophy* (D. Bodde, Trans.). Princeton, NJ: Princeton University Press.

Ferraro, G. (2001). *Cultural anthropology: An applied perspective* (4th Ed.). Belmont, CA: Wadsworth.

Fine, M., Weis, L., Powell, L. C., & Wong, L. M. (Eds.). (1997). *Offwhite: Readings on race, power, and society*. New York: Routledge.

Fine, M., Weis, L., Weseen, S., & Wong, L. (2000). For whom? Qualitative research, representations, and social responsibilities (pp. 107–131). In N. K. Denzin & Y. S. Lincoln (Eds.), *Handbook of qualitative research* (2nd Ed.). Thousand Oaks, CA: Sage.

Fletcher, J. J., Silva, M. C., & Sorrell, J. M. (2002). Harming patients in the name of quality of life (pp. 3–48). In N. Diekelmann (Ed.), *First, do no harm: Power, oppression, and violence in healthcare*. Madison: University of Wisconsin Press.

Foley, D., & Moss, K. (2001). Studying U.S. cultural diversity (pp. 343–364). In I. Susser and T. C. Patterson (Eds.), *Cultural diversity in the United States*. Malden, MA: Blackwell.

Foley, J. M. (2001). Foreword. In L. Evers & B. Toelken (Eds.), *Native American oral traditions* (pp. vii–xvi). Logan: Utah State University Press.

Fontana, A., & Frey, J. H. (2000). The interview: From structured questions to negotiated text (pp. 645–672). In N. K. Denzin & Y. S. Lincoln, eds., *Handbook of qualitative research* (2nd Ed.). Thousand Oaks, CA: Sage.

Foucault, M. (1972). *The archaeology of knowledge* (A.M.S. Smith, Trans.). New York: Pantheon.

Foucault, M. (1973). *The birth of the clinic.* New York: Pantheon.

Foucault, M. (1980). *Power/knowledge: Selected interviews and other writings, 1972–1977.* New York: Pantheon.

Foucault, M. (1994). *The order of things: An archaeology of the human sciences (Les mots et les choses)*. New York: Vintage Books.

Frank, G. (2000). *Venus on wheels: Two decades of dialogue on disability, biography, and being female in America*. Berkeley: University of California Press.

Frankenberg, R. (1996). "When we are capable of stopping, we begin to see": Being white, seeing whiteness (pp. 3–17). In B. Thompson & S. Tyagi (Eds.), *Names we call home: Autobiography on racial identity*. New York: Routledge.

Freund, P.E.S.; McGuire, M. B., & Podhurst, L. S. (2003). *Health, illness, and the social body: A critical sociology* (4th Ed.). Upper Saddle River, NJ: Prentice Hall.

Gadamer, H.-G. (1976). *Philosophical hermeneutics* (D. E. Linge, Trans., Ed.). Berkeley: University of California Press.

Gadamer, H.-G. (1989). *Truth and method* (G. Barden & J. Cumming, Trans.; J. Weinsheimer & D. G. Marshall, Rev. Trans.). New York: Crossroads Publishing.

Giroux, H. A. (1998). Insurgent multiculturalism and the promise of pedagogy (pp. 325–343). In D. T. Goldberg (Ed.), *Multiculturalism: A critical reader*. Oxford: Blackwell.

Goffman, E. (1961). *Asylums: Essays on the social situation of mental patients and other inmates*. London: Penguin.

Goffman, E. (1963). *Stigma: Notes on the management of spoiled identity*. London: Penguin.

Goldberg, D. T. (1998). Introduction: Multicultural conditions (pp. 1–41). In D. T. Goldberg (Ed.), *Multiculturalism: A critical reader*. Oxford: Blackwell.

Gonzales, A. A. (2001). Urban (trans)formations: Changes in the meaning and use of American Indian identity (pp. 169–185). In S. Lobo & K. Peters (Eds.), *American Indians and the urban experience*. Walnut Creek, CA: AltaMira Press.

Good, M-J. D. (1998). *American medicine: The quest for competence*. Berkeley: University of California Press.

Goode, J. (1998). The contingent construction of local identities: Koreans and Puerto Ricans in Philadelphia. *Identities* 5, 33–64.

Goode, J. (2001). Teaching against culturalist essentialism (pp. 434–456). In I. Susser & T. C. Patterson (Eds.), *Cultural diversity in the United States*. Malden, MA: Blackwell.

Goodman, A. H. (2001). Biological diversity and cultural diversity: From race to radical bioculturalism (pp. 29–45). In I. Susser and T. C. Patterson (Eds.), *Cultural diversity in the United States*. Malden, MA: Blackwell.

Goossen, I. W. (1995). *Diné bizaad: Speak, read, write Navajo*. Flagstaff, AZ: Salina Bookshelf.

Gore, R. (2003). The rise of mammals: Adapting, evolving, surviving. *National Geographic* (April), 2–37.

Gubrium, J. F., & Holstein, J. A. (1995). Biographical work and new ethnography (pp. 45–58). In R. Josselson & A. Lieblich (Eds.), *Interpreting experience: The narrative study of lives* (Vol. 3). Thousand Oaks, CA: Sage.

Gubrium, J. F., & Holstein, J. A. (2000). Analyzing interpretive practice (pp. 487–508). In N. K. Denzin & Y. S. Lincoln (Eds.), *Handbook of qualitative research* (2nd Ed.). Thousand Oaks, CA: Sage.

Hall, E. T. (1973). *The silent language*. New York: Anchor Press.

Hall, L.K.C. (1996). Eating salt (pp. 241–252). In B. Thompson & S. Tyagi (Eds.), *Names we call home: Autobiography on racial identity*. New York: Routledge.

Hallam, E., & Street, B. V. (Eds.). (2000). *Cultural encounters: Representing "Otherness."* New York: Routledge.

Hannerz, U. (1992). *Cultural complexity*. New York: Columbia University Press.

Heidegger, M. (1967). *Being and Time* (J. Macquarrie & E. Robinson, Trans.). Oxford: Basil Blackwell.

Heidegger, M. (1969). *The essence of reasons* (T. Malick, Trans.). Evanston, IL: Northwestern University Press.

Heidegger, M. (1971). *On the way to language* (Peter D. Hertz, Trans.). New York: Harper & Row.

Heidegger, M. (1981). *Nietzsche, Vol. 1: The eternal recurrence of the same* (D. F. Krell, Trans.). London: Routledge & Kegan Paul.

Hernández, A. (1997). *Pedagogy, democracy, and feminism: Rethinking the public sphere*. Albany: State University of New York Press.

Hicks, D. E. (1992). *Border writing*. Minneapolis: University of Minnesota Press.

Hirshberg, S., & Hirshberg, T. (1998). *One world, many cultures* (3rd Ed.). Boston: Allyn and Bacon.

106 KAVANAGH

Ho, M.-J. (2003). Migratory journeys and tuberculosis risk. *Medical Anthropology Quarterly* 17(4), 442–458.

House, D. (2002). *Language shift among the Navajos: Identity politics and cultural continuity.* Tucson: University of Arizona Press.

Hunt, N. B. (2002). *Shamanism in North America.* Buffalo, NY: Firefly Books.

Husserl, E. (1994). The phenomenological theory of meaning and of meaning-apprehension (pp. 165–186). In K. Mueller-Vollmer (Ed.), *The hermeneutics reader: Texts in German tradition form the Enlightenment to the present.* New York: Continuum.

Inwood, M. (1999). *A Heidegger dictionary.* Oxford: Blackwell.

James, A., Hockey, J., & Dawson, A. (1997). Introduction: The road from Santa Fe (pp. 1–15). In A. James, J. Hockey, & A. Dawson (Eds.), *After writing culture: Epistemology and praxis in contemporary anthropology.* New York: Routledge.

Janesick, V. J. (2000). The choreography of qualitative research design: Minuets, improvisations, and crystallation (pp. 379–399). In N. K. Denzin & Y. S. Lincoln (Eds.), *Handbook of qualitative research* (2nd ed.). Thousand Oaks, CA: Sage.

Josselson, R. (1995). Imagining the real: Empathy, narrative, and the dialogic self (pp. 27–44). In R. Josselson & A. Lieblich (Eds.), *Interpreting experience: The narrative study of lives* (Vol. 3). Thousand Oaks, CA: Sage.

Kavanagh, K. H. (2003). Mirrors: A cultural and historical interpretation of nursing's pedagogies (pp. 59–153). In N. Diekelmann (Ed.), *Teaching the practitioners of care: New pedagogies for the health professions.* Madison: University of Wisconsin Press.

Kaye/Kantrowitz, M. (1996). Jews in the U.S.: The rising costs of whiteness (pp. 121–137). In B. Thompson & S. Tyagi (Eds.), *Names we call home: Autobiography on racial identity.* New York: Routledge.

Kess-Gardner, J. (2002). *The incredible journey: The Jermaine Gardner story.* Baltimore: Incredible Journey Productions.

Kessler-Harris, A. (1992). Cultural locations: Positioning American studies in the great debate. *American Quarterly* 44(3), 302–315.

Kincheloe, J. L., & McLaren, P. (2000). Rethinking critical theory and qualitative research (pp. 279–313). In N. K. Denzin & Y. S. Lincoln (Eds.), *Handbook of qualitative research* (2nd Ed.). Thousand Oaks, CA: Sage.

Kingston, M. H. (1977). *The woman warrior.* New York: Vintage Books.

Kingston, M. H. (1980). *Chinamen.* New York: Alfred A. Knopf.

Kleinman, A. (1988). *The illness narratives: Suffering, healing and the human condition.* New York: Basic Books.

Knack, M. C. (2002). Southern Paiute letters: A consideration of the applications of literacy. *American Indian Culture and Research Journal* 26(3), 1–24.

Kottak, C. P. (2003). *Mirror for humanity: A concise introduction to cultural anthropology* (3rd Ed.). Boston: McGraw Hill.

Kumar, K. (Ed.). (1979). *Bonds without bondage: Explorations in transcultural interactions.* Honolulu: University of Hawaii Press.

Lamphere, L. (1992). *Structuring diversity: Ethnographic perspectives on the new immigration.* Chicago: University of Chicago Press.

Leacock, E. B., & Lurie, N. O. (1988). *North American Indians in historical perspective.* Prospect Heights, IL: Waveland Press.

Lee, G. (1992). *China boy.* New York: Penguin Books.

Lee, G. (1994). *Honor and duty.* New York: Alfred A. Knopf.

Lesage, J., Ferber, A. L., Storrs, D., & Wong, D. (Eds.). (2002). *Making a difference: University students of color speak out.* Lanham, MD: Rowman & Littlefield.

Lieberman, L., Kirk, R. C., & Littlefield, A. (2003). Exchange across difference: The status of the race concept: perishing paradigm—race 1931–99. *American Anthropologist* *105*(1), 110–113.

Lobo, S. (2001). Introduction (to overview of urbanism) (pp. 3–25). In S. Lobo & K. Peters (Eds.), *American Indians and the urban experience.* Walnut Creek, CA: AltaMira Press.

Lovejoy, A. O. (1996 [1930]). *The revolt against dualism.* LaSalle, IL: Transaction.

Mack, J. E. (2003). Deeper causes: Exploring the role of consciousness in terrorism. *IONS Noetic Sciences Review 64*(June–August), 10–17.

Madriz, E. (2000). Focus groups in feminist research (pp. 835–850). In N. K. Denzin & Y. S. Lincoln (Eds.), *Handbook of qualitative research* (2nd Ed.). Thousand Oaks, CA: Sage.

Mather, E. P., & Morrow, P. (1994). "There are no more words to the story" (pp. 200–242). In L. Evers & B. Toelken (Eds.), *Native American oral traditions* (pp. vii–xvi). Logan: Utah State University Press.

McGruder, A. (2001). Comic strip: *The Boondocks.* Universal Press Syndicate.

McLaren, P. (1998). White terror and oppositional agency: Towards a critical multiculturalism (pp. 45–74). In D. T. Goldberg (Ed.), *Multiculturalism: A critical reader.* Oxford: Blackwell.

M'Closkey, K. (2002). *Swept under the rug: A hidden history of Navajo weaving.* Albuquerque: University of New Mexico Press.

Mehta, J. L. (1976). *Martin Heidegger: The way and the vision.* Honolulu: University of Hawaii Press.

Menchú, R. (1984). *I, Rigoberta Menchú: An Indian woman in Guatemala* (A. Wright, Trans., E. Burgos-Debray, Ed.). London: Verso.

Merleau-Ponty, M. (1962). *Phenomenology of perception* (C. Smith, Trans.). New York: Humanities Press.

Merry, S. E. (2001). Racialized identities and the law (pp. 120–139). In I. Susser & T. C. Patterson (Eds.), *Cultural diversity in the United States.* Malden, MA: Blackwell.

Miller, C. (2001). Telling the Indian urban: Representations in American Indian fiction (pp. 29–45). In S. Lobo & K. Peters (Eds.), *American Indians and the urban experience.* Walnut Creek, CA: AltaMira Press.

Miller, W. L., & Crabtree, B. F. (2000). Clinical research (pp. 607–630). In N. K. Denzin & Y. S. Lincoln (Eds.), *Handbook of qualitative research* (2nd Ed.). Thousand Oaks, CA: Sage.

Mills, C. W. (1959). *The sociological imagination.* New York: Oxford University Press.

Mishler, E. G. (1979). Meaning in context: Is there any other kind? *Harvard Educational Review 49*(1), 1–19.

Momaday, N. S. (1993). From *The names: A memoir* (pp. 215–235). In P. Riley (Ed.), *Growing up Native American.* New York: Avon.

Momaday, N. S. (1997). *The man made of words: Essays, stories, passages.* New York: St. Martin's Press.

Montaño, M. (1997). Appropriation and counterhegemony in South Texas: Food slurs, offal meats, and blood (pp. 50–67). In T. Tuleja (Ed.), *Usable pasts: Traditions and group expressions in North America.* Logan: Utah State University Press.

Mwaria, C. (2001). Diversity in the context of health and illness (pp. 57–75). In I. Susser & T. C. Patterson (Eds.), *Cultural diversity in the United States*. Malden, MA: Blackwell.

Nash, J. (2001). Gender, ethnicity, and the new migration (pp. 206–228). In I. Susser & T. C. Patterson (Eds.), *Cultural diversity in the United States*. Malden, MA: Blackwell.

Nisbett, R. E. (2003). *The geography of thought: How Asians and Westerners think differently . . . and why*. New York: Free Press.

Olesen, V. L. (2000). Feminisms and qualitative research at and into the millennium (pp. 215–255). In N. K. Denzin & Y. S. Lincoln (Eds.), *Handbook of qualitative research* (2nd Ed.). Thousand Oaks, CA: Sage.

Olson, S. (2002). *Mapping human history: Discovering the past through our genes*. Boston: Houghton Mifflin.

Ong, A. (1996). Cultural citizenship as subject-making. *Current Anthropology 37*, 737–762.

Orr, L. (1991). *A dictionary of critical theory*. New York: Greenwood Press.

Oswalt, W. H. (2002). *This land was theirs: A study of Native Americans* (7th Ed.). Boston: McGraw-Hill Mayfield.

Palmer, R. (1969). *Hermeneutics: Interpretation theory in Schleiermacher, Dilthey, Heidegger, and Gadamer*. Evanston, IL: Northwestern University Press.

Patterson, T. C. (2001). Class and historical process in the United States (pp. 16–26). In I. Susser & T. C. Patterson (Eds.), *Cultural diversity in the United States*. Malden, MA: Blackwell.

Pickering, K. A. (2000). *Lakota culture, world economy*. Lincoln: University of Nebraska Press.

Punch, M. (1994). Politics and ethics in qualitative research (pp. 83–97). In N. K. Denzin & Y. S. Lincoln (Eds.), *Handbook of qualitative research*. Thousand Oaks, CA: Sage.

Quigley, D. (1997). Deconstructing colonial fictions? Some conjuring tricks in the recent sociology of India (pp. 103–121). In A. James, J. Hockey, & A. Dawson (Eds.), *After writing culture: Epistemology and praxis in contemporary anthropology*. London: Routledge.

Reiss, A. J., Jr. (1979). Governmental regulation of scientific inquiry: Some paradoxical consequences (pp. 61–95). In C. B. Klockars & F. W. O'Connor (Eds.), *Deviance and decency: The ethics of research with human subjects*. Beverly Hills, CA: Sage.

Richardson, L. (2000). Writing: A method of inquiry (pp. 923–948). In N. K. Denzin & Y. S. Lincoln (Eds.), *Handbook of qualitative research* (2nd Ed.). Thousand Oaks, CA: Sage.

Richardson, M. U. (2003). No more secrets, no more lies: African American history and compulsory heterosexuality. *Journal of Women's History 15*(3), 63–76.

Riley, D. (1988). *Am I that name? Feminism and the category of "women" in history*. Minneapolis: University of Minnesota Press.

Robinson, C. J. (1998). Ota Benga's flight through Geronimo's eyes: Tales of science and multiculturalism (pp. 388–405). In D. T. Goldberg (Ed.), *Multiculturalism: A critical reader*. Oxford: Blackwell.

Rose, A. M. (Ed.). (1962). *Human behavior and social processes: An interactionist approach*. London: Routledge & Kegan Paul.

Rosenberg, A. (1993). *Philosophy of social science* (2nd Ed.). Boulder, CO: Westview Press.

Ross, S. D. (1999). *The gift of kinds [the good in abundance]: An ethic of the earth*. Albany: State University of New York Press.

Sacks, K. (1994). How did Jews become white folks? (pp. 78–101). In S. Gregory & R. Sanjek (Eds.), *Race*. New Brunswick, NJ: Rutgers University Press.

Santiago-Irizarry, V. (2001). *Medicalizing ethnicity: The construction of Latino identity in a psychiatric setting*. Ithaca, NY: Cornell University Press.

Sapir, E. (1931). Conceptual categories in primitive languages. *Science 74*, 578–584.

Schutz, A. (1962). *The problem of social reality*. The Hague: Martinus Nijhoff.

Schutz, A. (1964). *Studies in social theory*. The Hague: Martinus Nijhoff.

Schutz, A. (1967). *The phenomenology of the social world*. Evanston, IL: Northwestern University Press.

Schwandt, T. A. (2000). Three epistemological stances for qualitative inquiry: Interpretivism, hermeneutics, and social constructionism (pp. 189–214). In N. K. Denzin & Y. S. Lincoln (Eds.), *Handbook of qualitative research* (2nd Ed.). Thousand Oaks, CA: Sage.

Silverman, D. (2000). Analyzing talk and text (pp. 821–834). In N. K. Denzin & Y. S. Lincoln (Eds.), *Handbook of qualitative research* (2nd Ed.). Thousand Oaks, CA: Sage.

Simpson, B. (1997). Representations and the re-presentation of family: An analysis of divorce narratives (pp. 51–70). In A. James, J. Hockey, & A. Dawson (Eds.), *After writing culture: Epistemology and praxis in contemporary anthropology*. London: Routledge.

Singer, M. (2001). Health, disease and social inequality (pp. 76–102). In I. Susser & T. C. Patterson (Eds.), *Cultural diversity in the United States: A critical reader*. Malden, MA: Blackwell.

Somé, S. (2000). A name is sacred and must be treated as such. *Parabola* 25(4), 19. Reprinted from *Welcoming spirit home: Ancient African teachings to celebrate children and community* (pp. 64–66). Novato, CA: New World Library. (Originally published in 1999).

Spinoza, B. de. (1988). *Collected works of Spinoza* (E. Curley, Trans., Ed.). Princeton: Princeton University Press.

Stam, R., & Shohat, E. (1998). Contested histories: Eurocentrism, multiculturalism, and the media (pp. 296–324). In D. T. Goldberg (Ed.), *Multiculturalism: A critical reader*. Oxford: Blackwell.

Straus, T., & Valentino, D. (2001). Retribalization in urban Indian communities (pp. 85–94). In S. Lobo & K. Peters (Eds.), *American Indians and the urban experience*. Walnut Creek, CA: AltaMira Press.

Susser, I. (2001a). Cultural diversity in the United States (pp. 3–15). In I. Susser & T. C. Patterson (Eds.), *Cultural diversity in the United States*. Malden, MA: Blackwell.

Susser, I. (2001b). Poverty and homelessness in U.S. cities (pp. 229–249). In I. Susser & T. C. Patterson (Eds.), *Cultural diversity in the United States*. Malden, MA: Blackwell.

Tan, A. (1989). *The joy luck club*. New York: Ivy Books.

Tan, A. (1992). *The kitchen god's wife*. New York: Ivy Books.

Tapper, M. (1999). *In the blood: Sickle cell anemia and the politics of race*. Philadelphia: University of Pennsylvania Press.

Taylor, C. (1998). The politics of recognition (pp. 75–106). In D. T. Goldberg (Ed.), *Multiculturalism: A critical reader*. Oxford: Blackwell.

Taylor, J. S. (2003). The story catches you and you fall down: Tragedy, ethnography, and "cultural competence." *Medical Anthropology Quarterly* 17(2), 159–181.

Thompson, B., & Tyagi, S. (1996). Introduction: Storytelling as social conscience—the power of autobiography (pp. ix–xvii). In B. Thompson & S. Tyagi (Eds.), *Names we call home: Autobiography on racial identity*. New York: Routledge.

Torrey, E. F. (1984). *Mind games: Witchdoctors and psychiatrists.* Northvale, NJ: Jason Aronson.

Tschaepe, M. D. (2003). Halo of identity: The significance of first names and naming. *Janus Head* 6(1), 67–78.

Tuleja, T. (1997). Introduction: Making ourselves up: On the manipulation of tradition in small groups (pp. 1–20). In T. Tuleja (Ed.), *Usable pasts: Traditions and group expressions in North America.* Logan: Utah State University Press.

Urciuoli, B. (2001). The complex diversity of language in the United States (pp. 190–205). In I. Susser & T. C. Patterson (Eds.), *Cultural diversity in the United States.* Malden, MA: Blackwell.

Wallace, C.D.C., & Torroni, A. (1992). American Indian prehistory as written in the mitochondrial DNA: A review. *Human Biology* 64(3), 403–416.

Wallace, M. (1991). Multiculturalism and oppositionality. *Afterimage* (October), 6–9.

Wallman, S. (1997). Appropriate anthropology and the risky inspiration of "Capability" Brown: Representations of what, by whom, and to what end? (pp. 244–263). In A. James, J. Hockey, & A. Dawson (Eds.), *After writing culture: Epistemology and praxis in contemporary anthropology.* London: Routledge.

Warnke, G. (2002). Social identity as interpretation (pp. 307–329). In J. Malpas, U. Arnswald, & J. Kertscher (Eds.), *Gadamer's century: Essays in honor of Hans-Georg Gadamer.* Cambridge, MA: MIT Press.

Waxler, N. E. (1981). Learning to be a leper: A case study in the social construction of illness (pp. 169–194). In E. Mishler, L. Amara Singham, S. Hauser, R. Liem, S. Osherson, & N. Waxler (Eds.), *Social contexts of health, illness, and patient care.* Cambridge: Cambridge University Press.

Wernitznig, D. (2003). *Going native or going naïve? White shamanism and the neo-noble savage.* New York: University Press of America.

West, C. (1990). The new cultural politics of difference (pp. 3–29). In R. Ferguson, M. Gever, T. T. Minh-ha, and C. West (Eds.), *Out there: Marginalization and contemporary cultures.* Cambridge, MA: MIT Press.

WHO. (1980). *International classification of impairments, disabilities and handicaps.* Geneva: WHO.

Whorf, B. L. (1956). A linguistic consideration of thinking in primitive communities (pp. 65–86). In J. B. Carroll (Ed.), *Language, thought, and reality: Selected writings of Benjamin Lee Whorf.* Cambridge, MA: MIT Press.

Willett, C. (Ed.). (1998). *Theorizing multiculturalism: A guide to the current debate.* Malden, MA: Blackwell.

Witherspoon, G. (1977). *Language and art in the Navajo universe.* Ann Arbor: University of Michigan Press.

Wood, P. (1975). *Classification of impairments and handicap.* Geneva: World Health Organization.

Young, R. W., & Morgan, W., Sr. (1994). *The Navajo language: A grammar and colloquial dictionary* (Rev. Ed.). Albuquerque: University of New Mexico Press.

3

Shared Inquiry

Socratic-Hermeneutic Interpre-viewing

CHRISTINE SORRELL DINKINS

In qualitative research studies, the researcher serves as the "instrument" through which data are generated. Just as the instrument in quantitative research must be appropriate to the research approach, so should the researcher in qualitative research engage in an interview approach that skillfully encourages and guides the participant to reveal data that have depth and clarity. The interview process must provide sufficient flexibility for the participants to uncover their own deeply held beliefs, yet the researcher must guide the interview so that it remains focused on the phenomenon of interest. The manner in which interviewers call forth participants' thoughts and feelings related to a phenomenon has a direct impact on the quality of the data obtained.

Despite of the considerable increase of phenomenological and other types of qualitative research studies in health care in recent years, most research references provide little guidance in the "how" of gathering data through an interview. The popularity of qualitative research methods has resulted in a growing number of texts related to qualitative health care research. An informal survey of many of these texts, however, indicates that very little space is given to the methodology of interviewing. Researchers/ authors discuss the interview process in general terms, without specific suggestions for how to adapt the process for different types of qualitative methodologies. In addition, specifics of the interview process appear to be a part of the research process that has been, for the most part, sorely neglected in published descriptions of qualitative research studies, with the notable exception of Geanellos (1999). It can be an extremely frustrating

experience for a novice researcher to attempt to determine how to structure (or un-structure) the interview. Yet, without careful thought to the
interview process, it is doubtful that rich data will be obtained.

Experienced qualitative researchers also struggle with how to design
the interview process. Over the past decade, however, many hermeneutic
researchers have come to adopt an interview approach that calls forth
long narratives from the respondent, with few interruptions or prompts
from the interviewer, in order to allow the respondents' stories to unfold
naturally (Benner, 1994). The interviewer often does not engage with the
respondent in a *dialogue,* or conversation. Instead, the interviewer avoids
"leading" the respondent, allowing the story to take its own course. This
approach has been effective in generating important data for many qualitative studies. However, it may not facilitate immediate reflection for
either the researcher or the participant on the ideas that emerge within
the interview. Such immediate reflection is more likely to occur when the
researcher creates a dialogue and is thus able to probe deeper and
deeper into the respondent's beliefs that shape her understanding of the
phenomenon of interest.

In addition to providing only limited or no opportunity for immediate
reflection, there may be a danger in the technique of interpretive interviewing that is being passed down from experienced scholars and teachers to their students. The danger is that the method may be becoming too
set, that in many cases of interpretive research, the "method" itself is
going unquestioned. Van Manen (1997, p. 28) notes that methodology
means the *logos* (study) of the *method* (way), so that methodology implies
"pursuit of knowledge" and a certain *mode* of inquiry is implied in the notion of "method." As qualitative research assumes increasing importance
in health care research, it is critical that researchers begin to question
how to incorporate a methodology in the interview that will enhance the
pursuit of knowledge.

Van Manen (1997, p. 30) suggests that the broad field of phenomenological scholarship should be studied as a set of guidelines for a principled
form of inquiry, neither rejecting or ignoring tradition, nor following it
unquestioningly. The purpose of this study is to raise these questions. In
considering the questions, an alternative approach to phenomenological
interviewing is presented: The Socratic-Hermeneutic Inter-view, in which
researcher and co-inquirer (the research participant) engage in a dialogue
that evolves through questions and responses that encourage researcher

and co-inquirer to reflect together on the concepts that are emerging and taking shape within the interview itself.

The Hermeneutic Interview

Although phenomenological interviews provide a framework for many types of qualitative studies, this discussion focuses on the hermeneutic phenomenological approach that has evolved from the philosophical traditions of Heidegger and Gadamer. Hermeneutic phenomenology is concerned with interpreting concealed meanings in phenomena. These common meanings are embedded in cultures that incorporate shared language, practices, and important practical knowledge about common day-to-day experiences (Sorrell & Redmond, 1995). The purpose of the phenomenological interview has primarily been perceived as a way to understand a phenomenon by drawing from the respondent a vivid picture of the "lived experience," complete with the richness of detail and context that shape the experience.

The term "lived experience" has become a common way of characterizing a hermeneutic study of interpretive research. Perhaps in the alignment of this term with hermeneutic research, the breadth of its original meaning has been ignored. Too often, "lived experience" seems to be characterized as a single experience described by a participant in an interview. Yet, Van Manen (1997, p. 9) reminds us that lived experience reflects the artistic, philosophic, communal, and poetic influences that, over the years, have united persons with the ground of their lived experience. Heidegger (1993a, p. 204), states that "perhaps lived experience is the element in which art dies." It is inherent in the phenomenological process to interpret this experience. Yet, experience is so immediate, elusive, and complex that it is difficult for any description to capture its essence (Van Manen, 1997). Thus, it is important that the researcher implement an approach to inquiry that facilitates apprehending the lived experience in its depths of artistic, philosophic, communal, and poetic influences.

In current phenomenological research practice, storytelling is believed to provide access to the lived experience. The story, or narrative, is a central focus for phenomenological interviews because the narrative structure helps respondents to reflect on specific experiences that help to avoid generalities (Benner, 1994). Benner (1994) states that narrative accounts of actual situations provide closer access to practical knowledge than do general questions about beliefs or theory. The interviewer shapes the interview around the narrative, attempting to gain insight into the phenomenon through the description of the experience.

Benner (1984) made an important contribution to the practice of phenomenological interviewing when she included guidelines in her *Novice to Expert* book for eliciting stories from respondents related to "critical incidents" that they had experienced. Critical incidents included such experiences as one in which an intervention made an important difference in a patient outcome, an incident that went unusually well or in which there was a breakdown, or an incident that was particularly demanding (p. 300). Benner provided specific prompts to guide the interview, such as encouraging the respondent to include details of the context of the incident, why the incident was deemed "critical," and the feelings and thoughts of the respondent during the incident (p. 301). Many qualitative researchers have adopted this approach to interviewing, in which they ask the respondent to focus on a specific incident that reflects the experience with the phenomenon, and to tell a story about that experience, including as many details of the context and the thoughts and feelings of the respondent as possible.

This widely adopted approach to interviewing has become the predominant method for hermeneutic inquiry, but hermeneutics, as Heidegger and Gadamer envisioned it, is not a *method* at all but a mode of understanding. Gadamer states in *Truth and Method:* "Hermeneutics has traditionally understood itself as an art or technique." But, he adds, "one might wonder whether there is such an art or technique of understanding" (1989, p. 265–266). Gadamer states the point more strongly later in the same work:

Given the intermediate position in which hermeneutics operates, it follows that its work is not to develop a procedure of understanding, but to clarify the conditions in which understanding takes place. But these conditions do not amount to a "procedure" or method which the interpreter must of himself bring to bear on the text; rather, they must be given. (p. 295)

Likewise, Heidegger argues that "every inquiry is a seeking," and that "every seeking gets guided before-hand by what is sought" (1962, p. 24). A consistent predetermined method, then, is problematic, because it cannot be guided in this way by what is sought. In fact, when Heidegger attempts to begin his hermeneutic of Being in *Being and Time,* he states that "the question about the meaning of Being is to be *formulated,*" and since the question "must be guided beforehand by what is sought, so the meaning of Being must already be available to us in some way" (1962, p. 25). Heidegger suggests here that what we already know about what is sought must inform our decision as to what question to formulate. Indeed, Heidegger spends much of his hermeneutic journey in this work and in others simply attempting to formulate the question.

According to Gadamer and Heidegger, then, not only can the hermeneutic method not be a set method, but the *question* must always be the primary consideration. In addition, Gadamer maintains that in "the art of asking questions . . . only the person who knows how to ask questions is able to persist in his questioning, which involves being able to preserve his orientation toward openness. The art of questioning is the art of questioning ever further" (1989, p. 367). This statement suggests that a limited number of primarily predetermined questions does not take the hermeneutic inquiry far enough. Questions must be pursued further and further; each seeming answer must be followed up with another question, and therefore, Gadamer argues, "the hermeneutic phenomenon . . . implies the primacy of dialogue" (p. 369).

If hermeneutics must give priority to the *question* and to the *dialogue,* it may be high time interpretive scholars turned to the philosopher who is a master of both: Socrates. Socrates' most shining student, Plato, left behind a legacy of rich philosophical works, written in dialogue form and designed to convey Socrates' method of inquiry. These dialogues, written by the founder of Western philosophy, serve as a reminder for us to return to discourse as our primary mode of philosophical inquiry. In fact, one of the most startling and important aspects of Socrates' character is that he does not believe he can successfully inquire after knowledge or wisdom by any means other than discourse.

Plato's works serve as models for modern readers in two ways: The works offer us first and foremost a model philosopher in the character of Socrates. For whether he is the lead speaker or merely a respondent to the questions of a more experienced thinker, Socrates is always a *philosophos,* literally a lover of wisdom, never tiring in his search for insight into the nature of his world around him. Second, the works also offer a model for philosophical inquiry, illustrating how such inquiry can and must be conducted through dialogue. By representing conversations between

Socrates and his co-inquirers, Plato grants the reader examples of how inquiry can be conducted, on topics ranging from the nature of friendship to the relationship between the soul and the body.

The difference between Socrates' method of inquiry, also called his *elenchus*, and the method of philosophers in the tradition that followed him, is that Socrates' inquiry is *shared* inquiry in the strongest sense. Socrates and his interlocutors search together for understanding, questioning each other's beliefs and helping each other to clarify their own thoughts. Because the inquiry is a shared one, Socrates puts himself very much into the inquiry. He expresses surprise when an interlocutor says something he didn't expect, he challenges beliefs that seem to conflict, and he acknowledges his own assumptions and allows them to affect the dialogue. He is never passive, and he never simply asks a question and lets the answer lie.

The Socratic mode of inquiry follows Heidegger's own guidelines laid down 2,400 years later. Heidegger cautions that in willing ourselves to let a phenomenon be, this act should not in any way be passive (1966, p. 61). Instead, as Gadamer explains Heidegger's hermeneutics, Heidegger believes "that the structure of Dasein is thrown projection, that in realizing its own being Dasein is understanding" and that therefore this "must also be true of the act of understanding in the human sciences" (1989, p. 264). For Dasein to understand its world, Dasein must understand that it is *part* of that world, and it must understand itself. For Dasein, to understand *is* to understand itself. As a result, Dasein must be an integral part of whatever inquiry it pursues. For current hermeneutic researchers, this means the inquirer must embrace the fact that she is an integral part of her inquiry. The interviewer must put herself into the interview.

This concept of bringing oneself into the interview coincides with the originary meaning of the term "interview." Originally, the term referred to a "mutual view of each other," as employed by Milton in *Paradise Lost* (*Oxford English Dictionary*). The term also originarily suggested "a looking into," and St. Augustine used interview to mean "a glimpse of something" (OED). Interview, then, in its original sense, is a viewing *of each other*, a looking into each other in which we hope to gain a glimpse of something otherwise beyond our ken. As it is used in modern-day language, though, interview implies a questioner and a respondent, with clearly defined roles, and an assumption that it is the respondent's beliefs that are being sought, not the questioner's. Such interviews are not a viewing of each other at all, but a viewing by one person of the other. If we link Heidegger's insistence on Dasein as part of the inquiry with the originary meaning of "interview," we see that an interview conducted as part of a hermeneutic inquiry must be an *inter-view* in which the researcher may reveal as much of herself as the participant does.

A second, perhaps even more important reason exists for the interviewer to bring herself back into the inquiry: The researcher must have an opportunity to identify and check her own assumptions. The caution against one's own assumptions intruding on phenomenological research is a well-known one, but the traditional phenomenological interview approach, in which the researcher takes a more passive role as the respondent's story enfolds, may fail to account for this danger. Gadamer warns that "all correct interpretation must be on guard against arbitrary fancies and the limitations imposed by imperceptible habits of thought, and it must direct its gaze 'on the things themselves'" (1989, pp. 266–267). Heidegger harbors the same concerns about inquiry, and suggests that "methodologically conscious understanding will be concerned not merely to form anticipatory ideas, but to make them conscious, so as to check them and thus acquire right understanding from the things themselves" (in Gadamer, 1989, p. 269). An inter-view that provides for shared inquiry helps both the researcher and the co-inquirer to reflect on their own assumptions and beliefs.

How are these "imperceptible habits of thought" and "anticipatory ideas" to be checked? How do we check something that is "imperceptible"? Gadamer's answer is that "our own prejudice is properly brought into play by being put at risk. Only by being given full play is it able to experience the other's claim to truth and make it possible for him to have full play himself" (1989, p. 299). To put our prejudices at risk is to expose them, to let them show. Socrates was quite aware of the danger of prejudices leading an inquiry astray, and he insisted on inquiry through dialogue for this very reason. If we have prejudices or "habits of thought" we have not even noticed ourselves, we need others to notice them for us, to point them out to us or to lead us to a point where we can notice them ourselves.

Dialogue, then, allows the researcher to acknowledge and embrace the fact that she is part of the inquiry, to check her assumptions with another inquirer, and to remain open to the possibility that her assumptions will be challenged in the dialogue. In addition, dialogue has a third

benefit: it encourages openness. Heidegger writes of openness to possibility, and he urges that when we wait for an answer, in that waiting "we
leave open what we are waiting for" (1966, p. 68). Gadamer acknowledges
that this call for openness poses difficult problems for the questioner:

Posing a question implies openness but also limitation. It implies the explicit establishing of presuppositions, in terms of which can be seen what still remains
open. Hence a question can be asked rightly or wrongly, according as it reaches
into the sphere of the truly open or fails to do so. We say that a question has been
put wrongly when it does not reach the state of openness but precludes reaching
it by retaining false presuppositions. It pretends to an openness. . . that it does
not have. (1989, p. 363–364)

   This concern with openness brings us back to Heidegger's insistence
that the formulation of the question is key. What "false presuppositions"
might underlie a researcher's choice of question? For instance, when researchers ask participants to recall an incident that for them captures the
essence of the phenomenon that is the subject under inquiry, what presuppositions lie in this question? On the surface, the question assumes
that the phenomenon *can* and *does* manifest in certain incidents. Many
possibilities are closed off by this assumption. For example, suppose that
the researcher is interested in learning about the phenomenon of caregiving within a family and therefore asks the participant to describe an incident that stood out in her mind as demonstrative of the essence of caregiving. The experience of caregiving is often such a long and not necessarily
consistent process that an "incident" may not capture the phenomenon,
which is always evolving. No doubt, the participant will be able to relate a
critical incident related to her caregiving experience, but will this incident be reflective of successive and connected stages of the caregiving
process? With such an extended process, will the one incident provide
adequate exposure to reflect on the wholeness of the phenomenon and
therefore result in a fruitful inquiry? Even if the participant is encouraged to describe several different incidents, the phenomenon may not be
best captured in "incidents" at all. Caregiving may be experienced in a
much more holistic way, as more than the sum of specific incidents.
   Once again, the importance of dialogue reveals itself. In a dialogue,
each question has the potential to be turned on itself, examined, and
even rejected. In a dialogue, the questions are led by the answers and by
what has been revealed of the phenomenon so far. The questions are led

by what Heidegger calls "the inconspicuous guide who takes us by the hand—or better said, by the word—in . . . conversation" (1966, p. 60). Socrates, too, perceived and respected this inconspicuous guide: He maintained that "the lover of inquiry must follow his beloved wherever it may lead him" (Plato, 1981c, 14b). In a dialogue, in which the inquiry itself guides the researcher, an assumption that leads to a flawed question, as in the example above, will be caught by the dialogue process. The participant as co-inquirer will be in a position to react to the question itself and change the direction of inquiry if necessary or appropriate.

Midwifing Understanding

To learn from Socrates' approach to dialogue as a way to understanding, we must first understand Socrates himself, since he, as Dasein, is an essential part of his own inquiries. Socrates believed that he was on a divine mission to help the citizens of Athens look inside themselves to seek out wisdom and understanding. Twice in Plato's dialogues, Socrates offers the image of a midwife as an analogy for how he sees himself and his relationship with his co-inquirers. In Athens, midwives were women who were unable to give birth themselves, and who were skilled not only in facilitating the birthing process but in making promising matches between men and women. These women enjoyed a high status in Athens.

Socrates explains to his friend Theaetetus that like a midwife, he himself is barren of wisdom, seeking only to help those who are pregnant with ideas. He can determine whether another is pregnant, and he can bring on the pains of delivery or relieve them. Also like a midwife, he knows which couplings of ideas are likely to produce fertile offspring. Compared to the art of midwives, though, Socrates believes his art is even more complicated—he must also distinguish between "phantoms" and "realities," between errors and "fertile truth" once he has delivered another's ideas (Plato, 1990, 149b–150c).

What Socrates is portraying here is his method of matching beliefs up against each other during an inquiry by process of his *elenchus*. In Plato's dialogues, one very consistent step in the elenchus is apparent: Socrates' inquiries move forward through the comparison of beliefs. Like a midwife, he matches ideas together in an attempt to produce fruitful offspring, that is, genuine insights. Socrates attempts to guide his co-inquirers to match up and compare their own beliefs about a given subject, and to realize when they have two or more relevant beliefs in conflict. That conflict can then be explored to determine which belief the co-inquirer privileges.

Socrates' trust in this matchmaking of ideas is based on his belief that every person has true understanding inside of him,[1] if he is only willing to search for it. This belief is a radical one for his time, and it is in direct conflict with the teachings of the Sophists, who were the dominant intellectuals and teachers-for-hire in Socrates' time. Even Socrates' own friend Meno challenges Socrates with a sophistic argument that has since become known as "Meno's Paradox":

How will you look for [something], Socrates, when you do not know at all what it is? How will you aim to search for something you do not know at all? If you should meet with it, how will you know that this is the thing that you did not know? (Plato, 1981, *Meno* 80d)

Socrates counters this dangerous argument, one that he sees as a threat to all inquiry, with a myth of recollection. He explains that the soul is immortal, and that at one time it lived in the realm of the gods. At that time, the soul beheld Beauty and Goodness and many other truths, but when the soul was born into a body, it forgot these wonderful things. Contrary to the Sophists' claims, then, human beings *can* learn, because "the truth about reality is always in our soul" (Plato, 1981d, 86b). Socrates admits that his myth is only one possible explanation, but he tells his friend that the important point to understand is that one can and should seek understanding. Even though Socrates admits the myth is conjecture, this aspect—that one should seek understanding—he clings to as something he cannot help but believe. Socrates confirms this belief in the *Theaetetus* as well, as he tells his companions that the search for wisdom is an inward one. Socrates explains that when students have continual discussions with him, they do not learn anything from him, but rather "they discover within themselves a multitude of beautiful things, which they bring forth into the light" (Plato, 1990, 150d).

Meno's paradox is remarkably similar to the puzzle Heidegger (1962) tackles in the beginning of *Being and Time*. How can we come to understand Being, how can we even formulate the question of the meaning of Being, without knowing what Being is? Heidegger's solution, of course, is the hermeneutic circle, and this solution is not so different from Socrates' myth of recollection. For Heidegger, an inquiry can make progress because everything ahead of us on the circle is already behind us as well. In other words, we can "recall" ideas we have not yet encountered. Heidegger's version has the advantage of two millennia worth of development of philosophical thought and language, so his solution and his explanation are more complex, but the essential idea is the same. We can look for that which we do not know, and recognize it when we find it, because that which lies in front of us is also already behind us. We must simply recall what we have forgotten.

Meno's paradox can inform current phenomenological research practice. Some researchers may argue that a researcher should be part of the culture she is examining, or have shared in the experience of the phenomenon. This argument raises valid concerns, particularly because of the problem of assumptions affecting the questions asked, as already discussed. In addition, though, as Meno would ask, how do these researchers find what they are looking for if they do not yet know that phenomenon? How will they recognize it when they find it? Socratic dialogue, the *elenchus*, is designed to help both the inquirer and co-inquirer "recall" their forgotten knowledge, or, in Heidegger's terms, to glimpse what is behind and ahead of them on the hermeneutic circle. Thus, for modern phenomenological research practice, the *elenchus* provides the best solution to the problem of Meno's paradox.

For Socrates, because he believes the truth about reality is always in our soul, any given individual need not have knowledge handed to him by another. A researcher, therefore, need not have understanding of a phenomenon given to her by a participant, but can find that understanding herself through the process of the shared inquiry. If the truth is in each person's soul, Socrates and his companions can find that truth together. For this approach to understanding to work, though, Socrates must hold a second belief: Each person, when he is honest with himself, can evaluate which beliefs he holds more dearly than others. Furthermore, Socrates believes that the more dearly held a belief is, the closer it is to genuine understanding. Therefore, if two or more people in a shared inquiry examine their beliefs, search out conflicts, and reject the beliefs which they hold less dear, they will move closer and closer to deeper understanding.

We must inquire as to why such inquiry can only be conducted through dialogue, as Socrates clearly believed. Socrates was put to death by Athens not because of his views but because he refused to stop conducting dialogues with the youth and men of Athens. Significantly, the gathered men of Athens, Socrates' jury, would not have objected, it seems, if Socrates simply would have gone home quietly and inquired after wisdom on his own, instead of troubling other men and discussing with the city's youth. In the *Apology,* Plato's dramatic retelling of Socrates' trial, though, Socrates never considers that option. To him, ceasing his questioning of the youth and of others constitutes ceasing philosophical inquiry altogether. For the same reason, he refuses the option of exile, understanding that few strangers of a foreign land would talk with him in the way he desires. He sees an end to such discussions as an end to his life of inquiry, and thus as an end to his life as a whole (Plato, 1981a, 37c–e). We are left with the conclusion, then, that *shared* inquiry serves as Socrates' only possible means of philosophical investigation. His love of dialogue is even acknowledged by his friend Phaedrus in the *Symposium,* who warns their mutual friend Agathon, "if you go on answering Socrates he will be utterly indifferent to the fate of our present business, so long as he has someone to [dialogue] with" (Plato, 1925, 194d).

As has been stated, Socrates possesses the unshakeable belief that each human being has within him an understanding of all matters important to the soul. But if each human being has within him understanding of all that is important, why is Socrates not able to spend his time alone, exploring his own internal wisdom? There must be something essential to shared inquiry that aids each inquirer in accessing the inner understanding within himself and others. We must then look to Socrates' *elenchus* for an explanation of how such an approach assists Socrates and others in this way, and why such an approach is not only better than non-dialogical inquiry but essential to the quest for ultimate understanding.

In the *Republic,* Socrates asserts to his friends: "our present discussion . . . shows that the power to learn is present in everyone's soul and that the instrument with which each learns is like an eye that cannot be turned around from darkness to light without turning the whole body" (Plato, 1992c, 518c). In other words, to make progress in an inquiry, an individual's entire soul must be turned toward that which he wishes to understand. Exploring the connections between beliefs is the way to turn the soul and to achieve this understanding, and Socrates' own dialogues, as portrayed by Plato, demonstrate that these connections and this turning of the soul can only happen when two or more people are conversing, examining each other's ideas.

When the young Socrates discusses the nature of philosophy with Parmenides, the older man, a far more experienced philosopher, advises Socrates on a method: "Examine the consequences that follow from the hypothesis" (Plato, 1997, 135e). He continues to explain that the other hypotheses "must be examined both relative to themselves and relative to any other you may choose" (136c). To inquire into something's nature, Socrates must elicit a hypothesis from a co-inquirer, then examine the consequences of that hypothesis.

In order to be able to deduce such consequences and then test their acceptability, Socrates must operate under the assumption that all of a person's beliefs are interconnected, that there will always be a way to relate a person's ideas about courage, for example, to other beliefs the person might have. Socrates describes this interconnectedness and the comparison which it enables to Theaetetus: "our first aim will be to look at our thoughts themselves in relation to themselves, and see what they are—whether, in our opinion, they agree with one another or are entirely at variance" (Plato, 1990, 154e). This assumption should not be a difficult one to accept for modern phenomenological researchers. It seems quite likely, for instance, that a respondent's views on personhood might be connected to her views of love, responsibility, and duty that she embodies in her practice.

Socrates' *elenchus,* then, proceeds by examining hypotheses or ideas, searching with his co-inquirer for implications and consequences of those ideas and then comparing those consequences with other beliefs the co-inquirer has. Socrates seems entirely comfortable rejecting, revising, or accepting ideas based on whether or not the consequences match with what he and the co-inquirer believe. In the *Phaedo,* he instructs his friends on the art of inquiry with similar advice, saying, "when you must give an account of your hypothesis itself you will proceed in the same way: you will assume another hypothesis, the one which seems to you best of the higher ones until you come to something acceptable" (Plato, 1981e, 101d–e). Socrates makes it clear here that one should privilege the hypothesis or idea which "seems to you best" as being the most likely to represent genuine understanding. The idea that "seems best" will be the idea that is consistent with other, connected, beliefs.

Socrates maintains that each person has within him not only beliefs about the world, but a hierarchy within those beliefs. There seems to be

a direct correlation between how difficult it is for a person to doubt or
deny a belief and how likely that belief is to represent his true understanding. If a co-inquirer comes across a belief of which he is not sure, for
instance an assertion about the nature of justice, he must then compare
this assertion with other beliefs by following through on its consequences.
If the assertion, as a result of this inquiry, comes into conflict with more
dearly held beliefs, then the assertion must be adjusted or rejected, if no
mistake has been made in deducing its consequences. Socrates seems to
have a particular talent for seeing these potential conflicts and helping his
co-inquirers to find and evaluate them. When his co-inquirer offers a definition of a key idea, for instance, Socrates begins to explore what will
hopefully be a fruitful line of inquiry, one that will at least lead to comparison with dearly held beliefs, even if it still ends in rejection of the definition. Socrates' description of his midwife abilities makes mention of this
talent when he reminds Theaetetus that midwives are also "marvelously
knowing about the kind of couples whose marriage will produce the best
children" (Plato, 1990, 149d). Socrates understands which questions will
gather together beliefs that can produce a test of a given assertion.

Typically, the *elenchus* proceeds as follows:

1. Socrates encounters someone who takes an action or makes a statement
   into which Socrates wishes to inquire.
2. Socrates asks the person for a definition of the relevant central concept
   (e.g., virtue, justice, friendship). The person, who has now become the
   co-inquirer, offers definition **D**.
3. Socrates employs analogies and examples; together, he and the co-inquirer
   deduce the necessary consequences **C** of the stated definition **D**.
4. Socrates points out a conflict between the deduced consequences **C**
   and a belief **B** that he suspects the co-inquirer holds. Socrates gives the
   co-inquirer a choice between rejecting the definition **D** or the belief **B**
   with which D conflicts.
5. The co-inquirer rejects definition **D** because he does not wish to reject
   B. The co-inquirer believed **D** when he stated it, but he holds **B** more
   dearly. Given the choice, then, **D** must go. **B** must stay.
6. Socrates asks the co-inquirer for a new definition, D_1.
7. Socrates and the co-inquirer repeat steps 3 through 6 several times.
8. The dialogue ends without Socrates and the co-inquirer finding a final,
   unarguable definition of the central concept in question.

Thus, when testing definition **D**, there are two possible results:

Rarely: **D**'s consequences are not found to conflict with any dearly held
  beliefs: **D** is accepted without qualification.
Commonly: **D**'s consequences are found to conflict with a dearly held
  belief: **D** is rejected or revised.

Examples of Conflicts with Dearly Held Beliefs

Clear examples of conflicts between beliefs are scattered throughout
many dialogues and occur in many different contexts. Socrates beauti-
fully illustrates the experience of such a conflict when he exclaims to
Theaetetus, "it seems to me that these three statements that we have admitted are fighting one another in our souls" (Plato, 1990, 155b). Later in
the same dialogue, after drawing out the necessary consequences of the
current statement under examination, Socrates and Theaetetus together
come to a startling conclusion that appears to be an inevitable result of
Theaetetus' statement: "Tell me," Socrates says, "if you are not yourself
astonished at suddenly finding that you are the equal in wisdom of any
man or even a god?" This is a statement that Theaetetus obviously cannot
accept, and he responds, "When we were working out the meaning of the
principle that a thing is for each man what it seems to him to be, it appeared to me a very sound one. But now, all in a minute, it is quite the
other way round" (Plato, 1990, 162c–d). This exchange is a classic example of how Socrates' interlocutor can think he believes one thing, but be
forced to abandon the belief when he is faced with its consequences and
those consequences' conflict with more dearly held beliefs.

In the *Crito*, we even witness Socrates himself expressing a conflict
with a dearly held belief that he cannot ignore. Socrates rejects Crito's arguments that he should escape from prison—thus avoiding execution—
for this very reason. After explaining to Crito the arguments that he must
instead accept, he concludes, "Crito, my dear friend, be assured that
these are the words I seem to hear, . . . and the echo of these words resounds in me, and makes it impossible for me to hear anything else"
(Plato, 1981b, 54d). Socrates cannot deny the much more deeply held
belief that tells him to remain where he is as the laws demand, despite
Crito's arguments to the contrary. Socrates' explanation of his reluctance
in terms of the words that "resound" in him is an eloquent description of
a belief Socrates cannot deny.

This process of comparing beliefs and identifying which are more
dearly held is paralleled in Gadamer's description of Heidegger's

hermeneutic method: "Rival projects can emerge side by side until it be-comes clearer what the unity of meaning is; interpretation begins with fore-conceptions that are replaced by more suitable ones. This constant process of new projection constitutes the movement of understanding and interpretation" (1989, p. 267). As an inquiry continues and under-standing develops, preconceptions that may not even have been noticed before are reevaluated, altered, or rejected, and replaced by "more suit-able ones." As the researcher and co-inquirer test their beliefs and their statements, they can reject or revise some while accepting those that en-hance their understanding and reveal the "unity of meaning" that Hei-degger believes is to be found in hermeneutic study.

The "Say What You Believe" Requirement

Because the *elenchus* functions by comparing and evaluating beliefs, Socrates' inquiries carry with them the essential prerequisite that each co-inquirer say what he believes to be true. If a co-inquirer takes an im-movable stand on a certain issue out of stubbornness, for instance, and thus refuses to acknowledge the consequences of his statement or their conflict with dearly held beliefs, the inquiry cannot move forward in a genuine search for wisdom. Socrates therefore states what is known as "the say what you believe" requirement many times throughout the dialogues, to reluctant and willing co-inquirers alike. Two typical state-ments occur in the *Crito* and the *Charmides*. Socrates asks Crito to "try to answer what I ask you in the way you think best" (Plato, 1981b, 49a), and he asks Charmides, "I suppose you could express this impression of yours in just the way it strikes you?" (Plato, 1992a, 159a).[2] Theaetetus is tempted to violate the requirement out of a desire to avoid contradicting himself. He is honest about this to Socrates, saying, "if I answer what seems true in relation to the present question, I shall say 'no, it is not pos-sible;' but if I consider it in relation to the question that went before, then in order to avoid contradicting myself, I say 'Yes, it is.'" Socrates then warns him against thinking this way: "if you answer 'Yes,' . . . the tongue will be safe from refutation but the mind will not" (Plato, 1990, 154d). Socrates makes it clear that if Theaetetus fails to observe the "say what you believe" requirement, their discussion will itself be false.

Just as Socrates insists with his co-inquirers, a phenomenological re-searcher employing Socrates' *elenchus* must insist that the co-inquirer say what she believes. If she says what she believes the researcher wants her to say, or if she says what she thinks most people would believe, or if she sticks to something she thought she believed when the consequences and conflicts demonstrate otherwise, the inquiry becomes false, and the phenomenon cannot reveal itself to either member of the shared inquiry.

Anticipating Conflicts Between Beliefs

Socrates is able to know which questions to ask because he anticipates the potential conflicts. When a co-inquirer makes a statement, Socrates expects that the co-inquirer probably holds certain beliefs, and Socrates recognizes that these beliefs will conflict with the current statement. This anticipation on Socrates' part can only be based on his own assumptions, and thus he brings himself into the inquiry. This activity closely parallels Gadamer's requirement of sensitivity in hermeneutic interpretation: "This kind of sensitivity involves neither 'neutrality' with respect to content nor the extinction of one's self, but the foregrounding and appropriation of one's own fore-meanings and prejudices" (1989, p. 269). Socrates is not neutral because he realizes he cannot be neutral, and so he foregrounds and appropriates his own prejudices, and allows them to have play in the dialogue.

By testing assertions, following them to consequences, and identifying conflicts between beliefs, Socrates can purge himself and his co-inquirers of false beliefs and begin to grasp the connections that will lead them higher in their quest. Gadamer observed that "it is the tyranny of hidden prejudices that makes us deaf to what speaks to us" (1989, p. 270). By helping his co-inquirer and himself identify and purge their false beliefs, Socrates helps both of them be able to listen to what speaks to them.

A phenomenological researcher who practices Socratic dialogue could thereby foreground and identify her own prejudices, giving her a chance to evaluate them, and she could also help the co-inquirer evaluate beliefs to find which are in tension and which are more dearly held. For instance, a participant in a study on living with dialysis is likely to have picked up on other dialysis patients' opinions on what it is like to live with dialysis, and she may also have been made aware of what others believe it *should* be like. She may unconsciously adopt some of these attitudes as her own as she assimilates into the culture of a dialysis unit or integrates into her own assumptions the described experiences of those awaiting a kidney transplant. When a researcher practices the *elenchus*, she can test the participant's statements against more dearly held beliefs the participant may have. When conflicts arise, the less dearly held belief can be abandoned or revised, clearing a way for better understanding, clearing away that "tyranny of hidden prejudices" that otherwise would make both researcher and participant deaf to what speaks to them.

The Socratic-Hermeneutic Inter-view

Socrates' ideas of shared inquiry help us to think about alternative approaches to phenomenological interviews that incorporate these ideas. A Socratic-hermeneutic interview can remain true to the goals of Gadamerian and Heideggerian hermeneutics by following the model of Socrates' teachings. One important insight we can gain from Socrates is that shared inquiry moves the focus away from "respondent" in the interview, toward a shared dialogue focused on reflections of both interviewer and interviewee as they share ideas, listen, and reflect together, thus forming an inter-view. Although Benner (1994, p. 111) suggested that a shared dialogue approach to interviewing be used to help show more clearly the participants' beliefs, this approach does not appear to have been widely used, in an effort to avoid "leading" the interviewee. However, the widely practiced approach of focusing a narrative around a given incident with minimal questions to interrupt the flow of the narrative may be more likely to limit the participant's perspective and to lead her than a shared dialogue would, for all of the reasons stated thus far. Without shared inquiry, the researcher's prejudices may remain hidden, and the participant is not in a position from which she can easily reject the premises of the questions. In a dialogue, though, the co-inquirer affects where the inquiry may lead, as opposed to being led by the mostly predetermined questions.

Further benefits of the *elenctic* method will become clearer if we examine specific options for steps in the inquiry. Definitions, analogies, implications, and consequences, the hermeneutic circle, and *aporia* are important in eliciting ideas from a participant in a Socratic-hermeneutic inter-view. None of these individual steps, however, is essential, and rarely would all be used in a Socratic-hermeneutic inter-view. As with the method itself, the specifics of the questions and paths should be led by the inquiry, and determined by what is appropriate and fruitful for the participant and for the subject matter.

Some of these steps, and the general approach of searching for conflicts between beliefs, may at first appear adversarial or off-putting, and researchers may worry that the process would be unpleasant or distressing for the participant. However, in describing Plato's dialogical method, Gadamer says it

consists not in trying to discover the weakness of what is said, but in bringing out its real strength. It is not the art of arguing . . . but the art of thinking . . . for in this process what is said is continually transformed into the uttermost possibilities of its rightness and truth . . . The speaker is put to the question until the truth of what is under discussion finally emerges . . . the process of question and answer, giving and taking, talking at cross purposes and seeing each other's point . . . performs the communication of meaning that . . . is the task of hermeneutics. (1989, p. 367)

Furthermore, the elenctic process is likely to elicit positive feelings in the co-inquirer. In Socratic-Heideggerian inter-views conducted for an ongoing study on the process of writing a doctoral dissertation (Sorrell & Dinkins, 2003), participants volunteered that the inter-view had been "enlightening" and "cathartic." One participant who was still in the dissertation process stated that the inter-view had helped her "think through [her] process" and "understand it better."

The Priority of Definition

Socrates always begins his inquiries by asking his co-inquirer for a definition of whatever the subject of their inquiry may be. Socrates insists on starting with a definition because be believes that he, or anyone else for that matter, cannot know that something is representative of a certain idea without first establishing what that idea in itself is. For instance, Socrates says to Euthyphro, "If you had no clear knowledge of piety and impiety you would never have ventured to prosecute your old father for murder on behalf of a servant" (Plato, 1981c, 15d), that is, you must know what piety is to be certain that your current act is pious. In the *Meno*, when Meno wishes to know whether or not the Greek trait of *arete*[3] is teachable, that is, when he wants to know something *about arete*, Socrates asserts, "I am so far from knowing whether *arete* can be taught or not that I do not even have knowledge of what *arete* itself is" (Plato, 1981d, 71a). In the *Laches*, Socrates asks about courage, "if we are not absolutely certain what it is, how are we going to advise anyone as to the best method of obtaining it?" (Plato, 1992b, 190b–c).

To employ the priority of definition concept in a Socratic-hermeneutic inter-view, a researcher would begin by asking the co-inquirer for a definition of the phenomenon being studied. For instance, she would ask "what is caregiving?" or "what does it mean to have Alzheimer's?" The co-inquirer should be encouraged to respond not with a dictionary definition or with what she thinks the concept is supposed to mean, but what it means *for her*, thus obeying the "say what you believe" requirement. Beginning with a definition is effective for several reasons. First, such a request carries with it no prejudices or assumptions, other than perhaps the basic assumption that the co-inquirer *can* say what the concept means for her. The dialogue is therefore starting on neutral ground and is ready to follow where the inquiry leads. Second, beginning with a definition is likely to give the researcher many fruitful avenues to follow for further inquiry. For example, in the aforementioned study of the dissertation process, when a participant, "Eleanor," was asked "what is a dissertation?" she responded:

It's coming up with an idea that's unique, beginning to form an argument for how to support that idea and seeing what follows from it, doing extensive research, not only around the idea but also around the implications, and then coming up with a way to identify again, after doing all that, what the idea really is, and to be able to express it and state it, and identify and defend it against helpful objections. I guess the other thing I would add is that in stating it, it's more than just finding a way to express the idea, after having done all the research, but also . . . you're *proclaiming* your ideas so that you're not merely saying, "here's what might be the case," you're saying, "I stand behind making this claim," so it's sort of also taking, I don't know if it's a *moral* stand behind it, but taking a stand behind the ideas that you have.

Based on this response, the researcher asked many follow-up questions, including "What do you mean by proclaiming?," "Say more about why it might be a 'moral' stand," and "Why is it important that the dissertation would be unique?" More follow-up questions inevitably resulted from the responses to these questions.

A third reason to begin with a definition is the reason given by Socrates himself when he is asserting the priority of definition: How are we to know that something is representative of a certain phenomenon unless we know that phenomenon first? If a researcher asks participants for an incident that represents a certain phenomenon to them, how sure can they be of their answer? Does that incident really represent the phenomenon? Since the participant has not necessarily thought about, and surely has not systematically inquired into, the phenomenon, how does she understand that this incident is representative? This is not to say that the incident *cannot* be representative, but simply that it might not be.

Finally, beginning with a definition is likely to avoid the problem that, as Weston observes, "Sometimes values may appear to vary just because we have different beliefs about the facts" (2002, p. 8). For instance, a health professional who is a co-inquirer may express great hesitancy toward getting involved in family disputes over care for the elderly, while a co-inquirer in another inter-view might be much more willing to get involved. The apparent difference between these two co-inquirers, though, could simply be that they have different "beliefs about the facts," i.e. different definitions of what it means to "get involved" in such cases. Without establishing a definition, then, the researcher may draw false conclusions about the different views of these two co-inquirers.

Analogies

The process of comparing beliefs only works for Socrates if he is able to find a way to help his co-inquirers understand the consequences of their statements and also the connections between those statements and their own dearly held beliefs. To this end, Socrates employs analogies to put questions and situations into contexts more familiar for the co-inquirer. In this way, he can help his co-inquirers see the patterns of their own beliefs.

When the young and inexperienced Menexenus comes to the odd conclusion that friendship can only exist between good and that which is neither good nor evil, Socrates helps him to think about his conclusion by making an analogy to medicine. "If we look attentively," he says, "we perceive that a body which is in health has no need whatever of the medical art or of any assistance, for it is sufficient in itself. And therefore no one in health is friendly with a physician on account of his health." Menexenus agrees, and the two soon realize that medicine is good, and a body is neither good nor evil, and so their most recent conclusion must have been wrong (Plato, 1961, 217a–b). Here, we see a boy who is easily confused when talking about concepts as complex as the nature of friendship, yet when Socrates offers an analogy, the youth is able to see his mistake right away.[4] His deeper beliefs about friendship are too far removed and too complicated for the boy to access directly, but by following a link to a conclusion easier to weigh against his own beliefs, Menexenus is also able to see that he does not believe what he thought he believed about friendship.

Socrates' co-inquirer here is incapable of thinking clearly about the concept at hand and its nature directly, and an analogy is required to help him better understand his own thinking and to better compare the current questions with his own beliefs. In a Socratic-hermeneutic inter-view, a co-inquirer may become stuck on a difficult question. While it is appropriate and recommended to give the co-inquirer plenty of time to think about the question, it may also be helpful to offer an analogy to assist the co-inquirer in thinking the question through. For instance, if a researcher asks, "how do you define authority in your relationship with your mother [for whom you are caregiving]", the co-inquirer may have trouble answering, or may even ask, "what do you mean?" The researcher could then give an analogy, saying, "well, for myself and my son, it's understood that my authority means he has to obey certain rules, but I also have to respect that he's almost 18 and wants and needs a certain amount of freedom." With this analogy as a starting point, the participant is more likely now to be able to answer the question about authority from her own perspective.

An analogy may sometimes help to clarify a co-inquirer's statement. Socrates sometimes must use analogies to help his co-inquirer clarify a point. By using such analogies, Socrates helps the co-inquirer explore what he really seems to believe about the concept in question and hence what he really means by his words. Euthyphro faces such a challenge no fewer than three times in his discussion with Socrates. When he argues that the pious is "what all the gods love," Socrates wants to know if he really means that the pious is loved by the gods because it is pious, or whether it is pious because it is loved by the gods. Euthyphro does not understand the problem, and so Socrates offers an analogy at a level that Euthyphro can more easily understand, comparing the question to the difference between carrying and being carried (Plato, 1981c, 10a–b). When Euthyphro later defines the pious as care of the gods, Socrates asks about hunting as the care of dogs to clarify what Euthyphro means by "care" (13a). Finally, when Euthyphro revises his claim so that the pious is now a matter of service to the gods, Socrates asks about shipbuilders and generals to pinpoint what sort of service Euthyphro has in mind (13e–14a). In each of these cases, the co-inquirer cannot find the means of clarifying his assertion until Socrates offers an analogy.

"Patricia," a participant in the study of the dissertation process, talked about an experience in which an analogy helped her understand and alter her own thinking. She had thought of the dissertation as a "black hole" that seemed to stretch deeper and deeper. It was her 10-year-old son who provided a useful analogy for her, calling it her "BIG paper." This analogy created a helpful sense of perspective for Patricia. When she would say goodnight to her son, he would ask for reassurance that she would be in "her special place," at the computer in the room next to his, working on her big paper. The analogy not only helped her to move the dissertation concept from a black hole to a manageable paper (even if it was BIG!), but created a meaningful connection in this phase of her life with her son (Sorrell & Dinkins, 2003).

Examples

In addition to analogies, Socrates often employs examples to test or explore the co-inquirer's statements. His companion can then examine his beliefs about these examples to determine whether or not their current status within the discussion is acceptable. Sometimes, Socrates can easily do this with simple matters of fact, as he does when young Lysis claims that his parents restrict his freedom because he is not old enough. Socrates points out the obvious fact that Lysis's parents let him read, write, and play the lyre. Only then does Lysis realize his mistake, and change his account of his parents' reasons to include the difference between restricting what Lysis does and does not understand (Plato, 1961, 209a). Socrates later, though, presents Lysis's friend Menexenus with an example as a consequence that is not a matter of fact, and that must be evaluated. When Menexenus claims that two can be friends when only one loves, Socrates presents the example of a man who is hated by his beloved. Faced with a concrete example, Menexenus is able to reevaluate his earlier claim, and he now believes that neither person in such a case can be called a friend (Plato, 1961a, 212b–c). Apparently, the idea of one member of a set of friends hating the other clashes with Menexenus' more dearly held beliefs, since he cannot accept that consequence.[5]

By offering an example, a researcher can help a co-inquirer to clarify her statement and explore it further. In the study on the dissertation process, "Louise" stated that after she had defended, she expected some sort of transition, some sort of letting-go by her advisor that she did not in fact experience, though she did not give further explanation. When the researcher asked, "maybe one thing you were expecting was that she would start treating you like a colleague?" Louise reacted strongly in the negative, and then exclaimed, "I thought she would say 'you can file.'" Louise then went on to explore the fact that this lack of ability to file her dissertation with the library, thus completing her degree requirements, was at the center of her frustration, and the fact that she simply wanted to be done when her advisor, from Louise's perspective, wanted the work to be book-quality first. In this inter-view, then, even though the researcher suggested an example that turned out not to be what the co-inquirer had in mind, the act of rejecting that example led to insights on what really had bothered the co-inquirer (Sorrell & Dinkins, 2003).

An example may also help a co-inquirer evaluate whether she really believes a statement she has made, because examples can help point out implications and consequences of a statement that the co-inquirer may not otherwise have noticed. For instance, in a pilot interview for the dissertation research study, the co-inquirer defined a dissertation as an example of research that had important implications for nursing practice. When queried by the researcher what she meant by "important implications," the co-inquirer explained that the dissertation should have an impact on the ideas and practices of others who would read it. The researcher then asked whether a dissertation that was for some reason ignored, and thus could not have "important implications," would still be a dissertation. The co-inquirer then questioned her original definition, since she did not want to agree that in such a case, the work would not still be a dissertation. Then she began to think about how many musicians wrote music that was ignored during their lifetimes but considered breakthrough compositions many years later. Thus, she circled back toward her original definition, adding that the implications for practice may be "ahead of their time" and may not be recognized as important until many years later. By making this adjustment to her own definition, the co-inquirer and the researcher both learned more about the co-inquirers' deeper beliefs about the nature of a dissertation (Sorrell & Dinkins, 2003).

Pointing Out Conflicts

In order to match beliefs with one another and test for conflicts, examples may often not be necessary. In a long inter-view, it is likely that apparent conflicts will arise on their own. When this occurs, the researcher should bring attention to the seeming conflict and explore it with the co-inquirer. In this way, they can determine if there is indeed a conflict, or if there is none, they can explore the relevant issues to find how they fit together after all.

In the dissertation research study, "Eleanor's" description of the complexity of the writing process illustrates how the dialogue helps to uncover inherent conflicts in beliefs. Eleanor stated:

It's kind of an odd thing, because the step that's most important, and the step that will truly make it happen, is the step where, that I have to make alone. So in a way, I think I've found it helpful, when I consider all the interactions I've had so far, I find it the most helpful when people seem to understand that. I think what I find most hindering is when I worry that people are trying to help by pointing out what I should do, by somehow making a list or direction for which steps to take.

Later in the interview, however, Eleanor described the type of communication she would like in an ideal advisor relationship:

As much communication as could be possible, and some means . . . to send along different thoughts, not only about the topic but also about the process and strategy.

In thinking through the apparent conflict between this desire for communication and her belief that a dissertation is a process undertaken alone, Eleanor realized that the "aloneness" she thought she needed was related to the fact that sometimes suggestions by others might not be helpful because, "I'm just seeing all the branches and not seeing what it is that holds them up," but if someone, e.g. an advisor, could help her clarify "what it is that holds up" the branches, she would not need to cling to her need to be alone in the writing process.

Interestingly, "Louise" noticed on her own a conflict in her beliefs, and explored that conflict to better understand her deeper beliefs:

But when my work was not polished the way she wanted me to, it was not me; I think she would take it personally. And it wasn't—now I see this with students when we get annoyed because they gave us a paper and it still has typos. It wasn't me being like, "I'm going to give her something sloppy and get it over with." No. I would spend hours and hours reading stuff, . . . [but] I could read a paper 10 times and I still won't catch all the mistakes.

Louise is aware that she has the same reaction to perceived sloppiness in her own students' papers as her advisor has to Louise's mistakes in papers, even though she is unhappy with her advisor for this reaction, and she is therefore able to identify the fact that she wants her advisor to understand that Louise is *not* like Louise perceives her undergraduate students to be, and is not simply being lazy (Sorrell & Dinkins, 2003).

Rewording a Co-inquirer's Statements

It is helpful for the researcher to restate the co-inquirer's beliefs in the researcher's own words. This helps to identify the researcher's assumptions and possible misunderstandings, and also helps the co-inquirer to think more deeply about the belief in an effort to clarify how the rewording may have been inaccurate. Although Benner (1994, p. 111) also suggested this technique, noting that it is helpful to give the participant at least two ways of paraphrasing what was said and keeping the question open for alternative interpretations from the participant, it does not seem to have found its way into common practices of phenomenological interviewing. In the inter-view with "Eleanor," the researcher attempted to paraphrase one of Eleanor's responses:

So it sounds like you're tying the uniqueness not so much to the importance of the product in the end being unique, the dissertation itself, but that that affects the process you go through, and somehow that makes it what a dissertation is supposed to be. Is that what I hear you saying?

Eleanor was not satisfied with the paraphrase, so she re-worded and expanded it:

Yeah, although the change I would make to that is that if you're, well, it's not going to be sufficient that if you use a certain process, you'll end up with a certain product, it's not that relation, but if you want to end up with the sort of product where you have produced something unique that engages the reader in a certain kind of thinking, and challenges them and challenges you as well, and if you want to end up with a product that *is* attempting to assert an idea and not just be an exercise, it seems to me that to end up with that product requires that you go through this process. So the process is linked with the product, but it's not sufficient necessarily to produce it either.

Another paraphrase that the researcher offered was also revised by Eleanor:

RESEARCHER: So meeting with an advisor in his office, it sounds like it connects him with all of that institutional, academia stuff? And that's where the intimidation is coming from, is that right?

ELEANOR: Yes, in part. I think the other part is kind of the fake sense of security that it's tempting to derive from what already has been put forward. . . . You're identifying a new idea and trying to look at it in a new way and hopefully move beyond just what is already in place in the machinery, and just kind of break free of the machinery, it's sort of a reminder that this machinery has a lot of power. It can get you jobs, it can get you acceptance, and so there's a lot of temptation to sort of succumb to that rather than maybe taking a less safe route that actually would be closer to discovery (Sorrell & Dinkins, 2003).

Asking About Ideals

When Socrates asked his co-inquirers for definitions, he and his companions were working under the assumption that the true nature of the concept under question was one and the same with its ideal nature. In modern times, that assumption no longer holds. When a researcher asks "what is justice?" the co-inquirer may respond in terms of what the ideal would be, but will more likely respond in terms of her actual experience. Both types of answers can lead to insights, and both should therefore be encouraged. When "Eleanor" was asked "How would you define the ideal relationship between an advisor and advisee for a dissertation?" her initial response was, "Ideal? Oh, that's a fun question." She then went on to discuss a relationship with plenty of room for what she termed "low-stakes" communication instead of only "high-stakes" communication. After she had gone into quite a bit of detail on the ideal relationship, the researcher and Eleanor inquired together on how that ideal matched up with her actual experience, and what they could learn from that comparison.

The Hermeneutic Circle of Socrates' Elenchus

The analogies and examples that make up such a large part of Socrates' question-and-answer process are complemented by the overall structure in which they occur. Socrates' belief that "the lover of inquiry must follow his beloved wherever it may lead him" (Plato, 1981c, 14b) often in fact leads him in circles, though potentially productive circles. This "circle" is similar to Heidegger's hermeneutic circle, the circle that he says is not "circular reasoning" in the vicious sense, but rather a "relatedness backward and forward" (1962, p. 28).

⋅ In almost all of the dialogues, Socrates utters a statement to the effect that he and his companions must examine the current question once again from the beginning. In the *Charmides,* he insists, "then start over again, Charmides" (Plato, 1992a, 160d);[6] in the *Theaetetus,* he tells his two companions, "the thing to do is to reconsider this matter quietly and patiently" (Plato, 1990, 154e); in the *Republic,* after nine books have gone by, Socrates still suggests, "let's return to the first things we said, since they are what led us here" (Plato, 1992c, 588b). In the *Euthyphro,* he says, "we must investigate again from the beginning what piety is" (Plato, 1981c, 15c); here, Socrates also implies that the necessity for such a backtrack is not simply his decision, but demanded by the discourse, as he observes, "our argument has moved around and come again to the same place" (15b–c).

This circular, back-and-forth approach is reflected in other ways, as well. In the *Phaedo,* Socrates reexamines the question at hand many times, following varied paths, and then goes back to combine two of them to make a further point: "It has been proved even now," he claims, "if you are ready to combine this argument with the one we agreed on before" (Plato, 1981e, 77c). Even at the end of this dialogue, though, when everyone seems as convinced as they are likely to become, Socrates insists, "our first hypotheses require clearer examination, even though we find them convincing. And if you analyze them adequately, you will, I think, follow the argument as far as a man can and if the conclusion is clear, you will look no further" (107b).

This practice of circling back to the beginning and reexamining the problem from a different angle is often necessitated by a hypothesis that has been rejected due to the clash of its consequences with dearly held beliefs, or when more exploration seems necessary. By encouraging his friends to continually reexamine the issue, Socrates helps them to form connections, to come to understand gradually why their most dearly held beliefs about justice, for example, *necessitate* belief in the claims currently under discussion. As Socrates and his co-inquirers follow the paths of their deeper beliefs, altering the path slightly each time, more of the connections are revealed to them, and their understandings of the connections are strengthened as each new angle is revealed. In this way, they can grow in their understanding of the belief in question.

More often, Socrates uses his hermeneutic circle to continue to explore issues that are much more unresolved. At this earlier stage, though, Socrates' circle works not only to reveal and reinforce the connections between more dearly held beliefs, but to expose false beliefs as well. As I have previously argued, Socrates seems to believe that the degree to which a belief is held dear reflects how likely it is to be a true belief. Thus, when Socrates and his co-inquirer are examining beliefs that are not held as dear, many of them may be false. When these beliefs are revealed as conflicting, rather than agreeing, with more dearly held beliefs, they can be purged; they can be gotten out of the way so that more promising connections can be explored.

Since this is Socrates' goal, his circular, back-and-forth approach is essential. In the spirit of Socrates' own method, an analogy may be appropriate here. When a person wishes to vacuum an entire carpet, he does so strip by strip. With each pass, he overlaps the most recent strip. In this way, he can be sure he has not missed any debris that may be in the carpet. Socrates' approach is just as careful, with similar motivations. By moving with his companions back and forth, beginning from the same place each time and following a slightly different though overlapping path, together they are more likely to find their own false beliefs and clean them out of the way. The repeated passes back and forth make it much less likely for them to miss any false beliefs.

This process—the back-and-forth continual examination that brings about the exposure and identification of conflicting beliefs at the early stage and the strengthening of dearly held beliefs at the later stage—is only shown to work through discourse, through *shared inquiry*. When the process mainly achieves purgation, it seems likely that the dialogue between two people helps to expose conflicts that one person alone might not have noticed. Once again heeding Gadamer's warning that "it is the tyranny of hidden prejudices that makes us deaf to what speaks to us" (1989, p. 270), these hidden prejudices must be exposed, and since the careful tracing and retracing from statement to consequence could still certainly leave gaps, two watchful minds are better than one in that respect. In fact, Socrates' goal and practice of discussing the same issue with many different people appears to be an extended version of his own repetitive method. In addition to reexamining a question many times with a given co-inquirer, he also examines an issue with many different interlocutors, thus traveling similar paths many times, testing and retesting his own beliefs.

The interview with "Eleanor" illustrates this circling back to the beginning. In her initial response to the question, "To you, what is a dissertation?" she stated:

It's more than just finding a way to express the idea, after having done all the research, but also, what it means to me is that the real dissertation is, you're proclaiming your ideas so that you're not merely saying, "here's what might be the
case," you're saying, "I stand behind making this claim," so it's sort of also taking,
I don't know if it's a moral stand behind it, but taking a stand behind the ideas
that you have.

As the interview progressed, "Eleanor" came back to the idea of "moral
stand" several times and, at the end, returned to it unprompted, apparently seeing the concept in a new light as an empowering force:

I'm digging a deeper and deeper hole for myself . . . so the way to try to get beyond that is to use the other sort of process we talked about. . . . I'd return to the
question about moral choice, in a way only by taking a chance and going ahead
and asserting an idea that isn't fully formed yet, and pursuing it (Sorrell & Dinkins, 2003).

This circling back and re-evaluating is also important in connecting
interviews with different co-inquirers as a research study evolves, as it facilitates identification of emerging themes and provides opportunities to
clarify whether they are common to inter-views with future co-inquirers.
In the first few inter-views for the dissertation research study, similar
ideas circled among the co-inquirers: the dissertation process as a deep
hole which one fears falling into permanently; the complex communication strategies needed between student and advisor; the influence of values on the dissertation process; and the importance of commitment in the
process. It was also evident that co-inquirers could easily contrast an ideal
with a reality. This helped to move beyond assumptions of the researchers
and suggested important questions to pursue in future inter-views.

The Interpre-view Process

The process of the inter-view itself embodies an interpretation, as co-
inquirers reflect and come to new, shared understandings. When Socrates engages in shared inquiry, the entire process of learning and discovery
happens within the dialogue. He does not retreat to a quiet place after
the dialogue to reflect on the inquiry and seek further revelation. Any
further investigation of the same central concept occurs in a dialogue
with another person or again with the same co-inquirer.

This practice of Socrates can inform modern phenomenological research. The current practice of collecting interviews tends to confine

most of the interpretive work to the process of looking back over transcriptions of interviews to identify themes and find what the phenomenon under study has revealed of itself. This practice fails to follow the model set forth by Gadamer and Heidegger in their own hermeneutic studies. In their works, the asking of the questions and the interpretation of the phenomena are part of one holistic cycle. Heidegger, for instance, does not ask questions of or about Being, then examine his findings afterwards. Similarly, in "What Calls for Thinking?" (1993b), his exploration of the question is largely one and the same with his interpretation of thinking.

The necessity of interviews for phenomenological research in the health sciences has given birth to the current separation between question and interpretation, but that separation is unnecessary. Just as Heidegger can interpret Being as he is questioning Being, so can a researcher interpret a phenomenon as she inter-views a co-inquirer. To leave the bulk of interpretation until after each interview or after all of the interviews is to invite back in the problems of the researcher's unnoticed biases. As already stated, the Socratic *elenchus* is designed to shed light on and check the inquirer's assumptions. As long as a researcher is engaged in *shared* inquiry, therefore, her assumptions are subject to constant testing and feedback. As soon as she steps away from her co-inquirer, though, she no longer has any such system of testing available to her. New assumptions or old ones are quite likely to slip into her interpretation, no matter how vigilant she remains.

The Socratic-hermeneutic inter-view avoids this problem, and it has another benefit as well: It allows the co-inquirer to be a much more central part of the interpretation process. The inter-view conducted in this manner avoids an artificial and undesirable separation between "expert" and "layperson" by accepting that the co-inquirer may have much to add to the ongoing process of interpretation. I do not suggest that no interpretation can or should occur once the researcher has finished the interview, for such a restriction would be too limiting. I do suggest, though, that the more interpretation that occurs during the inter-view and the more the inter-view and interpretation can become one holistic process, the more genuinely hermeneutic the research will be.

In fact, the concept of an *interpre-view* may help researchers avoid thinking of the inter-view and interpretation as two separate processes. Heidegger often coined words, and his reasons for this practice were twofold: First, it enabled him to avoid the pitfalls and limitations inherent in the use of traditional language; second, it allowed him to give readers a constant reminder of a new or re-imagined concept in the form of this fresh, new word. In this same way, the term *interpre-view* avoids the artificial separation inherent in the use of two words for what should largely be one process, and it serves as a reminder to researchers of the goals and purpose of the phenomenological research process.

The Hermeneutic Circle and Aporia

Socrates' back-and-forth approach works in concert with the lack of resolution, or *aporia,* experienced at the end of many of Plato's works, especially for the reader. While many of Socrates' co-inquirers may have the chance to follow up on discussions with him (as some in fact do in other dialogues, and others we can imagine may do "off stage"), the reader cannot. Plato ends many of his works not simply in *aporia* but in a way that dramatically brings attention to that aporia. Socrates or someone else suddenly has an appointment to keep, young Lysis and Menexenus are run off by their guardians, the *Symposium* is interrupted by revelers. Even the *Apology,* despite Socrates' sincere argument that a good man should not fear death, ends quite dramatically on a very unsure note: "Now the hour to part has come," Socrates declares. "I go to die, you go to live. Which of us goes to the better lot is known to no one, except God" (Plato, 1981a, 42a).

By calling such attention to the incomplete and unsatisfactory conclusion of the aporetic works, Plato leaves his reader even more unsettled than she may otherwise have been. When Socrates' co-inquirer runs off to an appointment, the reader is disappointed and left longing for more. This feeling is made even stronger in combination with Socrates' way of examining and reexamining each question. Such repetition begins to feel like an endless cycle, and when the cycle is suddenly cut short, the reader is driven to continue on her own. Again, an analogy may be helpful here. The works that contain this back-and-forth in combination with an aporetic ending are much like some of the western world's greatest pieces of music, pieces that are centered around a single, often complex, theme.[7] The theme is repeated many times throughout the piece, often appearing in varied form, and in the voice of different instruments. Often, after many versions of the theme—versions that tend to overlap each other—and once the listener has been drawn into the repetition, into the seemingly inevitable continuing cycle, the piece ends with the theme unfinished.[8] The accumulated effect of such a piece is that the hearer is left wanting more, a mixed feeling of disappointment and longing, sadness that the piece is over, but desire to continue the variations on the theme on her own. The effect of Plato's aporetic works is much like this, as the reader is left wishing that Socrates would explore the question further, but also feels driven to explore the issue on her own. Plato's design for these dialogues is thus very effective if his goal is in part to give the reader the experience of a Socratic inquiry.

Just as Socrates' dialogues end in aporia, most Socratic-hermeneutic interpre-views are likely to end in much the same way. It would be unreasonable to expect otherwise, to expect that by the end of an hour or even more, the co-inquirers would have the phenomenon entirely revealed to them. This aporia can be immensely helpful to both the researcher and the co-inquirer. The co-inquirer is likely to go home and think on the phenomenon more, thus gaining insights into her own life and experiences. The researcher should embrace the frustration and longing brought on by the aporetic void, and she should look inside herself to identify what she is still searching for. What is it that she wished they could have answered? What does she wish she would have asked? What connections were just starting to appear? By paying careful attention to this aporetic experience, the researcher can continue to be led by the ongoing inquiry, taking these questions and letting them guide her in her next interpre-view.

The Hermeneutic Circle Continues

The shared inquiry approach described in this manuscript provides an alternative way for hermeneutic researchers to uncover new understandings in interpre-views. In the dissertation research study described in this essay, co-inquirers seemed engaged in the interpre-view process. They did not appear to be intimidated by the consistent questioning of their beliefs and were comfortable rejecting or redirecting questions. An excerpt from the interview with "Louise" illustrates these observations:

INTERVIEWER: What made you feel stuck?
LOUISE: I never felt stuck in terms of, my dissertation—I always felt like it's not going fast enough, but I knew it was not like—I never had 4 months where it didn't work.

INTERVIEWER: So it went slow but not stuck.
LOUISE: Yes (Sorrell & Dinkins, 2003).

Co-inquirers also appeared comfortable in rejecting the researcher's attempt to clarify or reword what the co-inquirer said, as illustrated by the excerpts from "Eleanor's" interview above. In addition, Louise clarified the researcher's understanding of her perception that her advisor wanted to extend the relationship unnecessarily:

INTERVIEWER: She wanted you to keep working so that you would
    continue that relationship?
LOUISE: Not so much, but maybe perfect it for the book (Sorrell &
    Dinkins, 2003).

A statement by "Eleanor" illustrated how important it is for researchers to help co-inquirers separate their own views from those of others. In response to the question, "What is a dissertation?" she replied:

One thing I noticed when I started thinking about the question is I had
trouble separating it from what I believe other people think it should be
(Sorrell & Dinkins, 2003).

Co-inquirers tended to come back (often on their own) to defining central terms, and they seemed to be able to do so more clearly and thoroughly after having discussed surrounding issues with the researcher. Also, some ideas kept coming back during the interpre-view, even when not directly relevant to the question, suggesting that all the beliefs are interconnected. This interconnectedness is illustrated by "Eleanor's" description of how her fears of the dissertation spilled over into fears about her life:

The fear has gotten in the way as I do the dissertation. Then one thing that I've observed happening in my own life is that I take that sort of deformed process, it's not what it should be, a deformed process rather than what I'd like to be doing, and making a commitment, and . . . I end up applying it to other things in my life. So, to make a personal decision, such as when to begin adoption proceedings, once I make the decision and start to pursue the details, of course the details behave in a manner similar to the research. . . . And what I'll find is that sometimes I'll engage in the same malformed process, and I'll become very frightened by all of that and discouraged. . . . It almost ends up feeling like a virus that's replicating itself into other areas of my life, and so the stuck part ends up not only being . . . the hole I'm trying to get out of with the dissertation but trying to get out of the hole I'm in in the way I'm living in my life (Sorrell & Dinkins, 2003).

In summary, shared inquiry in the interpre-view process can help to uncover important beliefs and assumptions related to the phenomenon. Although the shared inquiry process requires the interpre-viewer to develop skills and comfort in the process, progress comes readily with experience. It is important that research assistants who will assist with interviews be trained in the shared inquiry process. It is hoped that this process will be used in future research studies to provide alternative approaches to generate rich data. Gadamer suggests the profound influence that can come from such a dialogue:

In a successful conversation they both come under the influence of the truth of the object and are thus bound to one another in a new community. To reach an understanding in a dialogue is . . . a matter of . . . being transformed into a communion in which we do not remain what we were. (1989, p. 379)

As the teachings of Socrates suggest, in a Socratic-hermeneutic interpre-view the researcher does not simply learn from the co-inquirer, nor does the co-inquirer learn from the researcher. Instead, they both "discover within themselves a multitude of beautiful things which they bring forth into the light" (Plato, 1990, 150d).

Acknowledgments

I would like to thank Dr. Jeanne Sorrell for providing background information for the introductory paragraphs, and for offering extensive feedback and support. Dialogues with Dr. Sorrell were essential in birthing, testing, and developing the ideas in this paper.

Notes

1. Because all of Socrates' co-inquirers were men, I will use male pronouns when referring to Socrates' own inquiries.
2. See also 1981c, 14e and 1992b, 193c.
3. *Arete* is a difficult term to define in modern language and culture. For the ancient Greeks, it referred to the quality of human excellence, encompassing the virtues of honor, courage, temperance, and many others.
4. Socrates uses a similar tactic to refute the claim that justice is "to give to each what is owed to him" in the *Republic* (Plato, 1992, 331e–334a).
5. Similarly, Laches cannot accept the consequence that a man who fights while in retreat cannot be courageous (Plato, 1992b, 191a).
6. See also 163d and 167b in this dialogue.

7. Including at least the *Parmenides, Lysis, Meno, Euthyphro, Symposium* (which features different people's accounts on the same subject and thus has the same effect), *Laches, Charmides* and *Theaetetus*.

8. Examples of such works include Barber's "Adagio for Strings," Ravel's "Bolero," the second movement of Beethoven's Seventh Symphony, and also many minimalist works.

References

Benner, P. (1984). *From novice to expert. Excellence and power in clinical nursing practice.* Menlo Park, CA: Addison Wesley.

Benner, P. (1994). The tradition and skill of interpretive phenomenology in studying health, illness, and caring practices. In P. Benner (Ed.), *Interpretive phenomenology: Embodiment, caring, and ethics in health and illness.* Thousand Oaks, CA: Sage.

Gadamer, H. (1989). *Truth and method* (2nd Rev. Ed.). Trans. Joel Weinsheimer and Donald G. Marshall. New York: Continuum.

Geanellos, R. (1999). Hermeneutic Interviewing: An example of its development and use as a research method. *Contemporary Nurse 8*(2), 39–45.

Heidegger, M. (1962). *Being and Time.* (J. Macquarrie & E. Robinson, Trans.). New York: Harper & Row.

Heidegger, M. (1966). Conversation on a Country Path about Thinking. In *Discourse on Thinking* (J. M. Anderson & E. H. Freund, Trans.). New York: Harper & Row.

Heidegger, M. (1993a). The Origin of the Work of Art. In D. F. Krell (Ed.), *Basic Writings.* San Francisco: HarperCollins.

Heidegger, M. (1993b). What Calls for Thinking? In D. F. Krell (Ed.), *Basic Writings.* San Francisco: HarperCollins.

Plato. (1925). *Symposium.* In *Plato: Lysis Symposium Gorgias.* (W. R. M. Lamb, Trans.). Cambridge: Harvard.

Plato. (1961). *Lysis.* (J. Wright, Trans.). In E. Hamilton & H. Cairns, *Plato: The Collected Dialogues.* Princeton: Princeton.

Plato. (1981a). *Apology.* In *Five Dialogues.* (G. M. A. Grube, Trans.). Indianapolis: Hackett.

Plato. (1981b) *Crito.* In *Five Dialogues.* (G. M. A. Grube, Trans.). Indianapolis: Hackett.

Plato. (1981c). *Euthyphro.* In *Five Dialogues.* (G. M. A. Grube, Trans.). Indianapolis: Hackett.

Plato. (1981d). *Meno.* In *Five Dialogues.* (G. M. A. Grube, Trans.). Indianapolis: Hackett.

Plato. (1981e). *Phaedo.* In *Five Dialogues.* (G. M. A. Grube, Trans.). Indianapolis: Hackett.

Plato. (1990). *Theaetetus.* (M. J. Levett & M. Burnyeat, Trans.). Indianapolis: Hackett.

Plato. (1992a). *Charmides.* In *Laches and Charmides.* (R. K. Sprague, Trans.). Indianapolis: Hackett.

Plato. (1992b). *Laches.* In *Laches and Charmides.* (R. K. Sprague, Trans.). Indianapolis: Hackett.

Plato. (1992c). *Republic.* (G. M. A. Grube & C. D. C. Reeve, Trans.). Indianapolis: Hackett.

Plato. (1997). *Parmenides.* (R. E. Allen, Trans.). New Haven: Yale.

Sorrell, J. M., & Dinkins, C. S. (2003). Shared inquiry: What do we know about the process of writing a doctoral dissertation? Unpublished research.

Sorrell, J. M., & Redmond, G. M. (1995). Interviews in qualitative nursing research: Differing approaches for ethnographic and phenomenological studies. *Journal of Advanced Nursing 21*(6), 1117–1112.

Van Manen, M. (1997). *Researching lived experience: Human science for an action sensitive pedagogy.* Albany: State University of New York Press.

Weston, A. (2001). *A practical companion to ethics* (2nd Ed.). Oxford: Oxford University Press.

4

Revealing Shape-shifting
Through Life-story Narrative

ROSE MCELDOWNEY

This chapter explores how using life-story narrative as a way of inquiry reveals the metaphorical construct of shape-shifting as an active process of teaching for social change in nursing. As well as revealing shape-shifting as teaching for change, I also show how life-story narrative research became a process of shape-shifting in and of itself. This study challenges the more traditional and, perhaps, accepted process of inquiry in which the researcher follows a "methodological recipe" (Polkinghorne, 1983). Providing an alternative process, the study serves as an exemplar of the seamlessness and reciprocity of phenomenon and method. Over two years, six participants and I as researcher, all nurse educators, sought to understand the "what," "why," and "how" of teaching for social change in new ways.

Because little is known about why and how nurse educators teach for social change, I undertook doctoral research to illuminate and give voice to the lived experiences of these six women nurse educators who teach for social change in Aotearoa[1] New Zealand (McEldowney, 2002). The research also breaks new ground in nursing education, but in hindsight the key decision was to use life-story narrative inquiry as a methodology and method to engage each of the participants in several in-depth conversations about teaching for social change.

The research is informed from a critical feminist perspective and is politically situated in two ways—teaching and learning cannot be neutral, and my choice of life-story narrative inquiry is a political act. I concur with Zeichner (1995), who says that teaching and learning cannot be politically neutral. By raising and critiquing issues of power, social justice, agency, resistance, and praxis in nursing education, my thesis is positioned in a counter-hegemonic way. Zeichner also says that as educators we

Need to act with greater clarity about whose interests we are furthering in our work because, acknowledged or not, the everyday choices we make as teachers . . . reveal our moral commitments with regard to social continuity and change. (1995, p. 12)

Using life-story narrative inquiry as the methodology and method to reveal the life-stories of the what, why, and how of teaching for social change *is* a political act. The six participants and I, the researcher, were able to reflect on and discuss their valuable and committed work for social change. They revealed how their lives have been shaped and how in turn they have shaped things in the present and for the future. Significantly, their stories and my analysis, interpretation and synthesis have contributed to the debate on counter-hegemonic teaching practices.

Although most research into social change occurs at the macro level (Freire, 1972; Murphy, 1999; Sztompka, 1993), it is also important to hear and understand nurse educators' inside stories (the micro level)— particularly what influences and motivates them to teach the way they do. Nurse educators' life-stories are notably absent in the discourses around teaching for social change (McEldowney, 2002). I also found no established or commonly accepted methods for framing a study that investigates the lives of those who are engaged in political activism in nursing education.

I present this chapter chronologically. First, I present the background about what led me to use life-story narrative as a way of inquiry in my doctoral research. In the second section, I position the use of life-story within the field of narrative inquiry as both methodology and method. Life-story narrative calls up (invokes) and calls forth (evokes) the lived experiences of the six participants as they teach for and with social change. As a feminist nurse educator, my approach to research is grounded in the belief that separating theory from practice "distorts the reality of the research process" (Munro, 1993, p. 163). This separation can result in the legitimisation of certain types of knowledge over others, for example: knowledges arising from quantitative research inquiry and what constitutes legitimate knowledge. In the third section, I focus on the research in action, beginning with an overview of the research journey that involved negotiating and establishing the life-story research process with the six participants (Anne, Eileen, Grace, Annie, Mary, and Miriam). The creation of, and rationale for using, a story map to negotiate the field of inquiry with these nurse educators is also presented. This process enabled us to journey together for up to two years and to hold the stories of their lived experiences over time. I also present some commentary on how I gathered their stories. The use of metaphor in narrative inquiry and the emergence of shape-shifting as a metaphor for transformation and change are also discussed. In the fourth section, I discuss the significance of how using life-story as methodology became a vehicle for revealing shape-shifting as teaching for social change. It is an example of how our research and teaching are intertwined. And finally, I discuss the implications and limitations of life-story narrative inquiry for research and scholarship.

Background

From my experience, those who teach for social change in nursing often consider themselves to be on the margins as they resist the hegemony of the center—that is, they challenge and seek alternatives to dominant or traditional educational practices. In so doing, they position themselves in opposition to colleagues who they perceive to be maintaining the status quo. They also teach in areas of the curriculum perceived to be more contentious in content and process, such as cultural safety,[2] women's health, psychiatric mental health nursing, and community development. I suggest that these areas are contentious because they raise issues about marginalization, power, oppression, hegemony, gender, race, class, and inequalities in access to education and healthcare. These issues can threaten other nurse educators who still cling to traditional pedagogies and hierarchical ways of teaching (Diekelmann, 1995, 2001; Ironside, 2001). For example, teaching about personal and structural racism can be a politically challenging place for both nurse educators and students as they constantly negotiate, impose, contest, and resist meaning according to their own subjectivities. In my experience, teaching cultural safety or feminist issues in healthcare often creates conflict for students who come from multiple and contradictory positions in relation to their own experiences of racism, sexism, and gender issues (McEldowney, 2003).

Because of their awareness (consciousness) of social justice and equity in nursing and teaching, those who teach for social change bring socio-political issues to the fore. They create space for students to dialogue, debate, and critically analyze these issues. Rather than inhibiting debate, they encourage questions such as what is happening here? why are things the way they are? what can we as nurses do about this? who gets to speak? who speaks for whom? who has the power? and, how might we change things in order to bring about fair and equitable health outcomes for our clients?

As well as participating in a democratic education process, nurse educators teaching for change are able to reflect on their own practice and research in order to make sense of their work with students. They are critically conscious of the need to call their own ideas into question, state their position about teaching for transformation and listen to others. Consequently, they are able to hold open the possibilities for making a difference in the lives of students. They are active, changing, and changeable agents who move between different ideas and world-views, and who shape and are shaped by the discourses of possibility. They are shape-shifters.

To date, nurse educators have not adequately documented or theorized about the socio-political aspects of their work. In our hegemonic institutions and in the day-to-day struggles that nurse educators mediate in teaching for change, their voices often go unheard or are silenced (Buresh & Gordon, 2000; Glass, 1998). Also they are often so busy that they do not have the opportunity to express their voices, except in the classroom. Colleagues do not always hear them when they attempt to engage in dialogue about some of the key socio-political issues that influence healthcare outcomes. Such educators want to hold these issues open for critique, but it can be tiring and diminishing to deal with the resistance that surrounds teaching for change and being on the margins, or "teaching against the grain" (Ng, 1995; Ng, Staton, & Scane, 1995).

It was always my intention that my doctoral research would contribute to the stories of teaching for social change because the research offers new ways of being political in the world. The research questions that I developed to guide the research process are: how do nurse educators' life-stories reflect their philosophies, goals, intentions, and practices as they seek to teach for and with social change? why are they teaching for and with social change? how are they teaching for and with social change? The questions evolved from narrowing the field to what is known or not known about the lives of nurse educators who teach for social change. It became evident from a review of the literature on these nurse educators that there was no specific literature anywhere that addressed these questions. However, several feminist educators do offer a critical feminist position on schooling, teaching, and learning that addresses issues of social justice, praxis, context, agency, counter-hegemony, individual voice, and difference (Ellsworth, 1997; Kenway, 2001; Weiler, 1988). Their critique has been strongly influenced by the liberatory pedagogical work of Freire (1972), theorizing on hegemony and agency by Gramsci (1971), neo-Marxist educators such as Apple (1993) and Giroux (1983), and the poststructural work of Foucault (1977). These notions are particularly relevant to the work of nurse educators teaching for social change. Also, some women educators have researched the lived experiences of women teaching for change by using a life-history approach (Casey, 1993; Coles & Knowles, 1995; Jipson et al., 1995; Munro, 1993, 1998; Weiler, 1988; Weiler & Middleton, 1999). By exploring ways in which theory and practice are interrelated, they found that asking women educators to share their experiences of teaching for change and addressing issues of social justice in their everyday practice gave rise to the development of indigenous knowledge. This feminist thinking helps shape what we think about education and also what we do. Weiler (1988) says that undertaking politically motivated life-history research provides the opportunity for participants to engage in reflection and dialogue as they talk about teaching for change and reveals the commitment to counter-hegemonic teaching practices.

Life-story narrative became my methodology and method of choice as a way of answering the research questions and for revealing the key constructs of shape-shifting as teaching for social change. Life-story narrative proved an appropriate methodology and method for several reasons. First, it was congruent with the research aims and the questions— why these nurse educators have a strong desire to teach in proactive radical ways, and how they make a difference. Second, life-story narrative helped me to illuminate and theorize about the practical knowing of the everyday lives of the six participants teaching for social change. Third, telling one's life-story is an in-depth process that reveals the participant's life as lived over time and within particular historical, social, cultural, and political contexts. Fourth, by naming their lives, the personal, professional, and political agency of the nurse educators who wish to teach in a counter-hegemonic way was revealed, thus ensuring that the research addressed a feminist concern of being collaborative and transformative (Munro, 1993). Kelly (in Maynard & Purvis, 1994) suggests that using the term "feminist research practice" is helpful in addressing feminist research concerns, such as what "questions we have asked, the way we locate ourselves within our questions and the purpose of our work" (pp. 14–15). These questions go beyond issues of method and are more about the methodology (theory, analysis, and interpretation) informing the research. I consider that theory, analysis, and interpretation are embedded and woven into the everyday lives and practices of nurse educators. Finally, I believe that using life-story narrative inquiry for this project has made a significant contribution to national and international research and literature on nurse educators teaching for and with social change.

Theoretically and conceptually, as a methodology and method, life-story sits within the qualitative framework of narrative inquiry.

Narrative Inquiry

Historically, narrative inquiry arose from the interdisciplinary work of qualitative researchers who argued that narrative helped make sense of one's own and others' experiences (Bruner, 1986; Coles, 1989; Polkinghorne, 1988, 1995; Ricoeur, 1981). In the early 1900s, Freud undertook psychoanalysis on case studies gathered from clients, which was considered to be the beginnings of using "life narratives for serious academic study" (Atkinson, 1998, p. 3). During the 1930s, sociologists linked to the Chicago School shifted to narrative because quantitative inquiry was considered too limited in understanding human experience and action (Riessman, 1993).

Autobiography or self-story as a genre in literature has been part of human inquiry since the 1930s (Ribbens, 1993), although there has been a move away from the idea of narrative sitting solely within the literary domain (Riessman, 1993). Roberts (2002, p. 3) suggests that there has been a "narrative, biographical or auto/biographical turn" that has produced a shift in social science inquiry. Narrative inquiry in the social sciences has developed substantively in the fields of history, anthropology, psychology, education, and sociology. Theoretically, and philosophically, narrative inquiry has been informed by history (White, 1973), phenomenology (van Manen, 1990), hermeneutics (Gadamer, 1976; Heidegger, 1999), and grounded theory (Strauss & Corbin, 1997). Over the past two decades, narrative inquiry has also been developed as a qualitative research methodology in nursing (Bailey & Tilley, 2002; Diekelmann, 2001; Frid, Ohlen, & Bergbom, 2000; Ironside, 2001; Koch, 1998; Sandelowski, 1991, 1995; Vezeau, 1994), and other health-related disciplines, such as medicine (Coles, 1989), psychotherapy (White & Epston, 1990), and social work (Church, 1995).

Marshall and Rossman (1999) say that life-histories and narrative inquiry (along with other methods, such as historical analysis, surveys, questionnaires and psychological testing) are secondary methods, each of which constitutes a "full and complete method in and of [itself]" and they have "a methodological literature explicating the nuances and subtleties" (p. 120). However, when studying a larger phenomenon, such as teaching for and with social change in nursing, in-depth interviewing (which I name "conversations") is considered a primary data collection source. Witherell and Noddings (1991) contend that narrative can also be powerful as an epistemological tool—that it is a way of knowing about ourselves and other knowers. The life-stories from the six participants in my study showed some of the ways in which stories can tell us what it is like to be involved in socio-political activity and teaching "against the grain." Given these theoretical and philosophical influences, I now make life-story narrative, as methodology and method, explicit in this chapter.

Polkinghorne (1983, p. 5) says that methodology is about the "examination of possible plans to be carried out—the journeys to be undertaken—so that the phenomena can be obtained." I consider that the methodology I used in my doctoral thesis sits within narrative inquiry, particularly life-story narrative as a way of inquiry. From my reading of the literature related to narrative inquiry, there appears to be a debate by social science researchers as to whether life-story is methodology or method (Geiger, 1990; LeCompte, 1993; Lieblich, Tuval-Mashiach, & Zilber, 1998), or both methodology and method (Clandinin & Connelly, 1998, 2000; Cortazzi, 1993; Middleton, 1993; Polkinghorne, 1995; Riessman, 1993). Riessman (1993, p. 1) says that "the study of narrative does not fit neatly within the bounds of any single scholarly field," so it could be considered as blurring the boundaries because of its cross-disciplinary approach to inquiry. Lieblich and colleagues (1998) consider that narrative methodology has not been given credence in qualitative inquiry, particularly in relation to models for analyzing and interpreting narratives and the classification of methods. Cortazzi (1993, p. 5) proposes that gathering and analyzing teachers' narratives "can be used as an innovative

methodology" to address research questions about how teachers themselves "see their situation, what their experience is like, what they believe
and how they think." Geiger (1990) offers a useful way to determine
whether life-story narrative is methodology or method or both. As a feminist oral historian, Geiger contends that no research method is inherently feminist. Personal experience methods such as autobiographical
and biographical approaches to storytelling "only become a *method* in the
hands of persons whose interests in it go beyond the immediate pleasure
of hearing/listening to the [story] being told" (p. 170). Further, she claims
that approaches to inquiry such as life-story "only become a feminist
methodology if its use is systemised in particular feminist ways and if the
objectives for collecting the data [stories] are feminist" (p. 170).

What I understand from these various positions is that narrative inquiry appears to be like an umbrella, that arches over different methods
that include the notion of a person or persons talking or writing about
their lived experiences or their lives and how they are lived. Examples include autobiography or self-story, biography through writing a story
about another person, oral history, life-history, and life-story in which
people talk about their lives. According to Hatch and Wisniewski (1995),
narrative

fit[s] into a larger category of related or synonymous terms such as autobiography,
biography, interpretive biography, autobiographical narrative, life-history narrative, oral narrative, life-narrative, personal narrative, stories, life-stories, self-
stories, personal experience stories, auto-ethnography, ethnographic fiction, personal history, oral history, case history, and case study. (p. 124)

As can be seen by this array of terms, while there is a similarity in the
aims and assumptions underpinning them, such as eliciting stories from
one's self or others in oral or written form, there has been development of
different emphases on the theories and methods engaged. I present a
vertical linear figure (see figure 1), which is a summation of narrative inquiry as a methodology in qualitative research, and includes the subfield
of life-story narrative as methodology and storytelling as the method for
gathering data for analysis and interpretation.

Clandinin and Connelly (1998, p. 155) suggest that "it is equally correct to say *inquiry into narrative* as it is to say *narrative inquiry*." That is,
narrative may be both phenomenon and method. Narrative may be used
to name "the structured quality of experience to be studied" or to name

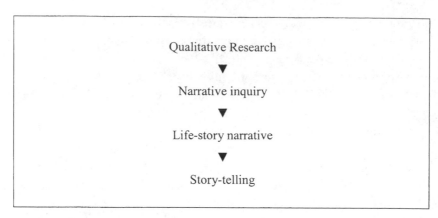

Figure 1. Life-story narrative as a methodology.

"the patterns of inquiry for its study" (Clandinin & Connelly, 1998, p. 155). Further, Clandinin and Connelly say that this difference can be preserved by "calling the phenomenon *story* and the inquiry *narrative*" (p. 155). Denzin (1989) and Cortazzi (1993) also name narrative as story. Revealing the structure and illuminating the patterns that emerge from stories is a common process of interpretive inquiry.

In her doctoral research, feminist educator Sue Middleton (1993) found no methodological recipe for gathering and interpreting the life-histories of feminist educators. Middleton says that the origins of her methodology were grounded in the ways she related to the women participants and the "way we made knowledge about our lives as women" (p. 65). She also likens storytelling and generating knowledge between the researcher and participants to the consciousness-raising process of giving voice to personal experiences during the feminist movement of the 1970s. Another important point Middleton raises is that she was not separate from the research process. She was "inside [her] own questions and methods, positioned within the object and the process of [her] inquiries" (p. 65). In this way, the researcher engaged in personal-experience methods such as life-story makes explicit her position about what is to be studied, why it needs to be studied, and how it is to be studied. This also follows the earlier comments from Geiger (1990) and Kelly (in Maynard & Purvis, 1994) about going "beyond issues of method" by focusing on feminist research objectives. For example, establishing and contributing to a new knowledge base of understanding women teachers' lives, accepting women educators' interpretations of their life-stories that reflect 'important truths,' deriving meaning from the stories, and not dismissing them as *"simply* subjective" (Geiger, 1990, p. 170).

In my doctoral study, I position life-story within the field of narrative inquiry as both methodology and method. Because I was focusing on the lives of women nurse educators and the meaning they give to their experiences, the research process was women-centered and positioned within a feminist qualitative field of inquiry. It also brings together a methodology that supports women educators in talking about their life-stories in their own voices; the use of storytelling as a method that holds open the subjective, partial, and contradictory nature of life-stories; a method that is collaborative and transforming; and a process of self-reflexivity as researcher to reveal biases, contradictions, the dialectic nature of life her-stories, and the emergent and evolving nature of my understandings about teaching for and with social change. As a critical feminist nurse educator, I make explicit my motivations for exploring the life-stories of the six women nurse educators by outlining professional and personal experiences of social and political activism that raised my awareness of the need to give voice to the various discourses that inform our work (McEldowney, 2002).

This presents a challenge to positivism and conventional scientific research in which the subjects are the objects of inquiry and the researcher is the "detached observer." Therefore, narrative inquiry has developed as a response to the restrictions of positivism and has disrupted dichotomies such as subject/object, knower/known, theory/practice, and method/process (Bunkle, 1992; Harding, 1986; Lather, 1991; LeCompte, 1993; Middleton, 1993). Narrative research (particularly the methodology of life-story research)

differs significantly from its positivistic counterpart in its underlying assumptions that there is neither a single, absolute truth in human reality, nor one correct reading or interpretation of a text. The narrative approach advocates pluralism, relativism, and subjectivity. (Lieblich et al., 1998, p. 2)

To this, I would also add six other underlying assumptions about narrative as inquiry.

First, narrative in research sits within the interpretive turn—the structure and patterns of material or text gathered is interpreted, reinterpreted, and given meaning from the subjective position of the researcher and often from the participants as co-researchers (Geertz 1983; Rabinow & Sullivan, 1987). Riessman (1993, p. 22) says "narratives are interpretive and, in turn, require interpretation." Second, stories elicited through narrative inquiry are contextually bound historically, culturally, politically, and socially. Lives are lived and stories are told about these lives within a particular historical, social, and political context. Third, there is a heuristic process inherent in narrative research as both the researcher and participant engage in uncovering meanings of lived experience to enhance understanding of the phenomena/phenomenon under inquiry (Moustakas, 1990). Fourth, temporality, or locating events or things in time, is an important aspect of narrative inquiry as the researcher and participants present stories that are an expression of a past (re-membered, re-viewed, and re-told), as well as an expression of a present and future life. Fifth, narrative inquiry "inhabits both social science and artistic spaces" which distinguishes it from other types of qualitative research inquiry (Blumenfeld-Jones, 1995, p. 25). In other words, the methodological approach that informs the inquiry arises from the social sciences and there is an aesthetic aspect to interpreting the stories that are gathered from the participants. Clandinin and Connelly (2000) consider narrative research as sitting within a "three-dimensional space" that is unbounded and therefore opens up "imaginative possibilities." Poetry, photography, or drawing can also convey narrative meaning. Sixth and last, there is the underlying idea of muthos developed by Aristotle (in *Poetics*) and expounded by Ricoeur (1991), which is central to the creation of stories and narrative inquiry. Muthos refers to the act of emplotment, which is a way of transforming several stories or subplots into one synthesised story. Ricoeur (1991, p. 21) defines emplotment as "a synthesis of heterogeneous elements."

In my doctoral research, I wanted to 'do science' differently and to disrupt the binaries of subject/object, knower/known, but also to provide a robust rationale for my choice of methodology and method. I positioned myself within the inquiry. The research questions were developed from my own positioning as a nurse educator, and I brought these subjective experiences to the research process. Consequently, I selected a methodology using life-story narrative as a way of unfolding and theorizing about the philosophy, goals, intentions, and practices of nurse educators. By taking this ideological and political position, I wanted to tell particular kinds of stories that are counter-hegemonic—that is, stories of social activism that have been silenced by those in power. For as Clandinin and Connelly (2000, p. 128) say, "the theoretical methodological framework for narrative inquiry includes a narrative view of experience with the participants' and researchers' narratives of experience being situated and lived out on storied landscapes." By eliciting the life-stories from the participants I became the interpreter whose task was to translate their stories in a way that speaks to a wider audience. I recognize that my accounts and interpretations are only partial as I selected particular discourses to illuminate the particular phenomena under investigation, that is, the "what," "why," and "how" of teaching for and with social change in nursing. McLaren (1993, p. 203) contends that "narratives can become politically enabling of social transformation or can serve as strategies of containment that locate 'difference' in closed epistemological discourses." He also suggests that we

use different kinds of narratives to tell different kinds of stories and that we sanction certain ones and discount others for ideological and political reasons. Our narrative identities determine our social action as agents of history and the constraints we place on the identities of others. (p. 203)

To summarize, narrative inquiry transcends disciplinary boundaries—for as Riessman (1993, p. 1) notes, it is "inherently interdisciplinary." It interweaves theoretical and empirical inquiry processes as a way of understanding lived personal experiences of people within certain historical, social, and political contexts. It is also situated within time and place. In the next section, I will present my rationale for choosing life-story narrative as the methodology and method, discuss definitions of life-story, and present key features that are foundational to life-story and story-telling.

Life-story Narrative as Research Methodology and Method

As a method of narrative inquiry in nursing research, story-telling's momentum has increased. Nurse academics and researchers have positioned narrative and story-telling as an integral aspect of interpretive scholarship for research, practice, and education (Bailey & Tilley, 2002; Baker & Diekelmann, 1994; Banks-Wallace, 1998; Diekelmann, 1993, 1995, 2001; Emden, 1998a & 1998b; Frid, Ohlen, & Bergbom, 2000; Giddings, 1997; Heinrich, 1992; Ironside, 2001; Johnstone, 1999; Koch,

1998; McDrury & Alterio, 2002; Sandelowski, 1991, 1995). A search of the ProQuest (CINAHL) database revealed that several nurse researchers have used life-story as methodology and method (Burkhardt & Nagai-Jacobsen, 1994; Clarke, 2000; Crisp, 1995; Forbes, Bern-Klug, & Gessert, 2000; Giddings, 1997; Hansebo & Kihlgren, 2000; Harden, 2000; Heliker, 1999; Lillemoen, 1999; Penn, 1994; Warman, 2001). A compelling reason for sharing life-stories of nurse educators teaching for and with social change is that they may encourage other nurse educators to share their stories. Diekelmann (1993, p. 6) argues, "telling stories publicly is political, critical, and transformative."

My decision to use life-story narrative for my doctoral research arises from both an experiential "doing" (ontological) position and a theoretical "knowing about" (epistemological) position. The "knowing about" and "doing" life-story narratives are embedded in my life as a woman, nurse, and nurse educator. I was interested in honoring the subjective life-story accounts of the six nurse educators who participated in the study. Each participant focused on her life, as it is lived, and on the meaning that she made of her teaching experiences for social change. Using collaborative theorizing, I wanted to build on existing knowledges to create new nursing knowledge (Diekelmann, 2001; Lather, 1991; Middleton, 1993).

The Experiential Ontological Position on Life-story

My interest in reading and writing stories began in childhood. My mother, in particular, encouraged me to read. Every Friday night we would go to the local library, where I would stock up with three or four books and then spend the weekend, and what ever other time I could snatch, buried in the stories. My parents and brother also read to me, so I was exposed to their interpretive accounts of the stories. They often embellished the stories by using a different tones of voice when portraying particular characters and using physical actions to add to the sense of drama and occasion. It also enabled me to "learn to listen" to the stories and ask questions if I needed clarification. The stories often covered both fictional and nonfictional accounts of people's lives. I would be transported into other worlds, imagining the lived experiences of heroes, heroines, and adventurers in mythical and real contexts. Fairy tales, myths, and legends have been used to transmit cultural patterns, values, and beliefs between generations through storying, painting, singing, and acting. Women writers such as Clarissa Pinkola Estes (1992) and Barbara

Kingsolver (1990) talk of the "underworld," which is the instinctive, intuitive self where the bones of life-stories are laid. Estes, a Jungian psychoanalyst and cantadora (storyteller), says that stories, myths, and fairy tales provide instruction to follow a path laid down, so that we may be led into our deeper instinctual knowing.

During my time at primary school I won a prize for a short-story competition. We were asked by the teacher to submit our stories and she would read them out to the class and students would then select the one they liked best. However, apart from that one brief moment of recognition it was to be some years before I returned to writing stories (narrative accounts of nursing practice). Professionally, nurses tend to lead storied lives. It is a way of transmitting the culture of nursing within groups of colleagues and between generations of nurses. My experiences of telling stories in practice or about practice have included: sharing information with colleagues about patients during handover at the end of a shift; taking an oral history from patients when assessing their health status and needs; participating in narrative therapy in a family-centered therapy unit; and attending narrative interpretive workshops with Professor Nancy Diekelmann at the University of Wisconsin–Madison. Further experiences in writing stories have developed over the last decade through academic study. My Master of Education thesis presented my lived experiences (autobiography) of resisting and accommodating oppression (McEldowney, 1995), and a chapter in *Teaching Practitioners of Care: New Pedagogies for the Health Professions* includes narrative exemplars arising from my practice as a nurse and nurse educator (McEldowney, 2003). It is because of these experiences that I have come to value the position of narrative, and in particular life-story as a qualitative research methodology. I consider life-story as a way of coming to understand the practices, values, and beliefs of nurse educators who teach for social change in nursing, and as a way of laying down a pathway that others may choose to follow.

The Theoretical Epistemological Position on Life-story

Numerous social science researchers have presented their views on life-story as a qualitative methodology and method (Atkinson, 1998; Clandinin & Connelly, 2000; Ellis & Flaherty, 1992; Hatch & Wisniewski, 1995; Lieblich, Tuval-Mashiach, & Zilber, 1998; Linde, 1993; Richardson, 1998; Riessman, 1993; Roberts, 2002). Life-story can also sit within the subfield or under the umbrella of narrative inquiry or the narrative study of lives (Atkinson, 1998; Josselson, 1996; Josselson & Lieblich, 1993, 1995, 1999; Lieblich & Josselson, 1994, 1997) as a form of narrative from life-history, oral history, and ethnography.

What distinguishes life-story narrative from other types of qualitative research? There are several features: a focus on the individual as participant; the personal dialogical nature of the research process; the practical nature of the findings appealing to a wider audience; and, an emphasis on the subjective nature of the research that goes beyond the empirical and scientific standards that "continue to dominate other qualitative methodologies" (Hatch & Wisniewski, 1995, p. 118). The central focus of life-story as part of the narrative research process is coming to understand the participants' individual lives and stories about their lives as lived (Clandinin & Connelly, 2000). Therefore, the stories become data as gathered from the participants, as narrators of their stories. Denzin (in Hatch & Wisniewski, 1995, p. 116) says that this research approach is focused "on the stories people tell one another," which distinguishes it from other qualitative methods, such as interviewing and participant observation. Among the various definitions of life-story as methodology, Atkinson (1998) defines it as

the story a person chooses to tell about the life he or she has lived, told as completely and honestly as possible, what is remembered of it, and what the teller wants others to know of it, usually as a result of a guided interview by another. (p. 8)

Linde (1993) refers to life-story as an oral unit of social interaction, which contains connections and coherence "created within each story and between the stories of the life-story" (p. 25). The act of speaking or writing life-story may occur in the present, but the life-story accounts told through stories over time about that which is past, are reflections recalled from memory. Cortazzi (1993) says that the story-telling process is about "reflection upon reflection" (p. 13).

Reflection was also part of the epistemological journey I engaged in when thinking about the processes and features of life-story as methodology and method. After I had read the texts on life-story, I would think about different positions that researchers had presented and would write in my research journal on reflections and insights. I include an excerpt from my journal on a reflection I wrote in March 2000:

Telling one's life-story is a conscious act of unfolding, re-membering, and re-discovering past events, that are significant and meaningful. It is a process of re-presenting significant events in a recursive and discursive way. As a person tells their life-story, they reflect on what stands out in their memory in response to a question or comment that the researcher has posed. This process can involve asking themselves key questions such as: why was that (person, event, time) important to me? in order to make sense of what happened and why has it "sat" in the subconscious or unconscious mind over time? The participants become the authors of their own life-story in the telling and re-telling of stories that matter to them. It seems that by telling their life-story the participants also create themselves by talking about what it is they do in teaching for social change. Their life is constructed through the telling of the story.

As well as reflecting and thinking through ideas about life-story, it was important for me to consider the difference between life-story and life-history because they were frequently included together in texts. I noted that some narrative inquirers consider life-story and life-history to be synonymous (Butt et al., 1992; Hatch & Wisniewski, 1995). But Goodson (1995) and Watson and Watson-Franke (1985) say there are differences that focus on the role of the researcher. Linde (1993, p. 47) claims there is a difference in the "reportability and relevance" of the oral materials (stories) that are gathered. According to Goodson, the important distinction is that life-story is about a personal reconstruction by the participant, whereas life-history starts off as a life-story the participant tells and the shift occurs when the researcher moves to include other evidence, such as "other people's accounts . . . documentary evidence and a range of historical data" (1995, p. 97). Watson and Watson-Franke (1985) say that life-history is a "retrospective account" of one's life that arises from the eliciting and prompting by another person. Linde (1993, p. 45) says that approaches to life-history can be more static than those from life-story. Life-history tends to focus more on a "fixed collection of [historical] facts," whereas life-story is a composition of meanings, and is more expressive of life as a lived experience.

Based on these distinctions, I identified life-story as the appropriate methodology for my thesis because I was not including other people's accounts about the participants or their practice. I define life-story as individual, contextually situated stories that the participants have told me in a series of conversations at a particular moment in time. The six participants brought or called forth to the present their stories that had been invoked (re-called, re-named, re-presented) from past experiences. Life-stories move beyond the personal by positioning the narrative accounts and interpretations within a broader contextual framework, such as the personal, historical, social, political, and institutional. Munro (in Hatch & Wisniewski, 1995, p. 117) warns that it is important not to decontextualise individual lives and says that life-story "requires an historical, cultural, political, and social situatedness in order to avoid the romanticisation of the individual, and thus reproduction of a hero narrative which reifies humanist notions of the individual as autonomous and unitary." In working with life-story, I also used these theoretical and practical considerations to inform the research design and process.

Research in Action

Following my choice and rationale for using life-story narrative as methodology and method, I needed to design the study so that it would be congruent with such a project. Feminist researchers, such as Anderson, Armitage, Jack and Wittner (1993) and Bloom (1998), say that women's life-stories are important in theory building. Because there was no indigenous material to use as a theoretical basis on how nurse educators teach for and with social change, I decided to have a series of conversations with six Pakeha/Tauiwi[3] women nurse educators throughout Aotearoa New Zealand, who reputedly taught for social change in undergraduate and postgraduate nursing programmes.

The features of life-story that guided me included focusing on the individual as participant; and, using a participatory, dialogical, and interpretive process of life-story, which would lead to more in-depth understanding of the phenomena under study. By sharing the stories, knowledge unique to the experiences of their lives as nurse educators teaching for change would be preserved and extended. By sharing their stories, the nurse educators would preserve and extend knowledge unique to their lives. The life-story accounts would provide the reader with an opportunity to engage in the story, analysis, and interpretation. By providing explicated texts, "common practices and shared experiences" are recognised and "an increased understanding of the meaning and significance of these explicated experiences" is offered from a critical interpretation (Diekelmann, 2001, p. 58). Life-story as methodology has the potential to contribute to nursing inquiry and knowledge by presenting lived experience as a way to "advance theoretical understanding of the human condition and commonalities in existential human experiences" (Johnstone, 1999, p. 136).

Beginning the Journey with the Research Participants

The first six women nurse educators who I approached volunteered to become participants. They were all involved in teaching for and with social change. One of my key recruitment assumptions was that the participants should be consciously teaching for social change. However, in some ways this is an ambiguous assumption, because so often what nurse educators do is grounded in the everydayness and tacit knowing of being a teacher. Here I was asking these participants to share their awareness of the "what," "why," and "how" of teaching for social change. Three of them indicated they were interested in spending time reflecting on their experience of teaching for and with social change. One said that it gave her an opportunity to take the time to think about her ideas and practices. Another said she was interested in the research process of life-story narrative because she was considering using it for her own postgraduate research. I then negotiated a time to meet with each of them to discuss the purpose, method and design of the project, the possible risks and time involved in being a participant, and my position as an interactive researcher (conversational story-telling rather than interviews). The participants were the story-tellers and I was the listener and recorder of the stories of teaching for and with social change. My role was to negotiate the process before, during, and after each conversation, ask clarifying questions, and, where mutual experiences emerged, to engage in dialogue. I will discuss this process further in the next section on using a story map to enter the field of inquiry, and the process of gathering the stories.

Using a Story Map to Enter and Negotiate the Field of Inquiry

Creating maps, or the act of mapping, is not confined only to the geographical notion of a spatial representation of terrain. Rather than confining mapping to those who use or make maps, such as cartographers, surveyors, geographers, and planners, it can also be regarded as "creative, sometimes anxious moments in coming to knowledge of the world, and the map is both the spatial embodiment of knowledge and a stimulus to further cognitive engagements" (Cosgrove, 1999, p. 2). How then did I

develop a story map to guide the participants and myself across the terrain and through a series of "cognitive engagements" and acts of gathering life-stories?

   While on paper the story map is represented two-dimensionally as an
interview framework, it is multidimensional, multitextured and multilay-
ered (see figure 2). When we read a map on a flat piece of paper we build
up an image in our mind by translating various signs and aspects into a
meaningful pattern in order to make sense of what is before us. This might
include remembering and recalling our knowledge of the location—have
I been there before? is there something familiar with which I can locate
my position? what is present in the foreground and background, such as
contours and patterns? what is the landscape like as a whole? The story
map is also a means of creating a space for our hearts and minds to speak.
The participants were called out to invoke (call forth) a better place, a
better community, a better world, a better universe ("the great invocation"), in much the same way as the archetypal shape-shifter. The relationship as/of the researcher with/to the participants, is significant in relation to the depth of insight that is invoked. The researcher may be able
to connect closely with the participant to invoke deep personal accounts
of his or her life. Cosgrove (1999, pp. 1–2) suggests acts of mapping involve exploring some of the "contexts and contingencies, which have
helped shape acts of visualizing, conceptualizing, recording, representing
and creating spaces."

   The story map (see figure 2), entitled "Creating the Space for Our
Hearts and Minds to Speak," was developed as a process for focusing on a
series of conversations recorded on audiotape and re-presented with each
of the participants over two years (1999–2001). It was praxiological by
nature—that is, an opportunity to reflect on their practice and unfold stories of teaching for change, while using creative forms to speak the story
(e.g., poetry, writing, photography), if the participant found this to be
symbolic of their experience. I had previously named "conversations" as
"interviews" in the application for ethical approval document. However, I
considered that "interviews" did not fit the idea of participants sharing
their life-stories, so I changed them to "conversations" because of the participatory nature of the researcher and participants conversing with one
another (Norrick, 2000). This occurred after I had developed the story
map and each of the participants had received a copy. If the researcher
wishes to invoke participants' stories of teaching for social change, then it

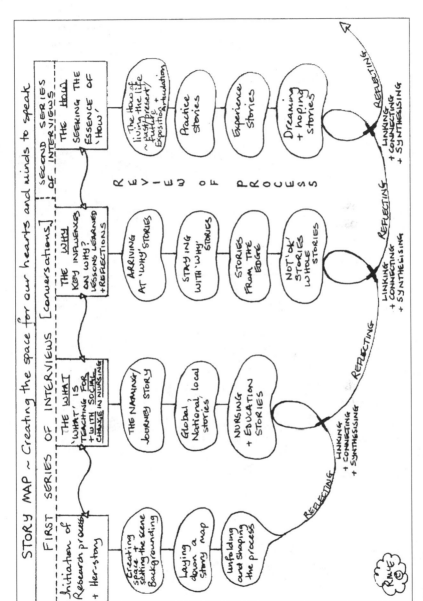

Figure 2. Story map.

seems more appropriate to have a conversation in which the participant has the space to talk about their experience and at each meeting can build on the previous conversation. Conversations seem to create a more conducive environment and equitable relationship between the researcher and the participant. Interviews tend to be more formal.

As we settled into the process of negotiating and exploring the terrain in relation to the research questions outlined on the story map, I recognised that there were times when we would converse about an aspect of teaching for social change that we were familiar with, or that required further exploration. One example was being involved in teaching cultural safety courses to undergraduate nursing students; a second example was nursing women in psychiatric inpatient units and trying to work with them in terms of a medical diagnosis but wanting to responsibly subvert the process by assisting the patients to leave safely as soon as possible.

The research questions were used as a guide for mapping and established the focus of the life-stories. I decided to frame it as a series of conversations. I grouped the conversations into two series with a pause between each series so that I could review the process. Within each series the research questions were identified and a suggested cluster of story ideas was linked to each question. Before embarking on the research questions in the first series, I began the research journey by laying down the story map and setting the scene for what might unfold or be shaped by the process. I also wanted the participants to provide me with some background into their lives—their family, schooling, becoming and being a nurse, becoming and being a nurse educator, and identifying key people or experiences that had influenced their lives. Sharing one's her-story can help establish rapport between the researcher and participant and also gives the participant an opportunity to be the author of her own life. I re-presented these her-stories as vignettes in my thesis as a way of introducing and backgrounding each participant (McEldowney, 2002). Once the her-story was laid down, we were then able to shift to the research questions. The participants returned to aspects of their her-stories at various times during the conversations when they remembered more detail about certain people or experiences. This added to the overall coherence and congruence of the life-stories.

The proposed story ideas outlined on the map were to provide a focus for the participant to reflect on in relation to the key questions and were always open to negotiation and interpretation. For example, in the first series of conversations I selected the "what" and the "why" questions as the focus; "what" is teaching for and with social change in nursing? and "why" teach for and with social change in nursing? In relation to the "what" question, I wanted the participants to consider what they considered teaching for and with social change meant to them. Did they name their socio-political work as teaching for social change, or was it something else? Did they have any specific stories from a global, national, or local context that would invoke and call forth examples of what teaching for social change meant for them, and were there any significant stories that they might share?

In relation to the "why" question, I wanted to explore what the key influences were about "why" they teach for social change, what were some of their reflections and lessons they had learned over time? The proposed story ideas for the "why" question include: arriving at the "why" stories; staying with the "why" stories; stories from the edge; and the "not okay" stories and whole stories. Arriving at the "why" stories and staying with the "why" stories refers to the participant's experience of why they became involved in wanting to teach for social change and what holds or compels them to stay teaching for change.

As teaching for change includes an element of resistance, I also wished to unfold stories from the participants about their experiences of being on the edge, or the "not okay" stories about times when they felt challenged or distressed by students and colleagues. The idea of asking them to talk about whole stories was to create the opportunity for the participants to unfold a more holistic perspective about why they teach for and with social change that reflects their personal, professional, and political position. It was also created as a space or pause at this stage of the research to review the process. During this time I was able to check with the participants once again if they were happy to proceed with the idea of the story map as a guide, or whether there were any other aspects they wished to include in the series of conversations.

The second series of conversations related to the "how" of teaching for social change—that is, seeking the essence of how the participants live their lives as nurse educators teaching for social change and asking them to articulate experiences as teaching and nursing practice stories and "experience as lived" stories. Some of the reflections included in seeking the essence of the "how" focused on the "what" and the "why" of the how. For example, what content and process did they include in their teaching practice that addressed socio-political issues in nursing, and why did they make certain choices or take a particular stand or position on these issues. The last cluster of stories in the second series focused on sharing the dreaming and hoping stories and was a way of arbitrarily bringing a sense of closure to the process. However, it was also a way of leaving the process open to a future of possibilities in which there is no closure, only pauses and rests on their life journey of teaching for change. This may seem paradoxical, but moments or pauses for dreaming and hoping about what has been, what is, and what might be, can create a space for reminiscing, contemplating, and reflecting about a journey. In a sense, the opportunity for sharing the dreaming and hoping stories created an oasis or resting place along the way.

The final aspect included on the story map was the praxiological processes of reflecting, linking, connecting, and synthesising. These are indicated as a reflecting loop at the bottom of each series of conversations with a nexus where the loop intersects (shown in darker tone in an x shape) representing the linking, connecting, and synthesising of the conversations throughout the research journey and beyond. The inclusion of these processes on the map was to ensure that the participants and I engaged in praxis-oriented research that involved reciprocal reflection and critique about the what, why, and how of teaching for and with social change in nursing. Because of the reciprocating nature of the questions, linkages, and connections between and across stories could be made. The idea of synthesising was that, as the researcher, I could reflect on previous conversations with the participants and carry them into the next conversation. This was achieved by listening to each of the participants' audiotapes and making notes on key ideas to emerge that could be followed up in the next conversation or whenever it might need to be recalled. I will give examples of this process in the next section, which focuses on laying down the map, gathering the stories over time, and reflections on the research in action.

Gathering the Stories From the Participants

The gathering of the stories through conversations with the six participants took place between 1999 and 2001. Organizing the date, place, and time for the conversations evolved through negotiation. As I had received ethical approval to gather data for a period of twelve months the majority of conversations took place during this time frame. However, three participants (Grace, Anne, and Eileen) requested and gave their verbal consent for me to have follow-up conversations with them during 2001.

Initially, I did not realize how time-consuming undertaking life-story research would be, but I became connected to the six women during this time as they shared their gift of stories about the hope and sadness, joy and despair of teaching for change. Estes (1993) says that

Stories reveal over and over again the precious and peculiar knack that humans have for triumph over travail. They provide all the instructions we need to live a useful, necessary, and unbounded life—a life of meaning, a life worth remembering. (back cover page)

Each of the participants was given a copy of the story map at the first conversation. We had an opportunity to discuss the layout and process. I was interested to know if they wanted to renegotiate the process of traversing the terrain and journeying through the cognitive engagements and acts of storying. All agreed to use the map, and at the commencement of each session I would check to see if anyone wanted to change anything or add to the process. The map provided a connecting and holding of ideas over time, particularly when a few months elapsed between conversations. Another important aspect to emerge from using the map and a life-story approach was that a pattern of reciprocity, constancy, and consistency in stories developed over time. Although the story map presented an arbitrary boundary around the questions, the participants would often move back and forth between same or similar stories. They would carry repeat stories across the "what," "why," and "how" questions and would sometimes focus on a story that was more related to another question that we would be addressing later in the series of conversations. For example, one of the participants, Anne, began talking about the "how" in relation to the dreaming and hoping stories during our first conversation, which was intended to focus more on initiating the research process, back-grounding and her-story. Anne says

And I think for me that's what keeps me going. The hoping of how you might picture things might be, if you persist away at the edges. (McEldowney, 2002, p. 60)

Several of the participants mentioned during the course of the conversations that the life-story process of inquiry had been significant for them. Annie thought that the conversations between us had given her an opportunity to reflect and find meaning in some of the events that had happened in her day-to-day life and were fundamental to

why I do what I do, how I do it, and why I keep on doing it. It's grown with having these conversations. It's only in conversing with you that this has got shape, so the whole internal process of what I do, why I do it . . . has now been given shape because it's out there, it's been heard and it's being responded to . . . and I find that absolutely amazing. (McEldowney, 2002, p. 62)

One of the key strategies I used to hold the stories over time and to assist the participants in reconnecting with the research process and content was to listen to the audiotapes and read the transcripts between conversations. This enabled me to begin an initial analysis of what the participants had shared in conversation and what I considered to be key ideas to take into their next one. I wrote the key ideas on paper and used them as a prompt at the beginning of each conversation. By carrying ideas across, there was an exponential process of building and developing over time, which gave rise to the depth and quality of the conversations. For example, after I had spoken with Eileen, during the second conversation, about what she thought teaching for social change meant for her, I began to engage with the text and summarized the key points as shown in table 1.

In the third conversation, Eileen found the process helpful and she was able to expand further on the ideas and to tell stories of specific instances that illustrated what she thought teaching for social change was about. But, it was during the process of thinking and reflecting on the participants' stories that an exciting moment occurred—the emergence of shape-shifting as a metaphor for transformation and change.

Shape-shifting as a Metaphor for Transformation and Change

Shape-shifting began to emerge from the participants' life-stories during our conversations and when I read over the transcripts during the initial stages of analysis. I had been thinking for some time about what teaching for change entailed and felt there was something embodied in the lives of the participants that had yet to reveal itself. One day while having some contemplative moments in the back garden at home, I started to say out loud "it's about changing and transforming things through

Extracted text from Eileen (Conversation 2)

- *social change is an extension of my life;*

- *being authentic in the classroom;*

- *my hope is to change minds by offering another pair of glasses;*

- *it's about me hearing what they are telling me;*

- *there has to be a congruency between what you say and what you do;*

- *it's about being vulnerable and authentic;*

- *believing what you do is important at the macro and micro level;*

- *holding the big picture;*

- *everyone has the right to be whoever they are, but the reality is that one person's right impinges on another's;*

- *hoping to privilege the position of the least powerful;*

- *how I use language is important;*

- *I make mistakes, don't get it right,*

- *that I'm a real person;*

- *don't want to be part of society that marginalises others;*

- *two major influences on thinking and practice — Marxist socialist influence and psychology;*

- *if the feelings change — the thinking changes as well . . .*

Table 1.

shifting and shaping . . . but what do I mean by that? . . . I know . . . it's shape-shifting!" Excited by the idea I went to the computer and searched for shape-shifting on the World Wide Web and Amazon.com, and found several texts (Jamal, 1987, 1995; McCafferty, 1997; Perkins, 1997). From this, I reexamined other literature that I thought related to the concept (Estes, 1992; Kingsolver, 1990; Starhawk, 1990). I felt as though the revelation had been called up from my "deeper instinctual knowing." It was sharing the life-stories with the participants that had invoked this response. I had experienced an epiphany, which van Manen (1997) describes as "the sudden perception and intuitive grasp of the meaning of something" (p. 364).

The concept of shape-shifting has been with us for centuries. In ancient times, shape-shifters, transformers, or change agents, were known as shamans (Estes, 1992; Jamal, 1987, 1995; McCafferty, 1997; Perkins, 1997). The shamanic women of old Europe established sacred feminine traditions and practices such as protecting women during and after pregnancy and childbirth (Jamal, 1987, 1995). Shamans were able to transform or metamorphose themselves into other life forms or allies, such as animals, birds, or trees. This process of shape-shifting enabled them to enter the body and mind of an ally, to create harmony between human life and these other life forms, to learn about survival, and to return to their human persona and teach about adaptation and change in their community (Jamal, 1995; Perkins, 1997). Later, with the emergence of Western science, shamanic practices were suppressed. Christian priests persecuted shamans, even burning them at the stake for their sacred and mystical beliefs.

Modern literature abounds with accounts of shape-shifting. Examples are found in folk, fairy, or spirit stories; in poetry and classic prose; and in science fiction (Estes, 1992; Jamal, 1985, 1997; Joyce, 1968; Perkins, 1997; Sams & Carson, 1988; Starhawk, 1987, 1990; Tuwhare, 1997). Today, shape-shifting is practised by many indigenous cultures, and maintained by Wicca (witches), wherever they live, and by Druids in England and Ireland (Jamal, 1997). Shape-shifting is also presented in various ways—on television through advertisements that entice us to transform our image and identity; in films and television programs such as *Star Wars* (destroyer droids and war droids), *Star Trek* (changelings), *Merlin* (King Arthur's fabled wizard), *The Mask, Batman,* and *Spiderman;* morphing video games; children's toys such as transformers; and music.

Several authors who have written about narrative inquiry and life-story methodology have discussed the use of metaphor in interpreting stories (Clandinin & Connelly, 2000; Polkinghorne, 1988; Riessman, 1993; Spivey, 1997; van Manen, 1990; Witherell & Noddings, 1991). Connelly and Clandinin (1988, p. 71) say that teachers' actions and practices are "embodied expressions of their metaphors of teaching and living." Metaphor is also used extensively in advertising to convey brand meaning

(Morgan & Reichert, 1999); by scholars, researchers and rhetoricians (Cameron & Low, 1999; Hawkes, 1972; Lakoff & Johnson, 1980; Mooij, 1976; Reagan & Stewart, 1978; Ricoeur, 1975); and in poetry, language, and communication (Cooper, 1986; Kittay, 1987; Richardson, 1990, 1998; Schon, 1983; Spivey, 1997; Steen, 1994). I identified three international doctoral research projects that used the metaphor of shape-shifting as magical transformation, crossing boundaries, transformation, transgression, and changing (Bathgate, 2001; Pulley, 1995; Swedlow, 1990). To my knowledge, no nurse researchers have explored the idea of shape-shifting in practice, either as educators or clinicians. However, nurses have written about using metaphorical stories as a psychotherapy technique (Billings, 1991), as an expressive tool to reveal stories about nursing and nursing roles (Hartrick & Schreiber, 1998), and as a way of explicating the use of metaphor in teaching abstract nursing concepts (Sutherland, 2001).

The word "metaphor" is derived from the Greek word *metaphora,* meaning "to carry over," and refers to a linguistic process in which "aspects of one object are carried over or transferred to another object, so that the second object is spoken about as if it were the first" (Hawkes, 1972, p. 1). In the fourth century B.C., Aristotle was perhaps the first to discuss metaphor as part of his treatise on the logic, rhetoric, and poetic modes of language.

Hawkes (1972, p. 9) says that the effect of metaphor used properly "is that by combining the familiar with the unfamiliar, it adds charm and distinction, to clarity." The best metaphors are those that bring images clearly and vividly to the eyes of the audience. The clarity comes by using everyday words; the charm from the resonance, playfulness, and pleasure in the choice of metaphor; and distinction arises from the surprising nature of the resemblances. Ricoeur (1975) refers to polysemy as the property of words in natural language having more than one meaning—that is, one name with several senses and resemblances—and metaphor is a creative use of polysemy. Hawkes (1972, p. 9) also adds that "metaphors must be fitting [and] in keeping with the theme or purpose." Eubanks (1999) presents a more contemporary approach to the aptness of metaphor. He considers that we "can develop a richer account of conceptual metaphor as a cultural phenomenon if we consider the patterned relationships between metaphors and other discursive forms—beginning with what [he] calls licensing stories" (p. 419). A licensing story is one that gives license to the appropriate and congruent use of a metaphor.

So why use shape-shifting as a conceptual metaphor that has resemblance to change and transformation? I consider shape-shifting to be the archetypal metaphor, as metaphor is symbolic of changing meaning (metamorphosis) and shape-shifting is symbolic of transformation and change (metamorphosis). It is a "pre-existent culturally [and conceptually] apt metaphor" (Eubanks, 1999, p. 421)—and perhaps one of the oldest and most deeply embedded ways of knowing. A conceptual metaphor is influenced by politics, philosophy, social attitudes, and individual constructions of the world. It can also be described in two ways—first, as a way of inventing discourse, and second, as underpinning culture (Eubanks, 1999; Lakoff & Johnson, 1980). Using the metaphor of shape-shifting provided me with a way to make meaning out of something that was not familiar. It enabled me to think about transformation and change in a different way and, as Aristotle says, "to get hold of something fresh." To understand the notion of shape-shifting, I had to link it to something that I could already identify with. As Hartrick and Schreiber (1998, p. 421) say, "by identifying the common essence between unknown and known phenomena, the understanding or knowledge of the unknown is extended." Transformative experiences in nursing can inform how and why we teach for and with social change. I describe these transformative moments as shape-shifting.

However, the view of shape-shifting as a shamanic or fictionalized process of metamorphosis was not necessarily apt as a conceptual metaphor for my thesis. Nisbet (1969, p. 4) acknowledges Wallace Stevens's position on the meaning and formation of words and the relationship "between metaphor and metamorphosis" that, "in the world of knowledge and meaning, [is] more than merely etymological." This position on metaphor is helpful in framing the way shape-shifting emerged as a phenomenon in teaching for social change. The participants, myself as researcher, and the process of using life-story narrative as a way of unfolding and revealing stories were not metamorphosing in the shamanic sense. Therefore, I re-mapped the conceptual metaphor of shape-shifting to be symbolic of transformation and social action in order to fit with my ideological commitment to the research—which was to illuminate the counter-hegemonic voices of the six nurse educators teaching for social change.

Shape-shifting is about moving, changing, transgressing, adapting, bringing about change through invocation and evocation, and changing

oneself in the process. Using life-story narrative and telling stories became a shape-shifting process for the participants and myself. For example, some participants found the process to be illuminating, a reflective
experience, and time for thinking about their practice. In one case it
made a difference to how a participant (Eileen) went back into the classroom to teach cultural safety. I include some of Eileen's comments from
our sixth conversation.

These conversations have fed into my own personal process rather than affecting
my practice directly. I think it's because they have been trying to get at values and
I've been reflecting quite deeply on those. A couple of weeks ago I was feeling
quite negative about some of the decisions that I've made and whether things
have been worthwhile and what of value have I achieved . . . and then thinking
that teaching for change has been one of the things of value that I can reflect on.
I certainly enjoy teaching cultural safety very much this semester . . . and I'm
sure this research process has contributed to that. It's given me a place to stand
back and reflect more deeply on it [cultural safety], and in believing it to be of
value. (McEldowney, 2002, p. 68)

Shape-shifting through the act of story-telling intertwines past experience with the present and gives a future of possibilities. "There is a
shape-shifting interchange between the storyteller and the audience,
even as the stories themselves are about shape-shifting" (Jamal, 1995,
p. xiv). We are forever changing, moving, and reshaping what it is we do
in our teaching and learning for social change.

Creating the story map enabled me to focus on a coherent and congruent structure and process for gathering the life-stories. It enabled the
participants and me to work within a multidimensional and dynamic
space and to hold and carry stories over between conversations. I also
kept a series of notebooks to record reflections on key ideas and questions that arose along the way and also created a file on the computer on
which I posted notes to myself as I was writing the research report.

One of the surprise findings while working with the data was how aptness emerged as another component of reflexivity. As a process of having
to work with shape-shifting as metaphor, the criterion of aptness needed
to be worked through reflexively, particularly in relation to interpretation
of the text. One of the things I wished to avoid was not forcing the metaphor of shape-shifting to fit my preconceived notions of teaching for
change, but rather let it emerge in an appropriate and apt way. However, I
did not deliberately set out to use metaphor when I entered the study, nor

did I have conscious knowledge about shape-shifting at that stage. Rather, it revealed itself through the life-stories of the participants. Therefore, I have illustrated shape-shifting to be an apt metaphor by describing the reflexive process I went through to consider its appropriateness.

I will now address the significance of the research process in revealing how using life-story narrative as methodology and method unfolded shape-shifting as teaching for social change.

Revealing Shape-shifting Through Life-story

Using the metaphor of shape-shifting brings new insight to the idea of teaching for social change in nursing. Before my research I had little awareness of shape-shifting. As I shared conversations with the participants, I began to recognise its emergence and significance. The relationship between life-story and shape-shifting is also significant. As the participants revealed themselves through their life-stories, they showed how they shape-shifted over time, how they chose to change and be changed, and how the act of telling stories about one's life brought about change through reflection on action. Their stories illuminated how they have thought about what they do, why they do it, and how they do it. I was struck by the congruence of this within their lives and practice, and was reminded of the way Starhawk describes the process of learning to become and be a shape-shifter. She says: "The way we define reality shapes our reality. It is only when we know how we have been shaped by the structure of power in which we live, can we become the shapers" (1987, p. 8). Each of the participants was clear about how they had been shaped and shifted by the structure of power, and how they could become shapers and shifters for social justice.

Shape-shifting can occur at different levels, such as cellular (losing weight), personal (changing self, becoming a different self, becoming an "other"), and institutional (creating different circumstances for teaching and nursing). It is the personal, or micro level of shape-shifting that this chapter addresses. By association, the participants have influenced educational and health institutions, so the macro level is also addressed. In a reciprocal way, they, too, have been influenced by institutions, such as school, church, hospitals, and educational institutes. The stories that the participants shared during the two years of data-gathering are life-changing shape-shifting stories—stories about events and relationships when they were children and adults. These events helped shape them as nurses and nurse educators. There is also a shape-shifting interchange between the storyteller and the audience, the audience and the storyteller—even as the stories themselves are about shape-shifting.

Life-story narrative as methodology is congruent with shape-shifting, because telling life-stories about making a difference or bringing about change is, of itself, "shape-shifting." Also, life-story narrative is suited to gaining insights into the "confusions, contradictions, and complexities" of everyday life and locating the significant turning points that are part of the influence for change (Russell & Korthagen, 1995, p. 141). Life-stories reveal shape-shifting processes over time. How this occurs is both contradictory and paradoxical, because the research process and content side of life-story are paradoxically positioned in relation to temporality. Life-story narratives reveal the participant's life as shape-shifter across a lifetime. Yet only fragments of a life are presented—in negotiated moments, as part of the research process. Further, the fragments depend on what the participants remember and the meaning they recount during those moments. Every experience, event, and relationship is not shared—only the memories and reflections that the participant wishes to reveal at the time. What their stories revealed, though, were consistent, integrated, and stable accounts of themselves within and across texts. Their self-identities and who they are as shape-shifters emerged from multiple texts across short periods of time. The stories revealed integrity between self-belief, social action, and commitment. This gave rise to an internalized congruence and coherence in their personal and professional lives that revealed elements of shape-shifting. Although there is an inconsistency between what is life-story and what occurs during the actual process of story-telling, one of the things that has been revealed is a consistency and stability of politicized commitment in their stories within and across texts. It is a series of stories that contribute to a life-story. There may be no connection or consistency in the storytelling. However, in this research I found the six participants to be consistent in what they told me, and often a story would be repeated over a number of conversations. By including a praxiological approach of reflecting, linking, connecting, and synthesising (see figure 2) the participants and I were able to hold stories across time.

Each of the participants has been through pivotal shape-shifting experiences that have transformed their lives. These experiences are exemplified in their her-stories and emerged powerfully in the story themes—the naming stories, the authentic self, crossing the boundary, creating safe space to be unsafe, and shape-shifting (McEldowney, 2002). The stories are, however, central to revealing the authentic integrated self of the participants that is expressed as: *who I am is what I do—what I do is who I am—I cannot not do this work—*and *I cannot do it apart from others.* Who they are as nurse educators and what they do is inexorably linked to who they are as people.

The political work of teaching for and with social change in nursing is an important part of their being. All participants expressed this at some time during our conversations. They have made a conscious life decision to work with change, although they do not consciously think about it in their day-to-day practice. It has become an embodiment of "who" and "why" they are, rather than a conscious act. Anne summed this up in her conversation about the "what" of teaching for social change:

I'm not consciously aware of working for social change, and because you live the life you don't always think about teaching and practice experiences as being stories for social change . . . that is the way you are . . . you are what you are, really. (McEldowney, 2002, p. 149)

Using the metaphor of shape-shifting through storytelling we intertwine the experiences of the nurse educators through life-stories of nursing practices that inform present-day reality. The old and new are melded and are brought to the present. It is by entering the experiences of the life-stories that the reader can begin to think about ways of knowing, being, and doing as exemplified by the participants—that is, it becomes a shape-shifting experience. By reading the journey of the nurse educator as shape-shifter through their life-stories, feelings of interconnection can be evoked. Through storytelling as shape-shifting we can learn about personal and professional change, how to transform and how to become shape-shifters teaching for social change.

Implications and limitations of life-story narrative inquiry for research and scholarship In this section, I present some of the key implications and limitations of using life story narrative for research and scholarship. How might we come to know and understand about teaching for social change differently because of this approach?

One of the exciting aspects of undertaking this study was that the stories of teaching for social change had not been talked about in public before. It also revealed how our research informs our teaching and how our teaching informs our research. Using life-story narrative inquiry surfaced and revealed how shape-shifting is borne through the life-stories of nurse educators' lived experiences and practice wisdom. The important aspect of life-story in this context is that it is connected to teaching, not so much to social activism. It is more about living the life and authenticity of self and the commitment and investment to teach for social change in nursing.

I am mindful that my interpretation of the participants' stories was influenced by my own life-story and personal encounters as a nurse educator who teaches for social change. I am also mindful that while a critical feminist perspective on schooling, teaching, and learning provided an initial theoretical framework for why nurse educators might teach for social change, the life stories and personal her-stories were more revealing about teaching for social change. Therefore, my theorizing about shape-shifting as teaching for social change has a connection between what is known and discussed in the literature, stories the participants shared with me over time, and what my thoughts, feelings, intuitions, and reflective awareness are about teaching for change. The participants also brought their knowledge, feelings, intuitions, and reflections into their life-stories as they theorized about the what, why, and how of teaching for social change. By not de-contextualising the participants' lives I avoided the heroine narrative—that is, holding the six participants as models of how one should be and teach for social change. That is why I included their personal her-stories, so that the reader could get a sense of who they are and why and how they have been shaped and shifted and become shape-shifters teaching for change. This is the way their lives have been and are lived. Nurse educators teaching for change move beyond a utopian view of the world and try to make changes within the reality of their everyday lives. They can also make mistakes and act in ways that are not okay. They can lose the way and close down others. They can get frustrated, angry, and need time out. But as shape-shifters nurse educators can recognise this as part of their authentic integrated selves and reflect on ways to be less into power—over students and as knowers of their work.

A significant challenge for researchers using life-story narrative as a methodology is the constant need to hold the participants' voices

as paramount. An aspect of my research that I reflected on was how
the participants' voices would be re-presented. Whose voice would be
privileged—mine or theirs? And who chose what stories were presented?
How can I say that it is their voices when there is an overlay of my voice?
I contend that "giving voice" is a misnomer unless we explain as researchers what it means in each of our projects. How can I give voice to someone else's stories—I can only interpret them from my own subjective position arising from experiences that may or may not be similar to their
experiences. Everyone's stories are unique, and the way they experience
and interpret them for others is also unique. However, I believe that the
participants and I shared voices and spoke together in conversation (co-
vocation), which I consider is a strength of the study.

Another challenge in using life-story narrative is the issue of temporality or locating things in time. It posed some questions for consideration
in my project. The participants talked in the present about current stories
or stories that were remembered, reviewed, and retold. Why did they select certain aspects of their lives to talk about? Is there such a thing as a
whole story and is what is being told an accurate account? I do not believe
there can be, because participants will only share what they want to and
what they remember and recall. Life stories are subjective, partial and incomplete. There was no objective or single truth that emerged from the
text, nor was there one correct reading or interpretation of the stories or
texts that arose from the study. What emerged were the ideas and stories
from a group of participants and the researcher as interpreter. They are
not generalizable to other nurse educators who teach for change. The binary of subject/object, knower/known, and method/process is disrupted
and laid open for critique and possibility. This raises an implication for
the application of findings from life-story narrative inquiry. What is required is further interpretive research (multi-site, multi-method) to investigate the micro level of teaching for social change in nursing because
it is important to situate the personal and intuitive knowing embedded
and arising from everyday practices as "legitimate" knowledge that contributes to a developing science for nursing education (Diekelmann &
Ironside, 2002). Research could also be extended beyond nurse educators who consciously teach for social change to those teaching professional practice and ethical issues in nursing. Would their values, beliefs,
motivations and commitments be similar or different? I suggest that the
discourses of possibility be opened up to other nurse educators to see if

and how they position themselves as teachers for change. However, one of the challenges in undertaking time-consuming research such as life-story narrative inquiry is that it does not tend to attract mainstream research funding. In these times of funding being linked to research outputs, is it feasible to undertake this type of research within a shorter time frame? The in-depth data collection process may preclude this from being considered.

And finally, how do we as nurse educators support and sustain shape-shifters as they engage in political counter-hegemonic work? How do we open up the silences that surround women's work in teaching for change? Weiler (1988) discusses the importance of providing mutual support and understanding for those educators who are engaged in political teaching activities. The participants in my study shared stories of how they are committed to working with difference every day as shape-shifters. To counter the silence we need to share our stories publicly about what it is we do as shape-shifters that makes a difference in order "to guide and extend continued reform and innovation across all levels of nursing education" (Diekelmann & Ironside, 2002, p. 380).

Conclusion

I commenced my doctoral research wanting to find out how and why nurse educators teach for and with social change in nursing. I also wanted to find out how their life-stories reflect their philosophies, goals, intentions, and practices as they seek to teach for change. I was fortunate to recruit six highly articulate, passionate, and committed nurse educators who were prepared to share their life-stories with me.

I am of the view that choosing a life-story approach for this inquiry was an appropriate way of seeking answers to my questions and thinking about my preconceived notions about teaching for social change. Life-story revealed and evoked the fascinating connections between personal life as lived and the participants' stances of activism in their everyday practices within their pivotal roles as nurse educators. The metaphoric emergence of the construct of shape-shifting revealed central aspects of the "what," "why," and "how" of teaching for social change, and showed the complex and inextricable links to the authentic integrated self of the participants as shape-shifters.

Shape-shifting experiences in the participant's lives have been pivotal and transforming in bringing about a desire and motivation to engage in a life-long commitment to "walk the talk" for social change. In their capacity as shape-shifters, the call to work within a pedagogy of discomfort positions them as agents of social and political action in educating for justice. This capacity is carried within their authentic integrated selves and is expressed as "who I am is what I do" and "what I do is who I am."

As an active process, shape-shifting presents new and different ways of thinking about the micro-level of teaching and learning for social change. Like the wise women shape-shifters who have preceded them over the centuries, Anne, Eileen, Grace, Annie, Mary, and Miriam have opened up pathways that others may choose to follow. Through naming what it is that they do, the agency of the participants is revealed in how and why they have shaped and shifted in their personal, political, and professional lives. By sharing these life-stories as shape-shifters, possibilities abound for how other nurse educators might build community and develop others as shape-shifters, further the socio-political critique of nursing and health care, and transform and challenge the status quo in counter-hegemonic ways.

Notes

1. Aotearoa is the Maori name for New Zealand and translated refers to "land of the long white cloud."
2. Cultural safety courses focus on addressing issues of personal and institutional power, and acknowledging and respecting difference in patients and clients to ensure that our practice does not demean, diminish, or disempower them (Ramsden, 1992).
3. Pakeha/Tauiwi refers to the identity of the participants—five are Pakeha and one is Tauiwi. Pakeha is the Maori (indigenous) word for European people born in New Zealand. Tauiwi refers to those who come from another place, i.e., born outside New Zealand and who have emigrated here.

References

Anderson, K., Armitage, S., Jack, D., & Wittner, J. (1993). Beginning where we are: Feminist methodology in oral history. In J. Nielson (Ed.), *Feminist research methods* (pp. 94–112). Boulder, CO: Westview Press.
Apple, M. (1993). *Official knowledge: Democratic education in a conservative age.* New York: Routledge.
Atkinson, R. (1998). *The life story interview.* Sage University Papers Series on Qualitative Research Methods Series, Vol. 44. Thousand Oaks, CA: Sage.

Bailey, P., & Tilley, S. (2002). Storytelling and the interpretation of meaning in qualitative research. *Journal of Advanced Nursing 38*(6), 574–583.

Baker, B., & Diekelmann, N. (1994). Connecting conversations of caring: Recalling the narrative to clinical practice. *Nursing Outlook 42*, 65–70.

Banks-Wallace, J. (1998). Emancipatory potential of storytelling in a group. *Image: Journal of Nursing Scholarship 30*, 17–21.

Bathgate, M. (2001). The shape-shifter fox: The imagery of transformation and the transformation of imagery in Japanese religion and folklore (Doctoral dissertation, University of Chicago, 2001). *Dissertation Abstracts International, 62*, 02A.

Billings, C. (1991). Therapeutic use of metaphors. *Issues in Mental Health Nursing 12*, 1–8.

Bloom, L. (1998). *Under the sign of hope: Feminist methodology and narrative interpretation.* Albany: State University of New York Press.

Blumenfeld-Jones, D. (1995). Fidelity as a criterion for practicing and evaluating narrative inquiry. In A. Hatch & R. Wisniewski (Eds.), *Life history and narrative* (pp. 25–35). London: Falmer.

Bruner, J. (1986). *Actual minds, possible words.* Cambridge, MA: Harvard University Press.

Bunkle, P. (1992). Becoming knowers: Feminism, science and medicine. In R. du Plessis, P. Bunkle, K. Irwin, A. Laurie, & S. Middleton (Eds.), *Feminist voices: Women's studies texts for Aotearoa/New Zealand* (pp. 59–73). Auckland, NZ: Oxford University Press.

Buresh, B., & Gordon, S. (2000). *From silence to voice.* Ottawa: Canadian Nurses Association.

Burkhardt, M., & Nagai-Jacobsen, M. (1994). Reawakening spirit in clinical practice. *Journal of Holistic Nursing 12*(1), 9–21.

Butt, R., Raymond, D., McCue, G., & Yamagishi, L. (1992). Collaborative autobiography and the teacher's voice. In I. Goodson (Ed.), *Studying teachers' lives* (pp. 51–98). New York: Teachers College Press.

Cameron, L., & Low, G. (Eds.). (1999). *Researching and applying metaphor.* Cambridge: Cambridge University Press.

Casey, K. (1993). *I answer with my life.* New York: Routledge.

Church, K. (1995). *Forbidden narratives: Critical autobiography as social science.* Luxembourg: Gordon & Breach.

Clandinin, J., & Connelly, M. (1998). Personal experience methods. In N. Denzin & Y. Lincoln (Eds.), *Collecting and interpreting qualitative materials* (pp. 150–178). Thousand Oaks, CA: Sage.

Clandinin, J., & Connelly, M. (2000). *Narrative inquiry: Experience and story in qualitative research.* San Francisco: Jossey-Bass.

Clarke, A. (2000). Using biography to enhance the nursing care of older people. *British Journal of Nursing 9*, 429–433.

Coles, A., & Knowles, G. (1995). Methods and issues in a life history approach to self-study. In T. Russell & F. Korthagen (Eds.), *Teachers who teach teachers: Reflections on teacher education* (pp. 130–151). London: Falmer.

Coles, R. (1989). *The call of stories: Teaching and the moral imagination.* Boston: Houghton Mifflin.

Connelly, E., & Clandinin, J. (1988). *Teachers as curriculum planners: Narratives of experience.* New York: Teachers College Press.

Cooper, D. (1986). *Metaphor.* Oxford: Basil Blackwell.

Cortazzi, M. (1993). *Narrative analysis.* London: Falmer.

Cosgrove, D. (Ed.). (1999). *Mappings.* London: Reaktion Books.

Crisp, J. (1995). Making sense of the stories that people with Alzheimer's tell: A journey with my mother. *Nursing Inquiry 2*, 133–140.

Denzin, N. (1989). *Interpretive biography*. Newbury Park, CA: Sage.

Diekelmann, N. (1993). Behavioural pedagogy: A Heideggerian hermeneutical analysis of the lived experiences of students and teachers in baccalaureate nursing education. *Journal of Nursing Education 32*, 245–250.

Diekelmann, N. (1995). Reawakening thinking: Is traditional pedagogy nearing completion? *Journal of Nursing Education 34*, 195–196.

Diekelmann, N. (2001). Narrative pedagogy: Hiedeggerian hermeneutical analyses of the lived experiences of students, teachers and clinicians. *Advances in Nursing Science 23*(3), 53–71.

Diekelmann, N., & Ironside, P. (2002). Developing a science of nursing education: Innovation with research. *Journal of Nursing Education 41*, 379–380.

Ellis, C., & Flaherty, M. (Eds.). (1992). *Investigating subjectivity: Research on lived experience*. Newbury Park, CA: Sage.

Ellsworth, E. (1997). *Teaching positions: Difference, pedagogy, and the power of address*. New York: Teachers College Press.

Emden, C. (1998a). Theoretical perspectives on narrative inquiry. *Collegian 5*(2), 30–35.

Emden, C. (1998b). Conducting a narrative analysis. *Collegian 5*(3), 34–39.

Estes, C. (1992). *Women who run with the wolves*. London: Rider.

Estes, C. (1993). *The gift of story*. London: Rider.

Eubanks, P. (1999). The story of conceptual metaphor: What motivates metaphoric mappings? *Poetics Today 20*, 419–442.

Forbes, S., Bern-Klug, M., & Gessert, C. (2000). End-of-life decision making for nursing home residents with dementia. *Journal of Nursing Scholarship 32*, 251–258.

Foucault, M. (1977). The political function of the intellectual. *Radical philosophy 17*, 12–14.

Freire, P. (1972). *Pedagogy of the oppressed*. Harmondsworth, UK: Penguin.

Frid, I., Ohlen, J., & Bergbom, I. (2000). On the use of narratives in nursing research. *Journal of Advanced Nursing 32*, 695–703.

Gadamer, H-G. (1976). *Philosophical hermeneutics*. London, CA: University of California Press.

Geertz, C. (1983). Blurred genres: The refiguration of social thought. In C. Geertz, *Local knowledge: Further essays in interpretive anthropology* (pp. 19–35). New York: Basic Books.

Geiger, S. (1990). What's so feminist about women's oral history? *Journal of Women's History 2*(1), 169–182.

Giddings, L. (1997). *In/visibility in nursing: Stories from the margins*. Unpublished Doctor of Philosophy thesis in Nursing, University of Colorado.

Giroux, H. (1983). *Theory and resistance in education: A pedagogy for the opposition*. South Hadley, MA: Bergin & Garvey.

Glass, N. (1998). Becoming de-silenced and reclaiming voice: Women nurses speak out. In H. Keleher & F. McInerney (Eds.), *Nursing matters* (pp. 15–23). Melbourne: Churchill Livingstone.

Goodson, I. (1995). The story so far: Personal knowledge and the political. In A. Hatch & R. Wisniewski (Eds.), *Life history and narrative* (pp. 89–98). London: Falmer.

Gramsci, A. (1971). *Selections from the prison notebooks*. New York: International Publishers.

Hansebo, G., & Kihlgren, M. (2000). Patient life stories and current situation as told by carers in nursing home wards. *Clinical Nursing Research 9,* 260–279.

Harden, J. (2000). Language, discourse and the chronotype: Applying literary theory to the narratives in health care. *Journal of Advanced Nursing 31,* 506–512.

Harding, S. (1986). *The science question in feminism.* Ithaca, NY: Cornell University Press.

Hartrick, G., & Schreiber, R. (1998). Imaging ourselves: Nurses' metaphors of practice. *Journal of Holistic Nursing 16,* 420–434.

Hatch, A., & Wisniewski, R. (Eds.). (1995). *Life history and narrative.* London: Falmer.

Hawkes, T. (1972). *Metaphor.* London: Methuen.

Heidegger, M. (1999). *Contributions to philosophy (From enowning).* (P. Emad & K. Maly, Trans.). Bloomington: Indiana University Press.

Heinrich, K. (1992). Create a tradition: Teach nurses to share stories. *Journal of Nursing Education 31,* 141–143.

Heliker, D. (1999). Transformation of story to practice: An innovative approach to long term care. *Issues in Mental Health Nursing 20,* 513–525.

Ironside, P. (2001). Creating a research base for nursing education: An interpretive review of conventional, critical, feminist, postmodern and phenomenological practices. *Advances in Nursing Science 23*(3), 72–87.

Jamal, M. (1987). *Shape shifters: Shaman women in contemporary society.* London: Penguin Arkana.

Jamal, M. (1995). *Deerdancer: The shape-shifter archetype in story and in trance.* New York: Penguin Arkana.

Jipson, J., Munro, P., Victor, S., Jones, K., & Freed-Rowland, G. (1995). *Repositioning feminism and education: Perspectives on educating for social change.* Westport, CT: Bergin & Garvey.

Johnstone, M-J. (1999). Reflective topical autobiography: An under utilised interpretive research method in nursing, *Collegian 6*(1), 24–29.

Josselson, R. (Ed.). (1996). *Ethics and process in the narrative study of lives.* (Vol. 4). Thousand Oaks, CA: Sage.

Josselson, R., & Lieblich, A. (Eds.). (1993). *The narrative study of lives.* (Vol. 1). Newbury Park, CA: Sage.

Josselson, R., & Lieblich, A. (Eds.). (1995). Interpreting experience. *The narrative study of lives.* (Vol. 3). Thousand Oaks, CA: Sage.

Josselson, R., & Lieblich, A. (Eds.). (1999). Making meaning of narratives. *The narrative study of lives.* (Vol. 6). Thousand Oaks, CA: Sage.

Joyce, J. (1968). *Ulysses.* Harmondsworth: Penguin.

Kenway, J. (2001). Remembering and regenerating Gramsci. In K. Weiler (Ed.), *Feminist engagements: Reading, resisting, and revisioning male theorists in education and cultural studies* (pp. 47–66). New York: Routledge.

Kingsolver, B. (1990). *Animal dreams.* London: Abacus.

Kittay, E. (1987). *Metaphor—its cognitive force and linguistic structure.* Oxford: Clarendon Press.

Koch, T. (1998). Story telling: Is it really research? *Journal of Advanced Nursing 28*(6), 1182–1190.

Lakoff, G., & Johnson, M. (1980). *Metaphors we live by.* Chicago: University of Chicago Press.

Lather, P. (1991). *Getting smart: Feminist research and pedagogy with/in the postmodern.* New York: Routledge.

LeCompte, M. (1993). A framework for hearing silence: What does telling stories mean when we are supposed to be doing science? In D. McLaughlan & W. Tierney (Eds.), *Naming silenced lives: Personal narratives and processes of educational change* (pp. 9–28). New York: Routledge.

Lieblich, A., & Josselson, R. (Eds.). (1994). Exploring identity and gender. *The narrative study of lives.* (Vol. 2). Thousand Oaks, CA: Sage.

Lieblich, A., & Josselson, R. (Eds.). (1997). *The narrative study of lives.* (Vol. 5). Thousand Oaks, CA: Sage.

Lieblich, A., Tuval-Mashiach, R., & Zilber, T. (1998). *Narrative research: Reading, analysis and interpretation.* (Vol. 47). Thousand Oaks, CA: Sage.

Lillemoen, L. (1999). The moral practice in nursing. *Vard-I-Norden-Nursing-Science-and-Research-in-the-Nordic-Countries 19(3)*, 11–17.

Linde, C. (1993). *Life stories: The creation of coherence.* New York: Oxford University Press.

Marshall, C., & Rossman, G. (1999). *Designing qualitative research* (3rd Ed.). Thousand Oaks, CA: Sage.

Maynard, M., & Purvis, J. (Eds). (1994). *Researching women's lives from a feminist perspective.* London: Taylor & Francis.

McCafferty, K. (1997). Generative adversity: Shapeshifting Pauline/Leopolda in *Tracks* and *Love medicine. American Indian Quarterly 21*, 729–751.

McDrury, J., & Alterio, M. (2002). *Learning through storytelling.* Palmerston North, NZ: The Dunmore Press.

McEldowney, R. (1995). *Critical resistance in nursing education: A nurse educator's story.* Unpublished Master of Education thesis, University of Waikato, Hamilton, New Zealand.

McEldowney, R. (2002). *Shape-shifting: Stories of teaching for social change in nursing.* Unpublished Doctor of Philosophy in Nursing thesis, Victoria University of Wellington, New Zealand.

McEldowney, R. (2003). Critical resistance pathways: Overcoming resistance in nursing education. In N. Diekelmann (Ed.), *Teaching practitioners of care: New pedagogies for the health professions* (pp. 194–231). Madison: University of Wisconsin Press.

McLaren, P. (1993). Border disputes: Multicultural narrative, identity formation and critical pedagogy in postmodern America. In D. McLaughlan & W. Tierney (Eds.), *Naming silenced lives: Personal narratives and processes of educational change* (pp. 201–235). New York: Routledge.

Middleton, S. (1993). *Educating feminists: Life histories and pedagogy.* New York: Teachers College Press.

Mooij, J. (1976). *A study of metaphor.* Amsterdam: North-Holland Publishing.

Morgan, S., & Reichert, T. (1999). The message is in the metaphor: Assessing the comprehension of metaphors in advertisements. *Journal of Advertising 28(4)*, 1–12.

Moustakas, C. (1990). *Heuristic research: Design, methods and application.* Newbury Park, CA: Sage.

Munro, P. (1993). Continuing dilemmas of life history research: A reflexive account of feminist qualitative inquiry. In D. Flinders & G. Mills (Eds.), *Theory and concepts in qualitative research: Perspectives from the field* (pp. 163–177). New York: Teachers College Press.

Munro, P. (1998). *Subject to fiction: Women teachers' life history narratives and the cultural politics of resistance.* Buckingham: Open University Press.

Murphy, B. (1999). *Transforming ourselves, transforming the world: An open conspiracy for social change.* London: Zed Books.

Ng, R. (1995). Teaching against the grain: Contradictions and possibilities. In R. Ng, P. Staton, & J. Scane (Eds.), *Antiracism, feminism, and critical approaches to education* (pp. 129–152). Westport, CO: Bergin & Garvey.

Ng, R., Staton, P., & Scane, J. (Eds.). (1995). *Antiracism, feminism, and critical approaches to education.* Westport, CO: Bergin & Garvey.

Nisbet, R. (1969). *Social change and history: Aspects of the Western theory of development.* New York: Oxford University Press.

Norrick, N. (2000). *Conversational narrative: Storytelling in everyday life.* Amsterdam: John Benjamin Publishing Co.

Penn, B. (1994). Using patient biography to promote holistic care. *Nursing Times* 90(45), 35–36.

Perkins, J. (1997). *Shape shifting.* Rochester, VT: Destiny Books.

Polkinghorne, D. (1983). *Methodology for the human sciences: Systems of inquiry.* Albany: State University of New York Press.

Polkinghorne, D. (1988). *Narrative knowing and the human sciences.* Albany: State University of New York Press.

Polkinghorne, D. (1995). Narrative configuration in qualitative analysis. In A. Hatch & R. Wisniewski (Eds.), *Life history and narrative* (pp. 5–23). London: Falmer.

Pulley, M. (1995). Beyond the corporate box: Exploring career resilience (job loss). (Doctoral dissertation, Peabody College for Teachers of Vanderbilt University, 1995). *Dissertation Abstracts International 57*, 02B.

Rabinow, P., & Sullivan, W. (1987). *Interpretive social science: A second look.* Berkeley: University of California Press.

Ramsden, I. (1992). *Kawa whakaruruhau: Guidelines for nursing and midwifery education.* Wellington: Nursing Council of New Zealand.

Reagan, C., & Stewart, D. (Eds.). (1978). *The philosophy of Paul Ricouer.* Boston: Beacon Press.

Ribbens, J. (1993). Facts or fictions? Aspects of the use of autobiographical writing in undergraduate sociology. *Sociology 27*(1), 81–92.

Richardson, L. (1990). *Writing strategies: Reaching diverse audiences.* (Vol.21). Newbury Park, CA: Sage.

Richardson, L. (1998). Writing: A method of inquiry. In N. Denzin and Y. Lincoln (Eds.), *Collecting and interpreting qualitative materials* (pp. 345–371). Thousand Oaks, CA: Sage.

Ricoeur, P. (1975). *The rule of metaphor.* (R. Czerny, Trans.). Toronto: University of Toronto Press.

Ricoeur, P. (1981). *Hermeneutics and the human sciences.* Cambridge: Cambridge University Press.

Ricoeur, P. (1991). *From text to action: Essays in hermeneutics, II.* Evanston, IL: Northwestern University Press.

Riessman, C. (1993). *Narrative analysis.* Sage University papers Series on Qualitative Research Methods Series, Vol. 30. Thousand Oaks, CA: Sage.

Roberts, B. (2002). *Biographical research.* Buckingham: Open University Press.

Russell, T., & Korthagen, F. (Eds.). (1995). *Teachers who teach teachers: Reflections on teacher education.* London: Falmer.

Sams, J., & Carson, D. (1988). *Medicine cards: The discovery of power through the ways of animals.* Sante Fe, NM: Bear & Co.

Sandelowski, M. (1991). Telling stories: Narrative approaches in qualitative research. *Image: Journal of Nursing Scholarship 23*, 161–166.

Sandelowski, M. (1995). *Focus on qualitative methods*. Chapel Hill, NC: John Wiley & Sons.

Schon, D. (1983). *The reflective practitioner*. New York: Basic Books.

Spivey, N. (1997). *The constructivist metaphor*. San Diego, CA: Academic Press.

Starhawk. (1987). *Truth or dare: Encounters with power, authority, and mystery*. New York: HarperCollins.

Starhawk. (1990). *Dreaming the dark: Magic, sex and politics*. London: Unwin Hyman.

Steen, G. (1994). *Understanding metaphor in literature*. New York: Longman.

Strauss, A., & Corbin, J. (Eds.). (1997). *Grounded theory in practice*. Thousand Oaks, CA: Sage.

Sutherland, J. (2001). Teaching abstract concepts by metaphor. *Journal of Nursing Education 40*, 417–410.

Swedlow, J. (1990). "Art to enchant": Shakespeare's magic (Doctoral dissertation, Brown University, 1990). *Dissertation Abstracts International 51*, 08A.

Sztompka, P. (1993). *The sociology of social change*. Oxford: Blackwell.

Tuwhare, H. (1997). *Shape-shifter*. Wellington: Steele Roberts Ltd.

Van Manen, M. (1990). *Researching lived experience*. Albany: State University of New York Press.

Van Manen, M. (1997). From meaning to method. *Qualitative Health Research 7*(3), 345–369.

Vezeau, T. (1994). Narrative inquiry in nursing. In P. Chinn & J. Watson (Eds.), *Art and aesthetics in nursing* (pp. 41–46). New York: National League of Nursing.

Warman, A. (2001). Living the revolution: Cuban health workers. *Journal of Clinical Nursing 10*, 311–319.

Watson, L., & Watson-Franke, M-B. (1985). *Interpreting life histories*. New Jersey: Rutgers University Press.

Weiler, K. (1988). *Women teaching for change*. New York: Bergin & Garvey.

Weiler, K., & Middleton, S. (Eds.). (1999). *Telling women's lives: Narrative inquiries in the history of women's education*. Buckingham: Open University Press.

White, H. (1973). *Metahistory*. Baltimore, MA: John Hopkins University Press.

White, M., & Epston, D. (1990). *Narrative means to therapeutic ends*. New York: Norton.

Witherell, C., & Noddings, N. (Eds.). (1991). *Stories lives tell: Narrative and dialogue in education*. New York: Teachers College Press.

Zeichner, K. (1995). Reflections of a teacher educator working for social change. In T. Russell & F. Korthagen (Eds.), *Teachers who teach teachers: Reflections on teacher education* (pp. 11–24). London: Falmer.

5

Combining Interpretive Methodologies

Maximizing the Richness of Findings

PHILIPPA SEATON

Introduction

Healthcare and human science researchers recognize the complexity and multidimensionality of human life and the consequent need for research approaches that investigate various aspects of life and health from diverse perspectives. To inform the research agendas in healthcare and the human sciences, contemporary studies are employing many different approaches to develop knowledge. Increasingly, multiple-methodology studies are seen as a way to provide the richness of data required to inform practice in healthcare and the human sciences. Multiple-methodology approaches have begun to pervade both social science (Greene & Caracelli, 1997; Teddlie & Tashakkori, 2003) and healthcare literature (Coyle & Williams, 2000). Typically, these studies have brought together paradigmatically and methodologically disparate approaches to inquiry, such as occurs in combining post-positivist and interpretivist approaches (Tashakkori & Teddlie, 1998). What appears to have been less common previously, but is now emerging, are approaches that bring together multiple interpretive methodologies either within a single study or through larger scale meta-analyses. Several authors cogently argue the need for using multiple qualitative methodologies in single studies and structured research programs (Morse & Chung, 2003), and for the metasynthesis of qualitative research studies that coalesce around specific research topics

(Sandelowski & Barrosso, 2003; Thorne, Joachim, Paterson, & Canam, 2002). These authors contend that such combinations would broaden the ability of qualitative research to guide healthcare practice. This is a compelling reason to expand the use and integration of multiple interpretive methodologies, and points to a need for further dialogue and debate regarding the commensurability of interpretive methodologies, and their underlying epistemologies and philosophies, in multiple-methodology research. This chapter therefore addresses some of the issues, challenges, and opportunities arising in the use of multiple interpretive methodologies in the development of knowledge for healthcare and the human sciences.

Terminology and Definitions

One of the issues that remains unresolved in combining methodologies in human science and healthcare research generally is that of consistency in terminology and definitions (Teddlie & Tashakkori, 2003). Before further discussion can take place here in regard to combining interpretive methodologies, attention needs to be paid to clarifying terms and definitions and the ways they will be used within this chapter. Teddlie and Tashakkori (2003) contend that common use of terms and definitions describing combining methodologies has been, to a certain extent, resisted by qualitative researchers, with some of these researchers maintaining that "codification" (p. 9) of terms and definitions is unproductive, and perhaps not even possible, across varying methodologies. In the debates focused around combining positivist and interpretivist methodologies, there appears to be a tendency for interpretivist methodologies to be gathered together under the term "qualitative methods" where "qualitative method is often portrayed in broad strokes that blur differences" (Gubrium & Holstein, 1997, p. 5) in methodologies. While the term "qualitative" signals the general direction of the contribution to knowledge, as Gubrium and Holstein (1997, p. 5) note, awareness of "the way the language of qualitative method shapes knowledge of social reality" is necessary, and this may be restricted when individual methodologies and their assumptions go unrecognized. This argument highlights an issue that is also significant in combining interpretive methodologies. It is important that the diverse nature of interpretive research approaches is acknowledged, and the individual methodological contributions valued, not just the overall nature of the qualitative enterprise (Gubrium & Holstein, 1997). This issue is important in combining interpretive methodologies in a rigorous manner, as will be discussed in more detail later in this chapter.

Terms found in the literature on combined research approaches include multi-method, mixed method, mixed model, triangulation, mixed methodologies, and multiple methodologies, each of which is used in variable ways by different authors and, in differing instances, may pertain to method, design or methodology (Teddlie & Tashakkori, 2003). Furthermore, using multiple methodologies implies a different activity from mixing methodologies, and nor are methods, methodologies and models synonymous. Methods are not associated only with specific methodologies, some methods may be used across different methodologies: for example, in-depth interviewing is a method of data collection used in many interpretive approaches. Such interviews, however, will be vastly different according to the influence of the underlying methodology (Wimpenny & Gass, 2000). Therefore, the use of the terms "multi-method," "mixed method," "mixed model," "mixed methodology," or "multiple methodology" interchangeably is confusing, and a desire by researchers for shared understandings of terms and definitions pertaining to combining methodologies is reasonable (Teddlie & Tashakkori, 2003) given this variety of meaning in the nomenclature appearing in the literature. While the current discussion cannot resolve this issue, for the sake of clarity the term "multiple methodologies" will predominantly be used here, given that the focus of this chapter is combining methodologies. However, there is a departure from this term in two circumstances: where methods rather than methodologies are specifically being discussed; and in the discussion of triangulation (although an argument is advanced as to why other terminology might be useful when combining interpretive methodologies, the term "triangulation" is almost universally used in the healthcare and human sciences literature; therefore, use of this term has been retained to avoid confusion from differing terminology in explicating this concept that is relevant to this discussion). This clarification of terms serves to locate the discussion in this chapter generally. However, fuller consideration of the definitional and philosophical issues specifically attendant upon the concept of triangulation in relation to multiple interpretive methodologies approaches follows the next section.

The tradition of Multiple-Methodologies Research

The debate surrounding the development of multiple-methodologies research that combines post-positivist with interpretivist methodologies has been more fully developed than has discussion of multiple interpretive methodologies. The former debate has produced a greater understanding of how paradigms may be brought together,[1] and an acceptance of their diverse applications in research (Patton, 2002). It is now acknowledged that a purposefully planned combination of differing methodologies, that maintains the integrity of each approach, has the potential to exploit the strengths of each individual methodology. The understandings that have arisen from the, often heated, debate over post-positivist and interpretivist paradigms (Tashakkori & Teddlie, 1998) also contribute to understanding the convergence of multiple interpretive methodologies, and as such, the relevant understandings as they pertain to combining interpretive methodologies are included in this chapter.

A key focus in using multiple methodologies has traditionally been the concept of triangulation, and as such, both its contribution to combining multiple interpretive methodologies, and the issues arising from adherence to the underlying assumptions of triangulation in combining interpretive methodologies are discussed here. Originally conceived in the science of land surveying (Patton, 2002) triangulation involves plotting a position by the use of three separate reference points. Subsequently applied within positivist and post-positivist research approaches to describe using multiple methods, data sources, theories, or researchers (Patton, 2002; Rice & Ezzy, 1999), triangulation underpins design decisions and is presumed to validate findings about a specific phenomenon by "showing that independent measures of it agree with it, or at least, do not contradict it" (Miles & Huberman, 1994, p. 266). Thus the purpose of triangulation within a positivistic paradigm is primarily confirmation of findings. In this way, researchers seek to balance strengths and weaknesses of different approaches to test for consistency in the findings from diverse sources or approaches (Patton, 2002; Shih, 1998); a purpose clearly consistent with the notion of truth espoused within positivist and post-positivist paradigms. Accordingly, the concept of triangulation has provided the justification for combining methodologies and methods in inquiries that conform to the tenets of the positivist paradigm.

However, such a purpose is antithetical to the philosophical under-pinnings of the interpretive paradigm and research approaches built upon it. Thus the concept of triangulation developed to include a further purpose: that of increasing the completeness of findings (Begley, 1996; Shih, 1998). Completeness aims to add depth and breadth to under-standing (Coyle & Williams, 2000; Shih, 1998). Bringing different meth-odologies together with the aim of completeness implies the researcher is intending to "reveal the varied dimensions of the . . . phenomenon being studied" (Shih, 1998, p. 633). Data gained are not expected to verify or confirm previously acquired data, but to contribute additional informa-tion and increase the completeness of the data (Begley, 1996; Greene & Caracelli, 1997). In this way, efforts have been made to shape the concept to be more congruent with the purposes of researchers who are seeking to understand more fully the complexities of human science and health-care practices. However, one should still exercise caution with regard to claims made for completeness of findings when multiple interpretive methodologies, with their focus on interpretation and meaning, are com-bined. A term such as completeness may still be construed as implying a finite state of knowledge that contradicts the claims of interpretive researchers who acknowledge both the relative nature of truth and the ever-present possibility of more than one warranted interpretation aris-ing in an inquiry as, for example, in a hermeneutic study (Baker, Norton, Young, & Ward, 1998; Diekelmann & Ironside, 1998) or a postmodern inquiry (Appignanesi & Garrett, 1999; Cheek, 1999; Davis & Glass, 1999; Foucault, 1979). It is with this distinction in mind that the justification for using multiple interpretive methodologies tendered in this chapter is one of maximizing the richness of findings, rather than arguing for confirma-tion of a truth, or claiming that completeness in findings is yielded by the use of multiple methodologies. Rather the understanding suggested here is that "no vision of a phenomenon is ever complete" (Sandelowski, 1995, p. 573). This view is consistent with several authors (Janesick, 2000; Rich-ardson, 1994; Sandelowski, 1995) who consider triangulation to be an in-adequate metaphor within interpretive inquiry, and instead support the idea of multifaceted crystals as a more appropriate metaphor for inter-pretive research (Janesick, 2000). These authors claim the notion of a crystal as a guiding concept offers infinite possibilities, "a greater degree of multidimensionality . . . and angles of approach" and a "deepened, complex . . . understanding of the topic" (Janesick, 2000, p. 392). This metaphor is thus particularly congruent with the purpose of combining interpretive methodologies for richness of information. Nor is this metaphor inconsistent with the strategies used for a triangulation described below, rather, it enables the use of these strategies to be extended beyond the three point notion of the triangle.

Bringing together multiple methodologies necessarily brings together one or more of the strategies that have been identified in the literature as types of triangulation. The first four are data, investigator, theoretical, and method triangulation (Denzin, 1989). The fifth type is interdisciplinary triangulation (Janesick, 1998). Multiple triangulations, which incorporate several of these strategies within one study, are also possible. Incorporating one or more of the aforementioned strategies in various combinations, this latter form of triangulation is akin to the multifaceted idea of crystallization suggested above, and captures the complexity that is inherent in bringing together multiple interpretive methodologies. The salient point being, where methodologies, as distinct from methods alone, are combined, then theory (whether implicit or explicitly recognized), data, and methods will be diverse, and possibly multiple investigators bringing varied expertise and perspectives may be required. How this will be dealt with needs to be a planned by the researcher. Choices of strategies also depend upon the substantive area being researched (Rice & Ezzy, 1999) and the degree of complexity inherent within this, the research questions being asked (Speziale & Carpenter, 2003), and the purposes of combining methodologies.

Data triangulation involves using multiple data sources to enhance the richness of findings (Patton, 2002). Tashakkori and Teddlie (1998) further discriminate between sources of data by introducing a distinction based on levels within the phenomenon, organization, or system being investigated, from which the data are gathered. For example, in an educational study of online teaching and learning, gathering data from individuals or groups at different levels might include sources at the administrative, academic, and student levels.

Investigator triangulation is predicated on the notion of different researchers bringing varied expertise to a study (Patton, 2002), the expertise being dependent upon the phenomenon under investigation, ways of thinking about the phenomenon, and the methodologies being employed. Thus investigators may bring either methodological or theoretical expertise (Speziale & Carpenter, 2003) and both similar and dissimilar perspectives of a phenomenon to the investigation. Rice and Ezzy (1999) point out that investigator triangulation may also include the participants as co-researchers in some forms of interpretive research, such as feminist or action research for example. When combining methodologies, as opposed to methods, the requirement for investigator expertise in the methodologies employed is necessary to ensure rigor in the ensuing research process.

Theoretical triangulation uses more than one theoretical perspective in the analysis of data (Rice & Ezzy, 1999). Primarily, when combining two interpretive methodologies, the respective epistemological underpinnings constitute a theoretical view of the knowledge generation that is possible, and thus provide a form of triangulation that the researcher must take into account when dealing with this influence on the findings that each methodology yields, and how these will be related to the other. A basis for such decisions is further explored in the later section on paradigmatic debates. Secondly, claiming that more than one theoretical perspective may be used in data analysis in interpretive research does not necessarily imply that theories are decided a priori and applied, but that more than one theoretical explanation or interpretation may emerge and "researchers investigate the utility and power of these emerging theories by cycling through data generation and data analysis until they reach a conclusion" (Speziale & Carpenter, 2003, p. 307).

Methods triangulation has been described both as between-methods and within-methods (Barbour, 1998; Begley, 1996; Kimchi, Polvika, & Stevenson, 1991). In the first type, different methodologies are combined: for instance, phenomenology and discourse analysis, as is evident in the example from Langridge and Ahern's (2003) study given later in this chapter. In the second type, more than one method, usually of data collection, is used within the same methodology. For example, in-depth interviews may be followed by focus groups (Darlington & Scott, 2002) or field notes. Savage (2000) provides another understanding of what has been described as within-methods triangulation, one moreover, that is salient to combining interpretive methodologies. Providing an example of using both thematic and narrative analysis on the same data, Savage contends that this process of analysis is not triangulation, as it is traditionally understood, but an engagement and re-engagement with the data through different perspectives. Savage's concern is with re-exploring data, thus illuminating alternative interpretations that may otherwise have remained hidden and viewing the findings yielded dialectically. Research is not always the tidy and linear process that is implied in textbook descriptions of process and procedures (D'Cruz, 2001), and interpretive researchers may need to be responsive to the demands of the research in progress for additional data collection. Thus, combining methods may not always be planned in advance, but may be deemed necessary as the study advances (D'Cruz, 2001; Speziale & Carpenter, 2003). This is not to suggest that methodologies may be set aside for only pragmatic reasons, but acknowledges that research is a process, and researchers need to remain sensitive to the needs of the research in addition to the paradigmatic underpinnings. Given this, it is argued here that researchers undertaking such convergence of methodologies or methods need to, in either case, clearly explicate for the reader what it is they have actually done in the conduct of their research (Koch, 1996).

Interdisciplinary triangulation is the use of multiple disciplines to inform understandings of both the methodology and the substance of the research (Janesick, 1998). For example, researching online nursing education would locate the project on the borders between the disciplines of nursing, education, and information and communication technology, with each of these disciplines having a place in informing the research. Thus, striving for richness may be undertaken in a variety of ways, with varying types of triangulation (or crystallization) included in the design of any one study, and several of these types of triangulation exist when interpretive methodologies are combined.

Both definitional and philosophical problems existing around the concept of triangulation have implications for the debate about multiple-methodologies studies in healthcare and the human sciences. Despite the widespread adoption of the term triangulation in the multiple-methodologies literature, the metaphorical implications of the term suggest that it is less accurate when used in relation to achieving completeness rather than confirmation of findings (Breitmayer, Ayres, & Knafl, 1993; Sandelowski, 2003), or as suggested earlier, in relation to information richness. The concept of triangulation is explicated in different studies through a variety of terms (for example, mixing, merging, or complementing), which themselves convey a variety of meanings. However, a common understanding of triangulation is often assumed despite this use of assorted terms suggesting otherwise (Sandelowski, 1995). A lack of clarity in what is combined, why it is combined, and what kind of combinations are involved demonstrates diverse understandings of triangulation, and appeals to very different ontological and epistemological underpinnings are often represented (Sandelowski, 2003). While such attention to detail in terminology may seem a minor issue, this lack of clarity among researchers has the potential to hinder development of multiple-methodologies research for healthcare (Twinn, 2003). This concern indicates a need for more discussion of, not only the paradigmatic and epistemological underpinnings and their suitability for combining, but also of the implications of various designs of multiple-methodologies research and the methodological consequences.

A further issue related to the term triangulation relates to the degree to which it is inappropriate in studies that are grounded in the interpretivist paradigm and methodologies. According to Sandelowski (1995) triangulation:

implies knowledge from which other knowledge can be derived. . . . In conventional descriptions of the "qualitative" paradigm, no such a priori knowledge or absolute reference points are presumed to exist. Moreover, different perspectives of *ostensibly* the same phenomenon do not add up to the whole of that phenomenon, nor is information obtained from different kinds of data easily compared or added up to yield the truth. (p. 571, emphasis original)

When richness of understanding is the goal of the research, and multiple interpretive methodologies are utilized in the research endeavor, using terms such as crystallization, combining, or confluence of methodologies may be more helpful than triangulation, as these terms encompass the meaning of bringing together for a common purpose, but allow the researcher to retain a commitment to the particular requirements of each interpretive methodology. Most importantly, researchers and scholars will assist the development of healthcare and human science knowledge and research designs appropriate to their disciplines through clearly articulating the assumptions upon which their design and research decisions are based in multiple-methodologies studies.

A commitment to maximizing the richness of findings in research is appropriate in many instances for the purposes of healthcare practice. Often these purposes require a response to the complex, multifaceted needs of health services and clinical practice (Foss & Ellefsen, 2002). Combining approaches provides a means of preventing the oversimplification of findings by highlighting the complexities, inconsistencies, and contradictions that arise from the use of multiple methodologies (Foss & Ellefsen, 2002).

Recently, Morse and Chung (2003) have made a case that while qualitative methods (that are often, but not exclusively, associated with interpretive-based methodologies) are particularly apposite for healthcare and nursing research, the use of a single qualitative method to address topics in nursing research works against nursing's holistic perspective. The ways in which these authors claim a single method research design "partitions reality" (Morse & Chung, 2003, p. 1) includes: delimiting the scope of the research by the focus on particular persons; limiting a researcher's particular research agenda by a single method; dictating a particular outcome through the use of one specific theoretical basis; and including, excluding, and legitimating various aspects of data according to the epistemological basis of the one particular method selected (Morse & Chung, 2003). Morse and Chung (2003) suggest overcoming these limitations by using multiple methodologies in one of three ways: through combining methods within a single study; in systematic research programs that over time have the potential to bring together multiple data sources, methodologies and methods, investigators, theories, and disciplinary contributions from single methodology studies in a more complex interpretation; or in metasyntheses of interpretive research. A commitment to evolving our understandings of healthcare and human sciences through diverse explorations drives each of these ways of combining methodologies, while avoiding the suggestion that our knowledge or understanding is ever complete (Savage, 2000).

Given the previous discussion of the purposes that combining methodologies might serve, and the foregoing rationale for multiple-methodologies research in healthcare and the human sciences, the subsequent sections of this chapter will explore, first, the ways in which the convergence and divergence of paradigms generally can be understood. Second, the contributions that interpretive methodologies can make from a philosophical perspective (rather than procedures and processes) as a basis for understanding how diverse world views might be combined, and in what ways they are incommensurable, will be described. And third, the issues and possibilities that arise from combining interpretive paradigms, epistemologies, and methodologies will be discussed.

Paradigmatic Debates in Multiple-Methodologies Research

The paradigmatic debate in the human sciences that has character-ized the mixing of post-positivist and interpretive methodologies sheds some light upon the concerns of combining interpretive methodologies. Epistemological, ontological, and axiological issues such as the relation-ship of the knower to what can be known; the nature of reality (Guba & Lincoln, 1994); and the role of values in research (Tashakkori & Teddlie, 1998) are central to the question regarding the commensurability and ac-ceptable use of any combination of multiple methodologies in research.

The stances discernable in the multiple-methodologies paradigmatic debate are discussed here to open these debates for consideration within interpretive multiple-methodologies research. The "a-paradigmatic" stance is predicated on the notion that paradigms and methods are dis-tinct and independent from one another (Teddlie & Tashakkori, 2003, p. 17). Teddlie and Tashakkori (2003) suggest that research in applied fields, including healthcare, has often taken this stance, ignoring the para-digmatic issues and using whatever methods appear appropriate to the question under investigation: a claim that is supported by the paucity of debate around the philosophical and epistemological issues involved in multiple-methodologies research, particularly in the nursing literature (Clark, 1998). Of those who do consider the paradigmatic underpinnings of research, at one end of a continuum, the "purist" stance (Greene & Caracelli, 1997, p. 8) assumes the "incompatibility thesis" (Teddlie & Ta-shakkori, 2003, p. 7). Researchers taking this view argue that the contrast between the ontological, epistemological, and axiological assumptions makes it meaningless to use multiple paradigms in a research study (Greene & Caracelli, 1997; Guba & Lincoln, 1994; Tashakkori & Teddlie, 1998) and thus proscribe the use of multiple methods in a single study. In contrast, those adopting a "pragmatic" position (Greene & Caracelli, 1997, p. 9), while accepting that paradigmatic differences exist, maintain that the primary focus should be on results rather than the underlying phi-losophies. The pragmatic researcher is not required to resolve theoretical contradictions, but rather, must respond to the practical needs of the re-search (Patton, 2002; Rorty, 1999). Pragmatism contends that at the level of methods, there is compatibility (Tashakkori & Teddlie, 1998), and pro-motes a focus on methods rather than philosophical and epistemological underpinnings. A fourth stance is the "dialectical" position (Greene & Caracelli, 1997, p. 8). A dialectic has been defined as a "discussion involving the juxtaposition or conflict of opposites" and a "process whereby contradictions merge to form a higher truth" (Moore, 1996, p. 297). As this definition suggests, a dialectical position argues that the differences between paradigms are of consequence, and can be used deliberately "both within and across studies toward a dialectical discovery of enhanced understandings, of new and revisioned perspectives and meanings" (Greene & Caracelli, 1997, p. 8). Finally a "complementary strengths" (Teddlie & Tashakkori, 2003, p. 19) position on multiple-methodologies research assumes that differing paradigms need to be kept separate within the inquiry (Brewer & Hunter, 1989; Morse, 2003). The aim of this stance differs from the purist view however, in that it is predicated on the notion that each paradigm has strengths or weaknesses that, used appropriately, can be brought together in a multiple methodologies study, where each will balance the other.

The purists' perspective, bounded by the assumptions of a single paradigm (Greene & Caracelli, 1997), criticizes a pragmatic viewpoint, claiming that to integrate methods without considering the underlying paradigm is unacceptable. Pragmatists, by contrast, consider a purist approach overly rigid, given that a paradigm is normative (Patton, 2002) and socially constructed by consensus of the scientific community to which it pertains (Clark, 1998). A consequence of the purist view is that an overly narrow standpoint may introduce "paradigm-derived biases" (Patton, 2002, p. 71) that limit the researcher to predetermined decisions about methods. On the other hand, Greene and Caracelli (1997) have argued, responding only to contextual demands potentially leaves research without epistemological guidelines with which to evaluate cultural, social, and political influences that may have an impact upon an inquiry. A given paradigm can provide an epistemological framework with which to view these influences and provide a structure for the researcher's decision-making, guarding against "conflation of the methodological with the ideological" (Miller & Fredericks, 2002, p. 983). While a dialectical or a complementary-strengths stance does not resolve the inconsistencies between paradigmatic viewpoints, it does provide a way for the researcher to consciously make research decisions without either ignoring or being overly rigid in regard to paradigmatic underpinnings, and thus such a stance can provide a path to possibilities in multiple-methodology interpretive research.

Central to the argument for a dialectical inquiry is the notion of maintaining the integrity of each paradigm and the differences between them, while finding productive common ground. According to Greene and Caracelli, in a dialectical approach:

Contrasts, conflicts and tensions between different methods and their findings are an expected, even welcome dimension of [multiple methodologies] inquiry, for it is in the tension that the boundaries of what is known are most generatively challenged and stretched. The analytic space created by the tension, however, must offer the possibility of co-ordination, integration and synthesis. (Greene & Caracelli, 1997, pp. 12–13)

Greene and Caracelli (1997) suggest that one way to reach integration and synthesis of knowledge claims from competing paradigms, is by paying attention to those characteristics of each paradigm that are different, but not necessarily contradictory, claiming that these characteristics are part of a continuum rather than dichotomous variables. Examples of these characteristics are: "particularity and generality . . . integrative synthesis and componential analysis . . . micro and macro perspectives" (Greene & Caracelli, 1997, p. 13). These authors argue that attending to these characteristics in a dialectical inquiry strengthens knowledge claims.

Given the practical imperative of healthcare and human science research in which the findings must address complex life situations that are themselves frequently inconsistent and contradictory, arguing that "paradigms are in contention is less useful than to probe where and how paradigms exhibit confluence and where and how they exhibit differences, controversies, and contradictions" (Lincoln & Guba, 2000, p. 164). This latter course allows multiple-methodology research to increase its contribution to healthcare and the human sciences. Appleton and King (2002) maintain that nursing researchers are often drawn toward the common features of methodologies, when using multiple methodologies, however, caution must be exercised to ensure that divergent features are also recognized and accounted for in all phases of the research process. Thus these varying stances illustrate the diverse positions possible in relation to paradigmatic commensurability that are applicable in combining interpretivist approaches. The features that define interpretivist paradigms that must be considered in bringing together various methodologies are discussed next.

Interpretive Methodologies

Meaning and understanding are central to all interpretive methodologies. However, as Rice and Ezzy (1999, p. 1) state, "qualitative research cannot be described in terms of a set of theories and techniques that always apply, rather, qualitative research draws on a variety of theoretical perspectives . . . including theories such as phenomenology, symbolic interactionism, cultural studies, psychology and feminism." A brief introduction to some widely used methodologies is given here, but no claim is made that this list is exhaustive, either in terms of methodologies that can be considered interpretive (only some examples are included here), or in the information about these specific methodologies. The purpose is to situate these methodologies philosophically, not to provide comprehensive definitions and details of the processes and procedures of each.

Phenomenology based on the philosophy of Husserl is descriptive. This approach is epistemological, and emphasizes individuals' construction of their everyday lives (Koch, 1995; Rice & Ezzy, 1999). The Husserlian phenomenological approach to researching phenomena assumes there is a so-called essence to all phenomena as experienced by human beings. The aim of phenomenology is for this essential structure of an experience to be understood (Pursley-Crotteau, Bunting, & Draucker, 2001; Sadala & Adorno, 2002; Todres & Wheeler, 2001) and described from the perspective of those who have had the lived experiences and are able to describe it (Rice & Ezzy, 1999).

Hermeneutic or interpretive phenomenology as a research approach derives mainly from the ontological philosophies of Heidegger and Gadamer, and is used to understand the meaning of being in the world (Baker, Norton, Young, & Ward, 1998; Benner, 1994; Diekelmann & Ironside, 1998; Pursley-Crotteau, Bunting, & Draucker, 2001), that is, human lived experience. This approach is predicated on the assumption that there is no truth "independent of interpretation" (Rice & Ezzy, 1999, p. 25) and that all experience is always already interpreted within the social and historical context (Heidegger, 1927/1962). The purpose of hermeneutic phenomenology is to achieve understanding of phenomena through interpretation (such as interpretation of narrative texts). Interpretation is aimed at uncovering or revealing hidden meanings (Palmer, 1969), and thus the interpreter uncovers new and different possibilities for understanding shared experiences and practices (Baker, Norton, Young, & Ward, 1998; Plager, 1994).

Grounded theory is based in symbolic interactionism, a theory concerned with understanding how the world is socially constructed, through illumination of "the relationship between individuals and society, as mediated by symbolic communication" (Milliken & Schreiber, 2001, p. 178). In symbolic interactionism, human behaviors are based in the meanings that things have for them (Baker, Norton, Young, & Ward, 1998; Pursley-Crotteau, Bunting, & Draucker, 2001) and thus to understand behavior, the meaning ascribed to the behavior must be understood (Milliken & Schreiber, 2001). Grounded theory research aims to generate a substantive theory of basic social process or social psychological process that relates the phases of the theory (Morse, 2001) and is derived from the empirical data (Speziale & Carpenter, 2003). A grounded theory approach includes interpretive, explanatory, and predictive purposes (Baker, Norton, Young, & Ward, 1998). A strength of this approach for healthcare and human sciences is that it may "yield a conceptual framework on which to base interventions" (Pursley-Crotteau, Bunting, & Draucker, 2001, p. 192).

Ethnography is a form of social research that involves interpretation of cultural behavior (Spradley, 1979). Originating in cultural anthropology, the core of ethnographic research is to understand the way of life of a particular cultural group from the perspective of that group by exploring "patterns of meaning that make up a culture and that guide and make sense of people's actions" (Rice & Ezzy, 1999, p. 13). Ethnography is based on the assumption that all groups of people develop a culture that structures the experiences of the group members (Polit & Beck, 2004). These groups may be broadly or narrowly defined, for example, in healthcare, nursing would be a broad culture, while the culture of the intensive care unit would be a smaller unit of study.

Feminist research involves primarily interpreting the subjective experiences of women, but is specifically ideologically driven to highlight gender discrimination in society (Polit & Beck, 2004; Rice & Ezzy, 1999) and has an emancipatory agenda (Wuest & Merritt-Gray, 2001). Central to feminist methodologies are the notions that research is political and reflexive in nature (Rice & Ezzy, 1999). Feminist research however, is not a singular research methodology, but embraces many variants that overlap with other research approaches, for example, feminist postmodernism, or feminist grounded theory (Wuest & Merritt-Gray, 2001).

Postmodernism is itself a contested term (Cheek, 1999), and there is considerable diversity among postmodern approaches (Rice & Ezzy, 1999). For the sake of clarity the explanation given here relies primarily on Cheek's (1999) exegesis of postmodern approaches to research in healthcare practices, as this provides a clear explanation of its relevance in the area of healthcare and as such is pertinent to this discussion. According to Cheek (1999), postmodern approaches are based primarily on the avoidance of universal truths or metanarratives, rejecting the notions of social coherence and causality, and instead retain a respect for fragmented and contradictory experiences and understandings through "emphasis on the plurality of reality" and "the multiplicity of voices, views, and methods present in any representation" (Cheek, 1999, p. 385). A central assumption is that reality is constructed through language, and writing (Rice & Ezzy, 1999) and that within these texts some views are privileged, and others excluded or marginalized (Cheek, 1999). Postmodern approaches thus aim to scrutinize and question even the most basic understandings and taken-for-granted assumptions in society.

These approaches can be seen to share several key features within their ontological and epistemological underpinnings, as well as differences that are a significant concern in multiple-methodologies research.

Ontological and Epistemological Underpinnings

Multiple interpretive methodologies possibly compete less overtly than the post-positivist and interpretivist combination of methodologies, as there is a degree of compatibility at the ontological level. Interpretive approaches do share several commonalities in their underlying philosophies. These approaches reject any notion of a foundational objective realism, either naïve or critical, and subscribe instead to a relativist view where reality is both local and constructed (Lincoln & Guba, 2000; Schwandt, 2000) and temporally and historically located. In interpretive philosophy, the world is a relational whole in which humans exist, and in which the self and the world cannot be separated (Palmer, 1969). That is not to say that there are not objects in the world separate from human beings: there are. But objects only have *possibilities* for meaning, not actual meaning, until humans experience them (Crotty, 1998). There is no meaning in the human world, separate to humans' knowing of it. Thus, there is a sense of human beings interpreting their world, their relationship with that world and those with whom they share their world. Interpretation, or understanding meaning, is thus constitutive of being human, rather than being something humans do (Polkinghorne, 1983). Central to that understanding is the uncovering of meaning through language (Gadamer, 1960/1994), and thus language defines what is represented (Sandelowski, 2003). Thus far, interpretivist methodologies, such as those described above, that derive from a view of reality as individually and culturally constructed, relativist, and multiple (Sandelowski, 2000) can be seen to have a basic point of compatibility for combining in an inquiry. For example, Wilson and Hutchinson (1991) noted the common commitments of Heideggerian hermeneutics and grounded theory to "qualitative, naturalistic, contextual, historic, intersubjective methodology to understand human responses and experiences from a variety of perspectives as they are transformed over time" (Wilson & Hutchinson, 1991, p. 267).

Beyond the ontological level of an inquiry paradigm is the axiological level, that is, the values espoused, and the epistemological aspect: the particular view of the way of understanding knowing and what is known, the relationship of knower to known, what constitutes legitimate knowledge (Crotty, 1998), and who is accepted as knowledgeable (Meetoo & Temple, 2003). However, paradigms as social constructions are not fixed, but instead evolve over time within a community of researchers and scholars (Clark, 1998). This can be seen in the paradigmatic debates, where some of the original proponents of the purist stance, such as Lincoln and Guba, have modified their position in recent times as interpretive inquiry has developed, and now recognize that paradigms with similar "axiomatic elements" (Lincoln & Guba, 2000, p. 174) may in some ways fit together. Lincoln and Guba (2000) have noted that elements of interpretivist, critical, and postmodern approaches resonate with each other and are commensurable in multiple-methodologies studies. Interpretivist research approaches assume broadly similar values in the "the relationship of researcher and what is studied, and the situational constraints that shape inquiry . . . the value-laden nature of inquiry . . . and [they] seek answers as to how social experience is created and given meaning" (Denzin & Lincoln, 2000, p. 8). However, while this evidence of a move towards a compatibility thesis that can inform multiple-methodologies interpretive research in particular is apparent, differences remain.

There are points of divergence among interpretive methodologies due to varying epistemological positions and axiological elements that suggest that assuming interpretive methodologies all belong to a single paradigm, and can be unproblematically brought together, is questionable. As opposed to the ontological level, at this level a greater degree of divergence is apparent between differing approaches. For example, feminist, critical or postmodern epistemologies show significant differences, such as in the acceptance or rejection of specific ideologies. For example, feminist epistemology holds that women are oppressed (Walter, Glass, & Davis, 2001), and while critical and postmodern epistemologies identify marginalized individuals, they lack this ideological commitment to only one group being the focus of the oppression. Similarly, whereas some values may resonate, other contradictory values need to be taken into account between different methodologies as these have the potential to generate tensions (Meetoo & Temple, 2003). Bringing together interpretive methodologies in research calls for the same adherence to understanding the effects of a particular perspective on research design and process decisions, and maintaining the integrity of each methodology, that bringing together overtly competing epistemologies and methodologies does. If they are to enhance the usefulness of interpretive research to nursing and healthcare, researchers need to recognize the ways in which they understand and bring together various methodologies. They also need to clearly identify and demonstrate the paradigmatic influences on their findings to the users of those findings, rather than assume a common understanding.

Draucker's study that combined grounded theory and hermeneutic phenomenology methodologies (Draucker, 1999, 2001; Draucker & Stern, 2000; Pursley-Crotteau, Bunting, & Draucker, 2001) provides an example of areas of commensurability and incompatibility in combining these two approaches. Draucker combined these two methodologies in a study of women's responses to violence, with the aims of obtaining both a description of the meaning of sexual violence in the women's lives through the hermeneutic interpretation, and a theoretical framework outlining the processes of healing using grounded theory methodology. Combining the findings from both phases of the project aimed to provide a comprehensive description of the women's responses to the experience of living through the violence, and allow recommendations for interventions to be developed. Draucker rigorously maintained the integrity of each methodology by keeping the conduct of each phase of the study separate (including separate groups of participants), and true to the tenets of the methodology, warning that violating the philosophical perspective of either method undermines the research project. Pursley-Crotteau, Bunting, and Draucker (2001, pp. 191–192), in reporting this study, noted that researchers using these two interpretive methodologies shared common beliefs in "knowledge as tentative and evolving, produce findings that are a result of an interpretive collaboration between researcher and participant, and seek to answer research questions that inform practice." However, they also noted significant differences in purpose: interpretive phenomenological researchers are "driven by ontological concerns and enter the hermeneutic circle to achieve understanding and grounded theory researchers are driven by epistemological concerns and analyze field data to develop substantive theory" (Pursley-Crotteau, Bunting, & Draucker, 2001, p. 206).

Accepting that, when approached with care, there are ways to engage with multiple methodologies to enhance nursing knowledge, what are the challenges and possibilities of combining interpretive paradigms, epistemologies and methodologies?

Challenges in Using Multiple Interpretive Methodologies

An understanding of the challenges in using multiple interpretive methodologics can be derived from two main sources. Firstly, from studies that employ multiple interpretive methodologies, and secondly, from the emerging qualitative metasynthesis literature that describes the methodological and analytic processes involved in such metasyntheses. The challenges these researchers face as they bring together the results of multiple studies by multiple authors, but relating to one topic, illuminate important considerations that may either be less obvious, or have gone unremarked in the reporting of a single multiple-method study (Thorne, Joachim, Paterson, & Canam, 2002).

Rather than assuming that using multiple interpretive methodologies is straightforward, this kind of research "can be seen to occupy a contested domain" (Barbour, 1998, p. 352). The paradigmatic influences described previously give rise to the many facets of research practice that ultimately affect the knowledge emerging from a study. These include epistemological issues related to the influence of disciplinary background, theoretical position, and methodological clarity proposed by Thorne, Joachim, Paterson, and Canam (2002), the practicalities of undertaking multiple-method research (Twinn, 2003), and the social agenda of the researcher (Barbour, 1998). These authors are all writing within the discipline of nursing, however the issues they raise are also applicable to other healthcare and human science research.

Epistemological Issues   Three overlapping disciplinary influences can be discerned in nursing research and scholarship, each of which has an impact upon multiple interpretive methodologies research. In the early stages of nurses' higher education, many who undertook research degrees at the masters or doctoral level did so in disciplines other than nursing, such as psychology, sociology, anthropology, or education. Consequently, while they may not always be easily discernable (Thorne, Joachim, Paterson, & Canam, 2002), disciplinary influences from these other human sciences may be brought to bear within nursing research, albeit for nursing's agenda. Nursing has now advanced to the stage of establishing its own body of knowledge, and preparing its own scholars, to the extent that it has established itself as a discipline in its own right, with its own disciplinary orientation. Thirdly, a new phase of disciplinary orientation towards research is now becoming apparent, which is the multidisciplinary approach that is becoming increasingly used in health research, and that may foreseeably bring a unique approach as it evolves, and with it nurse researchers who belong to different communities of practice versed in a new way of interdisciplinary thinking, with the potential for unique influences upon multiple-methodology research.

Researchers' differing disciplinary orientations encompass variations in accepted theoretical underpinnings and methodological approaches (Barbour, 1998) that influence the structure of the research problem, the question construction, data collection and analysis (Barbour, 1998; Thorne, Joachim, Paterson, & Canam, 2002), and dictate acceptable writing conventions for reporting findings and the dissemination of those findings (Barbour, 1998; Sandelowski, 2003), all of which influence the possible applications of research in nursing and healthcare practice. When researchers use multiple methodologies, it is important they reflect on the potential effects that their disciplinary backgrounds may have on the methodologies included in the study. In interpretive research in general, it is widely accepted that one criterion of rigor is for the researcher to provide the reader with a sufficiently detailed audit trail to ensure that the researcher's location within the research process is discernable (Koch, 1996). When researchers use multiple methodologies, this explication of process is equally, if not more, important. The disciplinary conventions brought to each aspect of the study must be clearly articulated and the relationship of one aspect to another demonstrated.

Although treated separately here for the purpose of discussion, in practical terms there is overlap between disciplinary and theoretical orientations. However, theoretical positions also have elements that are independent of disciplines (Thorne, Joachim, Paterson, & Canam, 2002) to the extent that they may be found across disciplines. For example, feminist theory plays a part in the research of many disciplines, as does critical theory or postmodernism. The extent to which the theory shapes the inquiry or parts of the inquiry, from framing questions through to gaining participants, data collection and interpretation varies (Barbour, 1998). For example, while they could all be broadly considered under the banner of interpretive research, feminist theory will inform research from the beginning, whereas some forms of phenomenology proscribe the use of any theory and specifically call for bracketing,[2] while in other approaches, theoretical positions may emerge, such as is intended in grounded theory research. It could be argued that without such differences there is no point to multiple-methodology research. In some views of combining paradigms, such as the dialectical stance, the notion of difference is regarded as both necessary and beneficial to the research, signaling the location for increasingly complex levels of interpretation (Greene & Caracelli, 1997). The challenge for multiple-methodology interpretive research is to retain the theoretical coherence of individual epistemologies and methodologies while combining them together in a single study or metasynthesis that comprehensibly interprets these multiple findings. As Barbour (1998) contends, "what is important is that we recognize when [different theoretical positions are] happening and that we remain alert to the implications for our interpretations and analyses" (p. 354). How and why the various theoretical lenses will be combined in the interpretation and findings needs to be determined in the research design.

Methodological Issues   Methodological issues are a third challenge to multiple interpretive methodologies. In both single multiple-methodologies studies and metasyntheses, there is an identified need for firstly, methodological clarification that determines ways in which interpretation can be carried out to bring together the multiple methodologies, and secondly, for specific descriptions in the published research of these research designs, methods, and specific ways of integrating findings to derive inferences (Sandelowski & Barroso, 2003; Sandelowski & Barroso, 2002). Descriptions that document the decisions made and the analytic processes undertaken allow the reader to evaluate the research and consequently judge the interpretation and the applicability of the findings to practice (Schreiber, Crooks, & Stern, 1997) or their contribution to scholarship in the healthcare or human science disciplines as appropriate. As long as the purposes and/or techniques of combining methodologies are not clearly described, then the challenge of developing multiple-methodology studies, and undertaking metasyntheses in research, remains difficult. Erzberger and Kelle (2003) caution, however, that the epistemological and methodological considerations of integration can only be understood within the substantive area under investigation, arguing that the research question should be the primary concern of researchers making these decisions. This suggests that interpretive multiple-methodology researchers need to find ways and forums in which to publish both general discussions of methodology (e.g., Baker, Norton, Young, & Ward, 1998; Barbour, 1998; Sandelowski, Docherty, & Emden, 1997) and specific descriptions of methodological processes within the context they were used (Plager, 1994). Although it is no easy task to explain the process and progression of interpretation (Barbour, 1998), such clarification will advance healthcare and human sciences research. An example of an article that describes the processes and analytic devices by which a particular metasynthesis was produced, thereby contributing through methodological transparency to developing and testing strategies of interpretation, is that of Sandelowski and Barroso (2003). These authors detail their use of strategies of integrating and interpreting findings (for example, sustained comparisons, translating in-vivo concepts, and using imported concepts) in a metasynthesis of findings about motherhood in HIV-positive women. All these ways of synthesizing findings are aimed at the "amplification of data and interpretive innovation" (Sandelowski & Barroso, 2003, p. 154), an aim that is consistent with the purpose of information richness for a given topic. In addition, such studies have a potential to increase access to qualitative research findings by both clinicians and researchers (Finfgeld, 2003).

Methodological slippage (Thorne, Joachim, Paterson, & Canam, 2002), blurring (Sandelowski & Barroso, 2003) or muddling (Morse, 2003) methodologies wherein the distinct processes of individual methodologies are not preserved when the methodologies are combined, constitutes a further risk. While systematically 'mixing' methods, through blending elements of the research process such as data analysis to form new designs has been advocated by some authors (for example, Teddlie & Tashakkori, 2003), blurring methodologies risks losing the individual contributions that each approach may have brought to answering the research question, and thus creates a methodological "quagmire" (Barbour, 1998, p. 356). In interpretive research the context and conditions of the research are crucial (Meetoo & Temple, 2003). Thus, while bringing findings together is valuable because this reflects social reality, which includes multiple perspectives, when combining interpretive methodologies, muddling methodologies is problematic. Distinctions among methodologies need to be carefully ascertained and maintained within an inquiry (Baker, Wuest, & Stern, 1992), as these differences will inform the interpretations, theories, and inferences drawn from the findings.

The "inherent good" notion raised by Twinn (2003, p. 552) in relation to positivist–interpretivist mixes also needs to be highlighted and questioned as a matter of rigor in studies that combine multiple interpretive methodologies. While there is evidence to support the argument that combining methodologies can provide valuable knowledge for healthcare, there is also a need to be careful about determining how multiple methodologies contribute to understanding a research question or phenomenon. Uncritical acceptance of the "inherent good" position that assumes multiple methods must be better than one, *should be regarded with caution*. While the "inherent good" stance makes a claim to rigor, it does not demonstrate rigor unless it is supported by detailed descriptions of how rigor has been achieved through multiple methods in a given study. Researchers are better advised to undertake "careful consideration of the research question and whether it lends itself to the design" (Twinn, 2003, p. 553) and then demonstrate for users of the research, wherein the value lies.

Beyond general methodological issues, other more specific methodological issues arise within interpretive multiple-methodologies studies.
One example of this is the relationship of the researcher and the participants to each other and the data that are produced. Within different
interpretive methodologies the role of the researcher varies in the degree
to which they co-construct the findings with the participants (Barbour,
1998; Lowes & Prowse, 2001). In participatory action research and some
forms of feminist research, for example, the researcher and participants
are regarded as co-researchers, and the design and methods accord with
this understanding. In other interpretive methodologies, researchers
view themselves as interpreting individual accounts in a way that honors
the participants' stories, but may be carried out by the researcher independently of the participants, as in phenomenological or narrative analysis, where it is not commonly the case for participants to be part of the
research team. In single method studies this issue is not problematic,
provided the decision made is appropriate to the research purpose and
individual methodology; however, in bringing together multiple methodologies in a study, attention needs to be paid to whether and how such
differences in epistemology are to be reconciled, as well as to their appropriateness to the phenomenon, the research question, and the purposes of the research.

Practical Issues   Some practical issues arise in bringing together multiple interpretive methodologies. These include the need for
skills in a diverse range of methodologies, which requires that researchers learn these new skills and gain expertise in the methodologies required (Morse & Chung, 2003) or that multiple researchers are brought
together. Both these courses of action have resource implications, for the
researchers personally and for the project. In combining multiple interpretive methodologies, researchers need the skills to work with varying
theoretical and methodological understandings, to be able to develop sophisticated and complex interpretations that account for the multiple
findings, and perhaps to work with multidisciplinary teams (Morse &
Chung, 2003).

High costs in time and resources attend any multiple-methodologies
study (Twinn, 2003) by virtue of combining methods, and perhaps, utiliz-
ing multiple investigators. The intensive in-depth nature of interpretive
research may make it particularly so, and due consideration should be

paid to this before a study begins in order to ensure a quality outcome where the important contributions of the combined methodologies are maximized, rather than one handicapped by inadequate resources that then contributes less to healthcare or human science knowledge.

Social Issues   The importance of social impact and an obligation to practical usability is highlighted by several authors writing in the field of interpretive research (Sandelowski, 2003; Sandelowski, Docherty, & Emden, 1997; Thorne, 1997; Thorne, Joachim, Paterson, & Canam, 2002). For nursing and healthcare research this point is particularly salient. Nursing is an applied discipline, and as such, understanding the influence of individual methodologies and the effects of combined methodologies in a given area of inquiry is important in determining the transferability of findings to the clinical arena.

The foregoing discussion is not meant to deter researchers from using multiple interpretive methodologies, but rather to encourage thinking about the paradigmatic, epistemological, and methodological issues that will enhance the use of multiple interpretive methodologies in nursing and healthcare research. Having examined challenges in undertaking research using multiple interpretive methods, it becomes apparent that in these very challenges lies much of the promise, and many of the opportunities for using multiple methodologies to maximize the richness of the findings.

Possibilities in Using Multiple Interpretive Methodologies

The promise and possibility of multiple interpretive methodology research lies for the most part in maximizing the richness of findings. Healthcare is complex and encompasses multiple experiences and understandings, and multiple methodologies inquiry is congruent with such a worldview, allowing for comprehensive and inclusive interpretations that represent the spectrum of experience (Morse & Chung, 2003; Thorne, Joachim, Paterson, & Canam, 2002). In addition, combining methodologies, through a dialectical multiple-methodologies approach in a single study, through research programs that combine findings systematically, or in metasyntheses, can help overcome the isolation of individual findings by bringing them into a larger interpretive context. As discussed earlier, bringing findings together dialectically opens up new possibilities for interpretation to find new meanings in the paradoxical, the puzzling, and the contradictory as well as the congruent, and through this, may bring new perspectives (Thorne, Joachim, Paterson, & Canam, 2002).

The iterative (rather than linear), circular nature of interpretive research is well established methodologically (Diekelmann & Ironside, 1998; Schwandt, 2000). Using this iterative approach for combining multiple methodologies reveals another possibility. A researcher who remains open to the needs of the research questions and responsive to the research process may combine methodologies in a research project, even as the study unfolds (Barbour, 1998; D'Cruz, 2001). An example might make this discussion clearer. One recent study that combines interpretive methods is Langridge and Ahern's (2003) study of advanced nurse specialization and education in Australia and its accompanying discussion of their reasons for, and methods of, combining interpretive methodologies. In this study phenomenology and postmodern discourse analysis were undertaken because "they each dealt with the perspective of a phenomenon characterized by contradictory and opposing realities" (Langridge & Ahern, 2003, p. 32). Originally in this project, Langridge and Ahern planned a phenomenological study of the experiences of advancing nurse specialists undertaking further education. However, as the study progressed, the researchers became aware during data analysis that there were external forces influencing the advancing nurse specialists and that they, as researchers, were unable, using a single methodology, to "sufficiently contextualize experiences in the broader social culture" (Langridge & Ahern, 2003, p. 32). Langridge and Ahern consequently decided to develop multiple methodologies based on the need to include other stakeholders with vested interests in educating these nurses. They chose to adopt a discourse analysis to analyze the data from those stakeholders involved who were critical of, or marginalized by, the advanced education system. Using both these methodologies, these researchers were able to provide both a rich description and a critique of the advanced nurse specialist education (Langridge & Ahern, 2003). Thus they demonstrated how they were constantly responsive to the needs of the research during its conduct and, in using multiple interpretive methodologies in this way, overcame the limitations they perceived in the research and enabled them to make the most appropriate recommendations for nursing.

Langridge and Ahern's (2003) study also demonstrates the potential of using multiple interpretive methodologies to advance methodological expertise within the discipline of nursing. These researchers contribute to this outcome firstly, through their explication of the way in which they conducted this research, the problems encountered and the decisions they made. Secondly, their study demonstrates the nature of multiple-interpretive-methodologies research in nursing as praxis—bringing together theory and practice in a way that evolves and informs the health-care research agenda. Schwandt (2000) has articulated the importance of this in social inquiry:

> Social inquiry is a distinctive praxis, a kind of activity that in the doing transforms the very theory and aims that guide it. In other words, as one engages in the "practical" activities of generating and interpreting data to answer questions about the meaning of what others are doing and saying and then transforming that understanding into public knowledge, one inevitably takes up "theoretical" concerns about what constitutes knowledge and how it is to be justified, about the nature and aim of social theorizing and so forth. In sum, acting and thinking, practice and theory, are linked in a continuous process of critical reflection and transformation (pp. 190–191).

Conclusion

Within contemporary research, interpretive methodologies used singly in studies provide the basis for most of the interpretive research and scholarship in healthcare and the human sciences, and make crucial contributions to the knowledge of most disciplines. There is no intention within this chapter to privilege multiple-methodologies inquiries over single-methodology research. The primary concern of the researcher must always be the phenomenon, from which the research question is derived, and only subsequent to this can decisions be made as to the most appropriate research methodology, design, and methods to fulfill the purposes of the research. However, interpretive research and scholarship are creative processes, and "methods and methodology are not always singular, *a priori,* fixed and unchanging" (Horsfall, Byrne-Armstrong, & Higgs, 2001, p. 5, emphasis original), and thus worldviews and methodologies will continue to grow and develop with the creativity and insight of interpretive researchers, as they consider emerging ways of investigating the complex social world. In this chapter, an argument has been presented for using multiple interpretive methodologies to increase the richness of research findings. There are many possibilities for advancing knowledge in healthcare and the human sciences, and developing healthcare research though such studies. However, there are also enduring paradigmatic, epistemological, and methodological issues and concerns that require further debate before there is a substantial or sufficient body of knowledge related to the use of multiple interpretive methodologies in healthcare and the human sciences. These concerns and tensions have been highlighted in this chapter. They are, however, considered as challenges rather than limitations. It is within these very tensions that the promise of multiple interpretive methodologies may be found. In exploring these issues this chapter argues for the primary importance of a match between the phenomenon, the research questions, the paradigmatic underpinnings, the logic of the method (Meetoo & Temple, 2003), and the research process. As researchers continue to develop interpretive research methodologies and ways of combining interpretive methodologies, the possibilities for advancing healthcare research will be expanded.

Acknowledgments

The author wishes to acknowledge and thank Professor Anne McMurray for her thoughtful comments on an initial draft of this chapter, and the anonymous reviewers for their helpful feedback.

Notes

1. A paradigm incorporates a set of assumptions, beliefs, and viewpoints regarding the social world, and how we know that social world. Such epistemological, ontological and axiological assumptions provide a frame for an inquiry.

2. Bracketing, such as is used in Husserlian phenomenology, involves consciously eliminating preconceived notions about a phenomenon. The researcher aims to disconnect from their assumptions about a phenomenon and in this way come closer to the essence of the phenomenon (Koch, 1995).

References

Appignanesi, R., & Garrett, C. (1999). *Introduction to postmodernism*. Cambridge: Icon Books.

Appleton, J. V., & King, L. (2002). Journeying from the philosophical contemplation of constructivism to the methodological pragmatics of health services research. *Journal of Advanced Nursing 40*, 641–648.

Baker, C., Norton, S., Young, P., & Ward, S. (1998). An exploration of methodological pluralism in nursing research. *Research in Nursing and Health 21*, 545–555.

Baker, C., Wuest, J., & Stern, P. (1992). Method slurring: The grounded theory/phenomenology example. *Journal of Advanced Nursing 17*, 1355–1360.

Barbour, R. S. (1998). Mixing qualitative methods: Quality assurance or qualitative quagmire? *Qualitative Health Research 8*, 352–361.

Begley, C. M. (1996). Using triangulation in nursing research. *Journal of Advanced Nursing 24*, 122–128.

Benner, P. (1994). The tradition and skill of interpretive phenomenology in studying health, illness, and caring practices. In P. Benner, *Interpretive phenomenology: Embodiment, caring, and ethics in health and illness* (pp. 99–127). Thousand Oaks, CA: Sage Publications.

Breitmayer, B. J., Ayres, L., & Knafl, K. A. (1993). Triangulation in qualitative research: Evaluation of completeness and confirmation purposes. *IMAGE: Journal of Nursing Scholarship 25*, 237–243.

Brewer, J., & Hunter, A. (1989). *Multimethod research: A synthesis of styles*. Newbury Park, CA: Sage Publications.

Cheek, J. (1999). Influencing practice or simply esoteric? Researching health care using postmodern approaches. *Qualitative Health Research 9*, 383–392.

Clark, A. M. (1998). The qualitative-quantitative debate: Moving from positivism and confrontation to post-positivism and reconciliation. *Journal of Advanced Nursing 27*, 1242–1249.

Coyle, J., & Williams, B. (2000). An exploration of the epistemological intricacies of using qualitative data to develop a quantitative measure of user views of health care. *Journal of Advanced Nursing 31*, 12;35–1243.

Crotty, M. (1998). *The foundations of social research*. St. Leonards, Australia: Allen & Unwin.

Darlington, Y., & Scott, D. (2002). *Qualitative research in practice: Stories from the field*. Buckingham: Open University Press.

Davis, K., & Glass, N. (1999). Contemporary nursing theories and contemporary nursing: Advancing nursing care for those who are marginalised. *Contemporary Nurse 8*(2), 32–38.

D'Cruz, H. (2001). The fractured lens· Methodology in perspective. In H. Byrne-Armstrong, J. Higgs, & D. Horsfall (Eds.), *Critical moments in qualitative research* (pp. 17–29). Oxford: Butterworth-Heinemann.

Denzin, N. K. (1989). *The research act: A theoretical introduction to sociological methods* (3rd Ed.). Englewood Cliffs, NJ: Prentice Hall.

Denzin, N. K., & Lincoln, Y. S. (2000). The discipline and practice of qualitative research. In N. K. Denzin & Y. S. Lincoln (Eds.), *Handbook of qualitative research* (2nd Ed.). (pp. 1–28). Thousand Oaks, CA: Sage.

Diekelmann, N., & Ironside, P. (1998). Hermeneutics. In J. Fitzpatrick (Ed.), *Encyclopedia of nursing research* (pp. 243–245). New York: Springer.

Draucker, C. B. (1999). Knowing what to do: Coping with sexual violence by male intimates. *Qualitative Health Research 9*, 588–601.

Draucker, C. B. (2001). Learning the harsh realities of life: Sexual violence, disillusionment and meaning. *Health Care for Women International 22*, 67–84.

Draucker, C. B., & Stern, P. N. (2000). Women's responses to sexual violence by male intimates. *Western Journal of Nursing Research 22*(4), 385–406.

Erzberger, C., & Kelle, U. (2003). Making inferences in mixed methods: Rules of integration.

In A. Tashakkori & C. Teddlie (Eds.), *Handbook of mixed methods in social and behavioral research* (pp. 457–488). Thousand Oaks, CA: Sage.

Finfgeld, D. L. (2003). Metasynthesis: The state of the art. *Qualitative Health Research 13,* 893–904.

Foss, C., & Ellefsen, B. (2002). The value of combining qualitative and quantitative approaches in nursing research by means of method triangulation. *Journal of Advanced Nursing 40,* 242–248.

Foucault, M. (1979). Interview with Lucette Finas. In M. Morris & P. Patten (Eds.), *Michel Foucault: Power, truth, strategy.* Sydney: Feral Publications.

Gadamer, H. G. (1994). *Truth and method* (J. Weinsheimer & D. G. Marshall, Trans.). (Rev. Ed.). New York: Continuum. (Original work published 1960.)

Greene, J. C., & Caracelli, V. J. (1997). Defining and describing the paradigm issue in mixed-method evaluation. In J. C. Greene & V. J. Caracelli (Eds.), *Advances in mixed-method evaluation: The challenges and benefits of integrating diverse paradigms* (pp. 5–18). San Francisco: Jossey-Bass.

Guba, E. G., & Lincoln, Y. S. (1994). Competing paradigms in qualitative research. In N. K. Denzin & Y. S. Lincoln (Eds.), *Handbook of qualitative research* (pp. 105–117). Thousand Oaks, CA: Sage Publications.

Gubrium, J. F., & Holstein, J. A. (1997). *The new language of qualitative method.* Oxford: Oxford University Press.

Heidegger, M. (1962). *Being and Time* (J. Macquarrie & E. Robinson, Trans). New York: Harper Collins. (Original work published 1927.)

Horsfall, D., Byrne-Armstrong, H., & Higgs, J. (2001). Researching critical moments. In H. Byrne-Armstrong, J. Higgs, & D. Horsfall (Eds.), *Critical moments in qualitative research* (pp. 3–16). Oxford: Butterworth-Heinemann.

Janesick, V. J. (1998). The dance of qualitative research design: Metaphor, methodolatry, and meaning. In N. K. Denzin & Y. S. Lincoln (Eds.), *Strategies of qualitative inquiry* (pp. 35–55). Thousand Oaks, CA: Sage.

Janesick, V. J. (2000). The choreography of qualitative research design: Minuets, improvisation, and crystallization. In N. K. Denzin & Y. S. Lincoln (Eds.), *Handbook of qualitative research* (2nd Ed.). (pp. 379–399). Thousand Oaks, CA: Sage.

Kimchi, J., Polvika, B., & Stevenson, J. S. (1991). Triangulation: Operational definitions. *Nursing Research 40,* 364–366.

Koch, T. (1995). Interpretive approaches in nursing research: The influence of Husserl and Heidegger. *Journal of Advanced Nursing 21,* 827–836.

Koch, T. (1996). Implementation of a hermeneutic inquiry in nursing: Philosophy, rigour and representation. *Journal of Advanced Nursing 24,* 174–184.

Langridge, M. E., & Ahern, K. (2003). A case report on using mixed methods in qualitative research. *Collegian 10*(4), 32–36.

Lincoln, Y. S., & Guba, E. G. (2000). Paradigmatic controversies, contradictions, and emerging confluences. In N. K. Denzin & Y. S. Lincoln (Eds.), *Handbook of qualitative research* (2nd Ed.). (pp. 163–188). Thousand Oaks, CA: Sage.

Lowes, L., & Prowse, M. A. (2001). Standing outside the interview process: The illusion of objectivity in phenomenological data generation. *International Journal of Nursing Studies 38,* 471–480.

Meetoo, D., & Temple, B. (2003). Issues in multi-method research: Constructing self care. *International Journal of Qualitative Methods 2*(3). Article 1. Retrieved 15 October 2003 from http://www.ualberta.ca/~ijqm/english/engframeset.html.

Miles, M. B., & Huberman, A. M. (1994). *Qualitative data analysis: An expanded source-book* (2nd Ed.). Thousand Oaks, CA: Sage.

Miller, S. I., & Fredericks, M. (2002). Naturalistic inquiry and reliabilism: A compatible epistemological grounding. *Qualitative Health Research* 12, 982–989.

Milliken, P. J., & Schreiber, R. S. (2001). Can you "do" grounded theory without symbolic interactionism? In R. S. Schreiber & P. N. Stern (Eds.), *Using grounded theory in nursing* (pp. 177–190). New York: Springer.

Moore, B. (Ed.). (1996). *The Australian pocket Oxford dictionary* (4th Ed.). Melbourne: Oxford University Press.

Morse, J. M. (2001). Situating grounded theory within qualitative inquiry. In R. S. Schreiber & P. N. Stern (Eds.), *Using grounded theory in nursing* (pp. 1–16). New York: Springer.

Morse, J. M. (2003). Principles of mixed methods and multimethod research design. In A. Tashakkori & C. Teddlie (Eds.), *Handbook of mixed methods in social and behavioral research* (pp. 189–208). Thousand Oaks, CA: Sage.

Morse, J. M., & Chung, S. E. (2003). Towards holism: The significance of methodological pluralism. *International Journal of Qualitative Methods* 2(3), Article 2. Retrieved 15 October 2003 from http://www.ualberta.ca/~ijqm/english/engframeset.html.

Palmer, R. E. (1969). *Hermeneutics*. Evanston, IL: Northwestern University Press.

Patton, M. Q. (2002). *Qualitative research and evaluation methods* (3rd Ed.). Thousand Oaks, CA: Sage.

Plager, K. A. (1994). Hermeneutic phenomenology: A methodology for family health and promotion study in nursing. In P. Benner (Ed.), *Interpretive phenomenology: Embodiment, caring and ethics in health and illness*. Thousand Oaks, CA: Sage.

Polit, D. F., & Beck, C. T. (2004). *Nursing research: Principles and methods* (7th Ed.). Philadelphia: Lippincott Williams & Wilkins.

Polkinghorne, D. (1983). *Methodology for the human sciences: Systems of inquiry*. Albany: State University of New York Press.

Pursley-Crotteau, S., Bunting, S. M., & Draucker, C. B. (2001). Grounded theory and hermeneutics: Contradictory or complementary methods of nursing research? In R. S. Schreiber & P. N. Stern (Eds.), *Using grounded theory in nursing* (pp. 191–210). New York: Springer.

Rice, P. L., & Ezzy, D. (1999). *Qualitative research methods: A health focus*. Melbourne: Oxford University Press.

Richardson, L. (1994). Writing: A method of inquiry. In N. K. Denzin & Y. S. Lincoln (Eds.), *Handbook of qualitative research*. (pp. 516–529). Thousand Oaks, CA: Sage.

Rorty, R. (1999). *Philosophy and social hope*. London: Penguin.

Sadala, M. L. A., & Adorno, R. D. C. (2002). Phenomenology as a method to investigate the experience lived: A perspective from Husserl and Merleau Ponty's thought. *Journal of Advanced Nursing* 37, 282–293.

Sandelowski, M. (1995). Triangles and crystals: On the geometry of qualitative research. *Research in Nursing and Health* 18, 569–574.

Sandelowski, M. (2000). Combining qualitative and quantitative sampling, data collection, and analysis techniques in mixed-method studies. *Research in Nursing and Health* 23, 246–255.

Sandelowski, M. (2003). Tables or tableaux? The challenges of writing and reading mixed methods studies. In A. Tashakkori & C. Teddlie (Eds.), *Handbook of mixed methods in social and behavioral research* (2nd Ed.). (pp. 321–350). Thousand Oaks, CA: Sage.

Sandelowski, M., & Barroso, J. (2002). Finding the findings in qualitative studies. *Journal of Nursing Scholarship 34*, 213–219.

Sandelowski, M., & Barroso, J. (2003). Towards a metasynthesis of qualitative findings on motherhood in HIV-positive women. *Research in Nursing and Health 26*, 153–170.

Sandelowski, M., Docherty, S., & Emden, C. (1997). Qualitative metasynthesis: Issues and techniques. *Research in Nursing and Health 20*, 365–371.

Savage, J. (2000). One voice, different tunes: Issues raised by dual analysis of a segment of qualitative data. *Journal of Advanced Nursing 31*, 1493–1500.

Schreiber, R., Crooks, D., & Stern, P. N. (1997). Qualitative meta-analysis. In J. M. Morse (Ed.), *Completing a qualitative project: Details and dialogue*. (pp. 311–326). Thousand Oaks, CA: Sage.

Schwandt, T. A. (2000). Three epistemological stances for qualitative inquiry. In N. K. Denzin & Y. S. Lincoln (Eds.), *Handbook of qualitative research* (2nd Ed.). (pp. 189–213). Thousand Oaks, CA: Sage.

Shih, F. J. (1998). Triangulation in nursing research: Issues of conceptual clarity and purpose. *Journal of Advanced Nursing 28*, 631–641.

Speziale, H. J. S., & Carpenter, D. R. (2003). *Qualitative research in nursing: Advancing the humanistic imperative*. (3rd Ed.). Philadelphia: Lippincott.

Spradley, J. (1979). *The Ethnographic interview*. New York: Holt Rinehart & Winston.

Tashakkori, A., & Teddlie, C. (1998). *Mixed methodology: Combining qualitative and quantitative approaches*. Thousand Oaks, CA: Sage.

Teddlie, C., & Tashakkori, A. (2003). Major issues and controversies in the use of mixed methods in the social and behavioural sciences. In A. Tashakkori & C. Teddlie (Eds.), *Handbook of mixed methods in social and behavioral research* (pp. 3–50). Thousand Oaks, CA: Sage.

Thorne, S. (1997). The art (and science) of critiquing qualitative research. In J. M. Morse (Ed.), *Completing a qualitative project: Details and dialogue* (pp. 117–132). Thousand Oaks, CA: Sage.

Thorne, S., Joachim, G., Paterson, B., & Canam, C. (2002). Influence of the research frame on qualitatively derived health science knowledge. *International Journal of Qualitative Methods 1*(1), Article 1. Retrieved 15 October 2003 from http://www .ualberta.ca/~ijqm/english/engframeset.html.

Todres, L., & Wheeler, S. (2001). The complementarity of phenomenology, hermeneutics and existentialism as a philosophical perspective for nursing research. *International Journal of Nursing Studies 38*(1), 1–8.

Twinn, S. (2003). Status of mixed methods research in nursing. In A. Tashakkori & C. Teddlie (Eds.), *Handbook of mixed methods in social and behavioral research* (pp. 541–556). Thousand Oaks, CA: Sage.

Walter, R., Glass, N., & Davis, K. (2001) Epistemology at work: The ontological relationship between feminist methods, intersubjectivity and nursing research—a research exemplar. *Contemporary Nurse 10*(3/4), 265–272.

Wilson, H. S., & Hutchinson, S. A. (1991). Triangulation of qualitative methods: Heideggerian hermeneutics and grounded theory. *Qualitative Health Research 1*, 263–276.

Wimpenny, P., & Gass, J. (2000). Interviewing in phenomenology and grounded theory: Is there a difference? *Journal of Advanced Nursing 31*(6), 1485–1492. Retrieved 30 January 2004, from *www.blackwell-synergy.com*.

Wuest, J., & Merritt-Gray, M. (2001). Feminist grounded theory revisited: Practical issues and new understandings. In R. S. Schreiber & P. N. Stern (Eds.), *Using grounded theory in nursing* (pp. 159–176). New York: Springer.

6

The Thinking of Research

ELIZABETH SMYTHE

What nature of thinking underpins research? Books on how to do research lay out the step-by-step tasks. Research articles report findings. This study, in contrast, takes on the challenge of uncovering the thinking of research. "The main characteristic of mental activities is their invisibility," suggests Arendt (1978, p. 71). Could it be that the thinking of research is so taken for granted, such a part of embodied experience, that it is seldom seen as "what it is?"

The impetus for this study was sparked when I presented a paper comparing phenomenology with scientific, quantitative methodology. In it, I drew from Heidegger's writing where he hailed research as useful and indispensable but suggested it was "thinking of a special kind" (1959/1966b, p. 45). He went on to distinguish between calculative thinking and meditative thinking:

whenever we plan, research, and organise, we always reckon with conditions that are given. We take them into account with the calculated intention of their serving specific purposes. Thus we can count on definite results. This calculation is the mark of all thinking that plans and investigates. Such thinking remains calculation even if it neither works with numbers nor uses an adding machine or computer. Calculative thinking computes. It computes ever new, ever more promising and at the same time more economical possibilities. Calculative thinking races from one prospect to the next. Calculative thinking never stops, never collects itself. Calculative thinking is not meditative thinking, not thinking which contemplates the meaning which reigns in everything that is. (Heidegger, 1959/1966b, p. 45–46)

My assumption that the thinking of quantitative research is calculative was met with passionate contestation. Colleagues who work in the

223

quantitative paradigm argued that they also engage in meditative thinking. Heidegger describes meditative thinking in this way:

meditative thinking does not just happen by itself any more than does calculative
thinking. At times it requires a greater effort. It demands more practice. It is in
need of even more delicate care than any other genuine craft. But it must also be
able to bide its time, to await as does the farmer, whether the seed will come up
and ripen. (Heidegger, 1959/1966b, p. 46–47)

I was called to conversation: conversation with myself; have I made unwarranted assumptions? Conversation with the writings of Heidegger and
related scholars; what are they saying about thinking? And, more importantly, conversations with experienced researchers to ask them to describe
stories and to put into words the invisible "thinking" of their research. This
is an interpretive phenomenological study of those conversations.

Putting Words to the Unsayable

The audacity of this search for the thinking of research is captured by
Gray: "To define thinking for someone else would be as hopeless as describing colours to the blind" (Heidegger, 1954/1968, p. xii). To define
thinking is to put words to the unsayable. Even to describe thinking is to
merely offer glimpses of momentary memories, or to parade the products of thought. Thinking itself remains buried in the ebb and flow of
every engagement with self and other. Let me not pretend that this study
will do more than point to a sense of "what might be."
    In the introduction to his translation of Heidegger's book *What Is
Called Thinking?* (Heidegger, 1954/1968) Gray offers some ideas from
which questions arise. He avers: "To be able to think does not wholly depend on our will and wish, though much does depend on whether we
prepare ourselves to hear that call to think when it comes and respond in
the appropriate manner" (p. xi). The theme, "Hearing the call to thinking," is a central one in the data analysis. According to Gray: "Thinking is
determined by that which is to be thought as well as by him who thinks"
(p. xi). The person who thinks is integral to the thinking that comes to be
revealed. The participants in this study are from different health disciplines and embrace a variety of methodological perspectives. Each is a

unique individual of time, place and history. Closely associated with "hearing the call" is the notion that each person will respond in a manner related to who they are and how they think. This theme reveals "Thinking as self." Thinking is not to be taken for granted: "Only the thinking that is truly involved, patient, and disciplined by long practice can come to know either the hidden or disclosed character of truth" (p. xi). How then do these health researchers tell us of their involvement, their patience, and their disciplined strategies of thinking? These strategies will be explored within the theme "Thinking as research."

Heidegger (1954/1968) seeks to describe the nature of thinking as experienced. "We come to know what it means to think when we ourselves try to think" (p. 3). Trying to think is never easy. Perhaps thinking is at its best when we cease trying and simply let the thinking come, but in doing so, do we lose the understanding of how it is to think? Is the richest thinking of research lost to the telling because in the deep concentration there is no space to think of the thinking itself? Is telling always "after the event," or diminished in some way because the talking distracts from the thinking?

Could research be likened to cabinet making? Heidegger asserts that to become a true cabinetmaker "he makes himself answer and respond above all to the different kinds of wood and to the shapes slumbering within the wood. . . . In fact, this relatedness to wood is what maintains the whole craft. Without that relatedness, the craft will never be anything but empty busywork" (1954/1968, p. 15). The poet Rainer Maria Rilke, in writing advice to a young poet offers these words: "Few things are in fact as accessible to reason or to language as people will generally try to make us believe. Most phenomena are unsayable, and have their being in a dimension which no word has ever entered" (1929/2002, p. 173). Can the cabinetmaker ever adequately put into words the essence of the skill that creates? Can the researcher, one expected to offer new understandings to practice, bring to word the skill of thinking that translates felt understanding into a saying of meaning? The themes presented in this study use these words as they seek to grasp meaning: "Hearing the Call to Thinking: Caring about Others"; "Thinking as Self: Shaping and Being Shaped by Thinking," and "Thinking as Research: Research as Thinking." Gathering these themes together is "Thinking as Being in Thought" and "Thinking as Thinking Itself."

Method

The embodied thinking behind this study arises from Heidegger-ian hermeneutic doctoral study, other postdoctoral work, and ongoing supervision of students using such methodology. I spend much time grappling with the writings of Heidegger. I engage in dialogue with the international hermeneutic community. I critique (and have critiqued) both my own work and that of students. The understandings have grown within me. In conducting this study my interest is already-there, leading me forward almost without thought. I am drawn to the participants, knowing already whom I would like to interview. As I hear their stories, they resonate with my tentative thoughts. As I dwell with the data the seeing comes. As I write the words they flow almost of their own making. I am in-experience rather than prethinking the next step (although some prethinking, such as gaining ethics approval, is necessary).

Following approval from the Auckland University of Technology Ethics Committee, New Zealand, I sent e-mails to ten experienced researchers within a health faculty. They came from nursing, midwifery, physiotherapy, and psychology backgrounds. Seven people immediately said "yes" to participation in the study. I proceeded to interview them one by one, usually in my office. I made an attempt to have a variety of methodological positions present, so I approached four additional people, who agreed to be part of the study. Three experienced nurse researchers from the United States of America crossed my path over the time of my study and generously agreed to participate.

Describing specific research studies identifies researchers to people who know their work. Therefore, we agreed that it would be more ethical to respectfully acknowledge the identity of all participants. The majority share a nursing background, unless stated otherwise. Professor Gregory Kolt is an experienced quantitative researcher from a background in physiotherapy and psychology. Dr. Peter McNair is a physiotherapist and biomechanist who leads a physical rehabilitation research center and is also an experienced quantitative researcher. Dr. Anne Barlow heads the Centre for Midwifery and Women's Health Research. She has developed expertise in evaluation research. Professor David Allen from the University of Washington with expertise in the critical/feminist/postmodern paradigms was a visiting scholar during the time of data collection. To my surprise the research study he chose to talk about was the quantitative challenges of a multimethod longitudinal study. Associate Professor Lynne Giddings is an eclectic researcher who did her doctoral studies at the University of Colorado. She tells her story of historical narrative inquiry informed by critical/feminist assumptions. Dr. Marion Jones uses ethnographic methods, informed by Bourdieu. Dr. Debbie Payne describes her preferred research methodology as Foucauldian Discourse Analysis. Dr. Deb Spence is an experienced hermeneutic researcher, drawing from the writings of Gadamer. Annette Dickinson has recently completed her phenomenological doctoral study. Barbara McKenzie Green is a keen grounded theorist. Professor Jo Walton reflects on her experience of working with a variety of methodologies. Professors Sharon Sims (Sherry) and Melinda Swenson both visited New Zealand and were visited by me in the United States of America. Sharon brings a background of grounded theory and Melinda one of phenomenology. Their recent work has involved "thinking together experiences" using phenomenology.

I began the interviews by asking the person to think of a research study that they had particularly enjoyed, or that "felt like them." From a phenomenological method perspective, it was important to situate the account of thinking within a story of a particular study. In this way the participant recounts specific experiences rather than more generalized statements. The studies themselves are not the interest of this paper. Rather, they serve as a context, an anchor, to keep the data as primordial (close to experience) as possible, so thinking may be captured as remembered within particular research moments.

I started the conversation by asking participants to tell the story of the study. My questions simply took the story from one step of the narrative account of the study to the next, always seeking to reveal the invisible thinking of the researcher. The researcher was prompted to stay engaged in the telling of the story. I listened for descriptive accounts of "thinking," at which point I encouraged a slowing down, to enable those thoughts to be said out loud rather than quickly skimmed over. Stories were crafted from the transcripts to bring forth a clear, uncluttered telling (Caelli, 2001). At times I added words to bring ease of reading, or moved parts of the story around to keep like things together. I tried not to change the meaning. On reflection a limitation of this study is the paradox that in "tidying" the data, I have removed indicators of thinking-as-experienced, such as: "I suppose . . ." "I think . . ." "I guess . . ." "Maybe . . ." (As an interpretive researcher, I am always aware of how conventions of data presentation call for continual thought.) Initial interpretations were returned to each participant. Some minor changes and clarifications resulted from that process. Data analysis has been through a process of writing, rewriting, and writing again (Van Manen, 1990). The first written interpretation closely considered each participant as a unique thinking researcher, situated within a particular methodology. The second layer of writing stood back to capture the common experiences or recurring themes that run across participants and methodologies. From that draft I brought new calls to understanding what was not-yet-thought. The writing was forever seeking the words that best captured the thinking. The final draft of this paper has been returned to participants for approval.

The Uncovering of Thinking

The hermeneutic tension between parts and whole (Gadamer, 1965/1982) underlies this exegesis of thinking. Within the experience of thinking there are no subheadings to categorize or arrange thinking. Thinking lives in rich, multidimensional ebb and flow, circling and recircling. Nevertheless, the written account demands a breaking down, and an order. I begin this discussion with the common experience that something prompts or calls researchers to thinking.

Hearing the Call to Thinking: Caring About Others

In the midst of the myriad opportunities that waft past each researcher, how is it that some linger, some demand close attention, and others go by almost unnoticed? What is it that calls interest and sparks the beginnings of a research study? For these researchers, caring and a social concern for participants often shaped their call to thinking.

GREGORY: There was a lot of literature out there to say that participating in physical activity is good for you. Then again, we also knew that for older people, quite often there are lots of barriers to their participating. So we identified that how we actually get people to do more of these activities is the difficult thing. We took a pretty careful look at the literature. That gave us a lot of information initially about how we can get people doing more walking. The thinking behind it was that research says that physical activity is great, but it doesn't actually tell you what you have to do to get people doing that activity. So there was, I suppose, a social conscience aspect there as well, with the need to be able to do something, to be able to apply these many research findings to an actual community.

For Gregory and his team the literature representing previous research studies indicated what had already been done, and more importantly, what was still to be thought. Nobody had yet discovered a way of ensuring that older people do more walking. From the collective research of the international community, this study was the next step. The call to thinking was shaped by careful searching and reading. Gregory signals, however, that it was more than that. Central to the thinking experience is a sense that unless research is able to have an impact on the issues it examines, then what is the point? For Gregory, caring about the health needs of others is a central concern in his thinking. Research needs to be worth doing for the sake of the community of interest. Peter talks of a study that arose from a sense of need:

PETER: The research that I am thinking about was one that is based around osteoarthritis. What made it happen was a real event. This study came about because there were a whole lot of people that got taken off a waiting list for joint replacements. They go back into the community, and the GP [General Practitioner] goes, "What do I do with them now?" We saw some six or seven hundred people, just being cut from lists.

As physiotherapists, Peter and his research team were distressed that hundreds of people with osteoarthritis were being left in pain and disability, no longer with even the hope of being on a list. The call to thinking was a human-to-human call of wanting to help. It seems they brought to their thinking a knowing of what it might feel like to be in severe pain, to struggle with physical disability, and then to have hope of help taken away. They respond to the silent yet anguished call to thinking. Anne heard a call in the midst of a conversation:

ANNE: Deciding to do the last study came out of a colleague's frustrations at not being able to get any funding just to paint and decorate the maternity unit, real basic stuff, and because of that she felt that the midwives were not being valued. I said to her, "What would be good would be an evaluation that was able to show how good the practice really is," and she thought that was a wonderful idea. That is how it started, out of a feeling over real practice concerns.

As Anne listened to her colleague's frustration and concern she heard the call-to-thinking of a midwife expressing a deep concern. No one seemed to care about the run-down state of the maternity unit. Anne saw the opportunity to bring her skill of evaluation research as a tool towards creating change. Her research could demonstrate the value of the unit and persuade funders that it was worthy of investment. Embedded in an ethic of caring for others, Anne's thinking embraced the understanding that the voice of research may be loud and strong. David also understands the political nature of research:

DAVID: When I was department chair of a psychiatric nursing program part of my portfolio was to get the department reconnected to the public mental health services. The U.S. was imprisoning the mentally ill at a vast rate, and so the jails and prisons are the largest mental health providers in the United States. So that then directed my attention to that phenomenon. I have an overall interest in trying to improve the care of people with mental illness and trying to keep them from going into prison in the first place, trying to get them out sooner, but in this case what we are trying to do is make the lives of those who are in it more tolerable. Politically, I am committed to maintaining this prison research because of an African American friend of mine who is much older, [who] says the problem is that "you" white liberals can leave. He is correct about that, and so a piece of me is committed to staying with the prison work. I could intellectually leave the prison study.

David was drawn into the issues of mental health and prisons as a task required of his department chair role. Once there he came face-to-face with enormous needs. The call to do research is relentless. This call to thinking is not about doing the research that is of his intellectual choice. It is rather a thinking that co-occurs and both shapes and is shaped by David's social commitment. Being able to walk away is too easy. Staying proves commitment. Lynne describes how her commitment arose:

LYNNE: I recall the first meeting with my Ph.D. supervisor; I came with two pages of possible research topics. Much later, I did a presentation on lesbianism to my research class, and it was the reaction of people in that group as I presented. I was standing there watching, the eyes turned down, seeing the whispering. I can remember at the time feeling my voice going to go, and having to reclaim it. In the following days and weeks, it was hearing the negative responses of students to bringing up the topic, let alone doing research on it, and that politically captured me. It was sort of like, "Wow," I thought, "All this is happening, nice people are doing not nice things"; and I thought, "Something has to be done." So that made me think about "how do people who are different experience injustice within the mainstream," and "how do they in fact survive, what do they do, what is it like?"

In her call to thinking Lynne had many research topics catch her gaze. Her thinking was influenced by her ongoing experiences. Of particular importance was an experience of standing before a group of peers and talking about lesbianism. She felt the emotional assault of social inequity and knew something was wrong. From her own "taste" of what it felt like to be treated as "different" she asked herself the question, "How do others survive?" The call to thinking for Lynne is a deep personal response to social injustice. It is her care for "others" that leads her thinking.

But not all researchers presented a clear and articulated "beginning of the thinking" in a particular study. Sometimes an interest in a phenomenon precedes the call for thinking in terms of a particular study. Other times, it is the availability of funding that calls out thinking. It can also be the case that thinking is called out as an inexplicable, unarticulated experience; that is one that occurs "somehow or other" as Jo describes:

JO: The study I am thinking about is an evaluation study of mental health services. I used to laugh and have coffee with the guy who was from the core liaison area, and somehow or other the idea came up that this service ought to be evaluated. And we decided that we would put this thing together.

Drinking coffee, laughing, talking together, and suddenly "somehow or other" thinking arrives and an idea is born and put together. The call to thinking is within the dynamic experiences of conversation-as-dialogue and being-together. Thinking arrives as a moment of conversation where thoughts enjoin and coalesce. Going-around-thinking finds the still point in which ideas become crafted by words, heads nod in agreement, and the way forward is chosen. Melinda and Sherry know this experience:

MELINDA: Here I am with a gerontology view and Sherry has a pediatric view, and how are we going to work together to do research in something that we both liked, and we can both relate to? And that's how we came to a study, which is called the Meaning of Home to Family Caregivers. I'd done a study on the meaning of home to elderly women, and I kind of missed it. I loved the literature and I liked reading about it, and so I wanted to continue to work on it somehow.
SHERRY: Part of my work that went into that made both angles a little bit newer. I had done a grounded theory study on families who were caring for technology-dependent children at home. It seemed to us that if you brought technology, the sort of medical gaze, into the home we could expand that notion of the meaning of home in this whole new context.

The call to thinking arrives again in the connecting conversations of Melinda and Sherry, who found a shared point of "caring-about" related to clients in their homes. They both shared the relevance of asking questions about technology within home healthcare. The call to thinking arrived within the relationship of positive regard to research together. With the synergy came expanded possibilities for thinking together.

These explicated stories challenge the assumptions made in some research texts that posit controlling the thinking behind a research question. The account of thinking as Gregory illuminated: searching the literature, finding the gap, addressing the practice need, is a necessary call to thinking but not sufficient to wider possibilities of thinking. This study revealed the call to thinking often comes not so much as a rational, predictable, analytic "thinking" experience as embodied moments of unpredictable knowing. Something clicks, resonates, and provokes a thought that arrives and illuminates the way forward of a new research study.

What calls thinking? Do we school doctoral students to reflect on the importance of their caring-about-others? Do we realize that such caring, left free to reveal itself, so often leads the way forward to the choice of a question? This study revealed how the interests and concerns of researchers and the plight of "the other" all shape and are shaped by the call to thinking. Study participants showed how as researchers social responsibility often "sustained" them and was an enduring practice in their lives.

Researchers in this study described the importance of thinking within their research experiences. Are there ways to enhance the thinking spaces and places for researchers? Are there research environments that encourage listening and responding to the call to thinking (Diekelmann, 2005)? Are the places where researchers conduct their scholarship rich, welcoming, thoughtful, and thought-provoking environments? Are they, in contrast, isolating and stressful spaces that close down on the call to thinking?

Heidegger (1927/1995) suggests we are in-the-world in a state of mind in which our moods are already there. We feel passionate, frustrated, excited before we translate such feelings to words. Our moods call us to thought, show us what matters, and capture our attention. The call cannot be manufactured within. It must arise of its own making. While a colleague may suggest ideas for research the moods hear those ideas before the logical, rational, cognitive self takes charge. To hear a call is to be attuned to the always-already-knowing self, to the bubbling mood, to the already-there excitement, passion, or concern. If the idea leads only to thoughts of practicalities, or generates a yawn, then it is merely an idea, not a call.

Research preparations, particularly the development of thinking as a skill and a process, often are influenced by textbooks. Does the textbook description of the research process privilege a rational, linear, and analytic approach to the-call-to-thinking that accompanies research? Is there a place in research preparation to explicate the common experiences of researchers as they are called to thinking? In this study, researchers often described how the call to thinking arises out of conversations or dialogues with colleagues where listening is attuned and held open and problematic. Do we have places in the preparation of new researchers or in our daily research environments that encourages this kind of dialogue? How and in what kind of environments do we spend our time as researchers? How much of what researchers do is committed to thinking and to creating and enhancing experiences that call-out thinking? Do we respect the importance of the call to thinking in our lives as researchers? Are we on watch for the flicker of excitement, or the discussion that grows into something where the pace of talking speeds, the faces flush, and time flies? Do we listen for the "Yes" that resounds with confidence and excitement? Do we ever stop to explore with the student the call to thinking and the experience of thinking that lie within and around their topic of research? Have we the courage to counsel a student out of a perfectly sound study opportunity when the student clearly describes no engagement with thinking or the presence of a resonating call to thinking?

According to Heidegger (1927/1995), humans are always already being called. How humans respond is the matter at hand. Doing a thorough review of literature and reflecting on the meaning and significance of extant research is one way to experience a call to thinking. Another is to seek out dialogues with others that are fertile converging conversations: thoughtful and thought provoking. Reflecting on past experiences and the implications of research all are possibilities in hearing the call to thinking. Perhaps more research is needed on this very important common experience of researchers—the call to thinking? Perhaps more complexity could be added to the assumptions about how to call-out thinking; specifically that a review of literature, precedes and gives rise to thinking that leads to the identification of a research problem.

Through studying how successful practicing researchers actually experience thinking in the conduct of their day-to-day research, the complexities of thinking practices such as the call-to-thinking can be identified and understanding extended. As well, ongoing critiques of current

approaches to thinking can be increased and further explicated. For example, are analytic approaches to thinking privileged because they reflect
the research process? Is thinking circumscribed by the research process?
The call to thinking lies in the mystery of a knowing that comes. To take
away the mystery by a circumscribed method or research process may be
to undermine something of essence to the thinking of research.

When the person comes from a place of care for the other, wanting to
help, striving to give voice, the call to thinking experiences both shapes
and is shaped by their concerns for social justice and well-being. It is
a breathing-thinking, knowing-what-matters experience. In contrast, I
have a picture of the "arms-length" researcher enacting the initiation of
a study by a thoughtful review of the literature as per the prescribed
method. While that in itself may generate a call, it may also be merely a
task in a series of methodical steps. In this study, researchers describe the
experience of being-called. Such thinking does not come on demand. It
can only arise if the embodied self is already engaged and thinking. To
dispense with the call may be to miss out vital underpinnings of the thinking experience.

Thinking as Self: Shaping and Being Shaped by Thinking

In hearing the call, does the researcher pause to consider the many
possible ways of responding to the call, or do they simply proceed as self-
being-self? Is their mind already running ahead and envisaging how the
study might proceed? In other words, does the call coming to their
unique-receiving-self shape the thinking down a certain path? And, how
does thinking shape the call?

GREGORY: The other thing that informed us taking that approach was that that
sort of area had been identified as a national health priority. We were very conscious of trying to attract some national funding. The sort of research we are talking about needed significant funding or else there was no way we could have
done it. It also stemmed quite clearly from a fair bit of earlier work I had done, so
the research was a logical next progression.

Thinking is always situated and contextual. Gregory knows that research funding matters, for without adequate resources the type of research he is involved with cannot proceed. His team keeps in front of
their thinking the national health priorities and considers ideas through

that lens. These are pragmatic decisions that make the research both possible and manageable within constraints of time and money. His support to the department for a part of his salary, financial support of research assistants, or his ability to keep current with his interests all shape his thinking and are shaped by his thinking. Thinking is a temporal and historical experience. For Gregory, this study links closely to previous thinking he has done. He knows the literature. He is already in-the-thinking of previous and present issues. The thinking of the research is already on-the-way before the study begins. The self prepares the way for self and others discerning what is realistic and possible. Peter also describes how thinking connects:

PETER: One of my research themes is osteoarthritis and rehabilitation and we already had a study going at a hospital, which was looking at a program of exercise, advice and education just prior to surgery. We were confident, based on what we had seen in our previous study, that we could make a difference to these people with severe osteoarthritis. We could improve their strength. We could decrease their pain. We could improve their function. We could improve their quality of life. What we did not know was how long the improvement lasted. So part of this study was to look at the effectiveness of our exercise program with these people, and then look at the detraining effect, and therefore be able to gauge when these people might need booster sessions along the way, to be able to monitor their progress over time.

The call to thinking arrived when hundreds of people were dropped off a waiting list. This event for Peter aroused a desire to "make a difference." The themes in this osteoarthritis study are neither linear nor discrete but rather describe common experiences that co-occur. Peter's research team was already conducting a research exercise program at this hospital. They already knew the research program was making a difference. A new context for thinking was now presented to involve these people in a study that moved on from earlier work. They would now explore how long a training program gives people relief. The thinking was circular and embraced everything they had already achieved. Further, the thinking generated attended to providing evidence for the ongoing efficacy of such programs. This thinking was utilitarian and it was in everybody's interests to embark on the new study. The thinking here is situated, historical, and circular; complete and neverending. Anne suggests there is also a personal dimension:

ANNE: I think that underlying my interest in evaluation research is some sense of wanting to improve things. At the end of the day I keep coming back to issues around social justice and equality; issues around the purpose of things that are there for public good that do not always do public good. I never really thought of it particularly in moralistic terms until perhaps in the last year. It is very seductive of course when you are in a helping profession and you have somebody come along and say, "Look you know, we cannot be heard here," and so I don't think you end up impartial. I don't believe you can ever be truly separate from what it is you are doing.

Anne offers how an interest in social justice shapes her thinking but also how she as a person is shaped by this kind of thinking. She cautions herself to be wary of thinking, recognizing the seductive nature of giving voice to the silent for the public good. Yet at the same time there is a sense of understanding that it is important for her to be involved in a quest to improve healthcare. The issues of social justice and equality clearly shape her thinking and sit comfortably with her sense of self and who she is becoming. David describes how he pays attention to the shape that will best serve the task:

DAVID: The increasing prevalence of poststructuralism was already showing up in my work and in my courses, and it became increasingly obvious that it was going to be really useful as a theoretical framework and as technology with respect to the prisoners. This piece of the study I think you would have to call a kind of quasi-experimental design. It is a way of trying to harness a traditional measurement technology to a justice study with a lot of risks in it.

For David, "being David" is to take on a poststructural openness to doing whatever needs to be done. Within the interview he acknowledged thinking that a quasi-experimental design is not a method he is particularly experienced in, but it is a good way of attacking this justice study. Poststructuralism frees him from thinking any one approach and rather places the focus of his thinking on what he seeks to achieve through the research. He sees poststructuralist thinking shaping in his "being." It is becoming the way he frames his outlook on things; another way research thinking shapes and is shaped by the researcher. Lynne knows that she reacts to situations in a way that resonates with her strong political beliefs:

LYNNE: It was my political, "it's not fair" that got me involved, because I tried to name or give voice to racism and heterosexism in the classroom. My family tells the story of me as a five-year-old deciding that something wasn't fair at school. It didn't matter that it was the teacher in authority. If something wasn't fair, I reacted against it. Once I get a sense of something not being fair, for me not to do something, I couldn't live with myself. You cannot let it go. If I don't do something, well, then I feel bad.

For Lynne there is a fairness monitor that shapes her thinking. When it rings an alarm she has no choice but to respond. To do nothing is to live with the guilt of ignoring the injustice. The up-welling of the need to challenge injustice in her thinking is not daunted by authority or by the derogatory attitudes of others. The self and who she is becoming shapes her thinking and knows what must be done. Marion talks of how the self "likes":

MARION: I think I was sold on Bourdieu on reading the title A *Theory of Practice*, because it was practice that I was talking about and everything else that I was reading was detracting from practice. I liked his concept that power is everywhere and stop putting it into particular boxes from the perspective that it is always negative, which it isn't. That appealed to me. His multidimensional processes allowed me to look at all of the data in a multidimensional way and try and get the value and worth out of it that demonstrated that nothing was simple. It allowed me to look at how an interplay of dimensions of peoples' thinking could give me a richer and deeper descriptive possibility of what was happening. How they understood it, how they created the tensions and how they could actually make that interplay work for them and not against them.

The call Bourdieu put forth resonated with Marion's own thinking. She was "sold" by the title. She "liked" his work. More than that, it allowed her to make sense of the world of practice in a manner that was congruent with her own thinking and experience. Do we read philosophers to find a new way of thinking and understanding the world, or do we search until we find an approach to thinking that puts into words what we already know? Or is it both? That is, perhaps what the researcher already knows shapes and is shaped by what philosophers or other texts say. Debbie talks of how she also was drawn to a particular philosopher:

DEBBIE: I had used Foucault in my master's thesis and knew that I always wanted to read further, but in my everyday life to actually sit down and read Foucault is not something I would do as a normal activity. Embarking on this study would create a legitimate structure for me to actually get to grips with his writings. I remembered my experiences during pregnancy and being labeled an "elderly primigravida." It seemed to me that my experience fitted his notion of subjectivity and labeling, being identified as one particular kind of person.

Thinking often shows up as reading, writing, and dialogue. The call to thinking for Debbie emerged as the opportunity to read more closely the writings of Foucault. The experiences of doctoral research would help her create an opportunity for further reading-as-thinking to achieve a greater depth of understanding. The dissertation topic followed. Her thinking embraced the personal experience of being labeled and held open a Foucauldian analysis. This was thinking in which the self was integrally interwoven. Deb, in contrast, needed to first find the philosopher she would draw from:

DEB: I looked at grounded theory for a while. I went to a workshop, which I didn't entirely agree with from a philosophical standpoint. I also found the method quite prescriptive. It just seemed to be a tremendous amount of minute work, in which case you risked losing the bigger, more significant picture somehow. Another probably stronger tug was critical social science. I knew that there were power elements inherent in my study topic, but I had experienced being a participant in another study and having the researcher "misinterpret," or differently interpret, my data by using a particular critical social lens. I guess you gradually start to piece together what matters to you about research, as well as what will work with your research question. I didn't want to go right back, if you like, in the Heideggerian sense of something that was primordial. Gadamer's work was ideal. It was all about understanding and bringing that to language. This is something that was not happening, and is not happening, in nursing. It is like a key that unlocks the door really.

Deb's thinking shapes and is shaped by her investigation of several methodologies until she discovers a place that resonates. She is very clear about why other methodologies don't appeal. In Gadamer she found her "ideal" guide. In her thinking, she knew what mattered to her. Gadamer gave her the key to thinking in a manner that felt congruent with her own sense of how to think through her topic. Barbara similarly explored methodologies, and where Deb rejected grounded theory, Barbara liked the thinking and what it could achieve:

BARBARA: I toyed with a number of methodologies. What I wanted to do was to be able to explore service processes so that people could see what gets in the way and what facilitates certain ways of working. And I liked grounded theory for that. I thought if I can reveal the processes of the work of registered nurses then that would help us to look at why things were, or were not, happening. I went to Glaser's website, I read all the books. I read and read and read. I worried it. I thought about it, I struggled with it. I struggled with some peoples' comments about it like: "Oh, he is just a post-positivist." Other people said, "But you are a critical social theorist, you are always into power. Why are you doing this? This will drive you crazy. Grounded theory will drive you crazy." But I still wanted to develop process, and nothing else could. I could not see how I could do it another way.

For Barbara, making the decision to use grounded theory challenged her thinking and was an experience rich in tension. Other people could see the thinking of a critical social theorist in her and tried to guide her in that direction. Some challenged the thinking of grounded theory, putting their own biases forward. Through all this Barbara is thinking what she wants the shape to be, and only grounded theory could do that. While in her thinking she explored other ways, she knew that for her to explore her topic in the way she knew it needed to be done, nothing else would do. Annette could have chosen grounded theory but did not:

ANNETTE: In choosing my methodology I knew that I needed to do something that was familiar, but I knew that even though I quite liked grounded theory, it hadn't really answered the question I had put in my master's study. I was totally scared of phenomenology by the papers I had done. And I was very sure that if I wanted to do something over three years it had to be of some meaning, and to feel comfortable. I went back to the grounded theory again, because everybody said to me, "You are crazy changing methodologies for a Ph.D.," and I thought, "No, it isn't going to do it for me this time round." I mean I hoped that phenomenology wasn't going to work, because it looked too hard! I struggled with the philosophy. And the other bit I found really hard was that there wasn't a step-by-step structure, which tells you to do this, and this, and this. Now that seems quite freeing but at the time it felt quite scary and hard.

Annette's thinking is shaped by her past experiences but also her present concerns. She chose phenomenology, even though she didn't particularly like it and found reading philosophy difficult. Having a very clear sense of what she wanted for her thinking, she knew that scary though it was, she needed to embrace a methodology that would let her thinking explore her topic in a particular way. In contrast to others who chose their methodology first, Annette's passion for thinking was her topic. She could live with a methodology if it took her thinking to the place she wanted to explore. She, like others, experienced her thinking as a "restless to and fro, between yes and no" (Heidegger, 1959/1966a, p. 75). Jo, also, is more drawn by the topic than the methodology:

JO: For me, research depends on the question. I am not wedded to any methodology. If the question fascinates me, the method ought to follow. I did grounded theory with my masters degree. It's pretty boring. The conceptual stuff is quite okay, but it is so laborious. I am not methodical enough; I am not good enough at keeping notes. And I couldn't do a Ph.D. in that because I couldn't manage the volume. I like the hypothesising sort of bit in it, but all of the other stuff, no.

One grounded theory experience convinced Jo that her thinking and her way-of-being does not sit comfortably with the methodical nature of the data analysis. She knows the type of thinking she likes, but is not hooked into one methodological approach. It is the question that grabs her thinking. Once she has the question in front of her, then she thinks about the "how."

Thinking is also an experience of the body, an embodied experience. Melinda describes how she found and felt immediately at home in her preferred thinking and methodological approach:

MELINDA: I can tell you the day I figured it out. I was starting my doctoral program, and I took a course called Qualitative Methods. The teacher was Egon Guba, and his book had just come out, it was about '86, and this little man started talking about this kind of research. The minute the class ended I bought the book. I went home and read the whole thing in about a day and a half. And I ended up with a dissertation I liked writing every single minute. It was hard, and I worked on it and it took a while, but I liked it, and I liked it when it was done.

Melinda's thinking was captivated by the man, by his book, by the ideas, and by the experience of doing the research. She liked this kind of thinking, even when it was hard. There was an embodied connection that resonated. She discovered an at-homeness in her thinking and had found her place-to-be. Sherry took a more convoluted path in which thinking is an epiphantic (epiphany) experience:

SHERRY: Back in 1982, we had a course in qualitative methods taught by a nurse gerontologist, named Margaret Diamond. It was one of those sorts of epiphanies where I realised what it was I had always hated about quantitative research. It was that moment of realisation that I could do it, and I could do it well, but I didn't like it because it didn't speak to me. It wasn't the kind of question I wanted to ask. But I never knew until that moment that you were allowed to ask a different kind of question. So that was an eye opener, but I was in the nursing educational administration program, and there really weren't any people who were particularly good at qualitative methods. From that I just kept reading and thinking there was more than just description. That is when I got interested in grounded theory, and my next couple of studies had a crack at that. But, you know, I am the kind of person who is always searching for the thing that is a better match for me, and grounded theory, while it was lots better than the quantitative description, at that place in my life there were too many strictures to what I can ask and how I can ask and what I can do with it after I have asked. So I think, for me, it was a natural progression of letting go of the restrictions, and understanding them and being able to use them and then letting go of them.

Sherry uses the word "epiphany" to describe her thinking and the moment of insight that quantitative research was "not her." Her thinking is shaped by an *augenblicht* (or moment of vision). Later she came to see that the thinking embraced by grounded theory was not sitting comfortably. In this way Sherry's experiences shape her thinking. Her choices were within experience and thus influenced by the people with whom she had contact. Looking back she sees herself as a "kind of person" whose thinking is always exploring a "better match" methodologically. As such there are times that are good fits for thinking and other times that are not such good fits. Her thinking has led her to let go of the approaches that limit and constrain her thinking.

The participants in this study reveal that it is not possible to take the person or personal experiences out of thinking. There can be no such thing as an objective experience of thinking. Further, the person is always within a unique context of possibilities, which is similarly influential. Doors open, exciting the thinking of the person who is researcher. Imagination for the researcher is caught together with a seamless interweaving of the thinking of "how." An idea does not fall into a value-neutral, experience-equal, calculating mind. Mind itself is an analytic construct. As experienced, each researcher in this study described embodied experiences of thinking within and about research that enticed or discouraged.

Thinking cannot be dictated or willed. A person both shapes and is shaped by thinking. For those who go looking for a methodology that connects with "their" thinking there can be a moment of epiphany. Since methodologies reflect particular approaches to thinking, the finding self

at home in a particular method is possible. For others, the thinking passion for their research question will take them into scary methodologies
and approaches to thinking because the question is all important. This is
the restless to and fro of thinking. When the research books counsel one
to identify the question first, they miss the uniquely self-initiating thinking of doing research. Each person will find his or her own way to thinking. Each will experience thinking and be guided by different influences:
people, possibilities and contexts. And as they become experienced researchers, their thinking will recognize that "knowing self" is the vital
step in the research journey.

   This study showed that research thinking is not one-dimensional,
solely analytical, and directed toward methodological selection and questions or outcomes of research. Selecting first a problem (phenomenon)
and then matching a method to the hypotheses or the phenomenon of
study implies a simplicity to thinking that is not described in these stories.
Likewise, a corresponding relationship between what is studied and how
it is studied is not borne out in the interpretive phenomenological analysis of these stories. Rather, what commonly shows up is how thinking—
for example, about selecting a method—is shaped by past experiences,
epiphanies, embodied understanding, and many complex and nuanced
insights as well as the nature of the phenomenon to be studied. Research
literature names the particular method chosen. Perhaps there is also a
place for narrative accounts of how the thinking-of-the-researcher came
to embrace a particular instrument or method. Contemporary research in
healthcare and the human sciences explores complex issues. It is time to
acknowledge that the thinking that underpins research is just as complex.

Thinking as Research: Research as Thinking

   Hearing the call-to-thinking, shaping and being shaped by thinking,
and thinking-as-research all co-occur, but they show up in different ways
and at different times for researchers. Gregory reveals the thinking-as-
research in the scientific paradigm:

GREGORY: What we are going to do with our data is very prethought, very predetermined. Often what happens during data analysis is you might come up with
some further ideas you would explore, but generally speaking I think it is important to determine how we are going to treat the data, and that will determine how
we are actually going to collect the data. So at the end of the study analysing the
data, I do not want to kick myself and say why didn't I ask that in that way? If I

would have I could have done this data analysis differently. We also thought it very important to involve biostatistical experts at a very early stage, so that we could get advice on how to collect the data, and how to set up and manage the data collection so that it is easily useable later on. We have managed to set up client databases where we can flick from screen to screen and simply enter the data as we take it over the telephone, which obviously saves many hours.

Gregory describes an approach to thinking that is analytic and pre-scriptive. Thinking is planned in advance, for once the outcomes of think-ing are in place, it can be too late to make changes. This kind of research thinking goes ahead in structured ways in the journey of design and data collection. Entering the information from the telephone conversation straight into the database shows the effectiveness of prethought strategies. There is a sense of a carefully focused analytic thinking that attends to a designed study running like clockwork. Peter continues in the same vein:

PETER: We were comparing a group of individuals who got about four or five weeks of high, intensive exercise to current standard practice at the hospital, which was not getting any exercise but just getting a sheet about what was going to happen to you. We were looking at: Can you exercise people with that level of severity of osteoarthritis? Can you give them an exercise program and see a dif-ference in them in terms of function, and pain level? And then, given that you might see a difference in them, when they go to operation do they then come out of hospital earlier? Is their time in hospital shorter? Do they have fewer complications? Is the first six days to weeks after they have gone home easier? Do they see the doctor less? But what we were thinking was that we can give them these four or five weeks of exercise, but like all exercise there is detrain-ing. When you stop exercise, you just gradually come back to your baseline levels. At this time nobody knows, we just do not know how long that is going to take.

Peter provides an example of analytic research thinking in the form of a linked progression of questions. The "what if ?" needs to be prethought. Having found the things for "thinking about" the design can then be set in place. There is a real sense in thinking-these-questions that Peter knows and attends to in the context of his study, specifically the care and treatment of this client group. He has to. Analytic thinking is rational and calculative; it seeks to identify cause and effect. Unless he has thought about all the questions to ask, his design will be flawed. This kind of thinking comes in advance of the data collection. Anne, with her evalua-tion research, shows how in thinking ahead as a research activity she is also shaping and being shaped by her thinking about "what works" and "covering her bases."

ANNE: You think about What is this service? What are the aims of this service? What is it that this service is wanting to achieve? You work back from that to What are the barriers? What things already exist to support it? What are you actually trying to achieve within the service, and how would you know whether you had achieved it or not? I suspect that very experienced evaluators get a repertoire that they pull from and they probably cut and paste their ideas into what it is they are doing. I think there is a bit of intuition there as well about what might work and what might be better in certain things. Planning is important. In terms of chronological time, you would be at least halfway down your timeline, maybe even longer, before you actually started. That is because you need to set the scene, and talk to so many different people, and sort out that you have got the questions and where you are going, and is it the right direction, have you covered all the bases. Maybe you don't always get it right. Sometimes things can change along the way, like the accessibility, or the practicality becomes apparent to you and you suddenly know that no, you cannot do those questions, it is not going to work, and that will just have to be a limitation, and you just get to a place where you feel that everything is all lined up and ready to go.

For Anne, preparation is the key to the thinking behind successful evaluation research. Thinking about the design takes at least half the time. Anne describes a process of actively thinking and investigating the field of interest to ensure that the appropriate questions are asked. She recognizes that with more thinking experiences, the questions may be easier to identify. She further acknowledges the place of intuition and situated contextual thinking in making plans, and accepts that the changing nature of every situation means no plan-for-her-thinking is ever sure. Nevertheless for Anne contextual-thinking-as-planning underpins the experience; though for others contextual thinking has more of a primacy. David gives an example of the kind of thinking that guides his research:

DAVID: As I read the literature that has looked at this phenomenon, they have attributed the psychosocial dysfunction to sensory deprivation, but when you are on these prison units it is very clear that there is not a lack of sensory stimulation. If anything, there is an overload. So as we begin to think, if something was producing increasing disability what was producing it, the features of the environment we are most interested in are interactions between guards and prisoners, and the relationship between the prisoners and the physical environment. In addition to the measurement of light, and the scaling of changes in functions, we are also doing an ethnographic study of the interactions between guards and prisoners and the ways in which the guards and prisoners interpret their interactions. So there is an ethnographic process going on because we do think that a part of the de-skilling of prisoners is related to the lack of sustained social interactions. I mean, prisoners will say, "I have forgotten how to talk." And we want to understand the interactions amongst some prisoners and amongst some guards. We are trying to simultaneously deal with the social environment, and the physical environment in this study, which is a central piece of this challenge.

Thinking-as-research and research-as-thinking show up in David's account. To know the experience of being in prison, he has to spend time experiencing the environment and thinking and listening to the people who are not free to leave. He has to be open to a thinking that challenges taken-for-granted assumptions and understandings. The challenge for thinking in this research is for David and his team to find a design that will address both the physical and social environment. It is like a disordered array of jigsaw pieces with no picture to guide. One senses thinking that wrestles with challenge and identifies strategies toward getting it right. This thinking is both research and a path to research; that is, thinking-as-a-special-kind-of-research. All thinking is open to possibility as a plan unfolds.

Thinking-as-research in more qualitative approaches, often shows up in the conversations directed to the experience of data analysis. Lynne describes her experience:

LYNNE: I had 26 multiple interviews. I got immersed in listening to and reading their stories. What I found was that when you listen to an interview you deal with the emotion, but if you immerse yourself, the emotion becomes part of your emotion and your thinking. I found myself getting very upset, and that is probably to be expected because that is what hooked me in.

Thinking as listening is a central research practice for Lynne that she cannot separate herself from emotionality. Getting upset is a kind of engagement that accompanies her thinking-as-research and reveals the pain of injustice. Her mood and her thinking are one. She knows that being immersed in the data is opening herself to the experiences and thinking of others, and in doing so, experiencing her own emotional pain. The pain speaks and is felt in the thinking that accompanies data analysis. Thinking as research is an embodied experience. Marion describes a more investigative type of thinking:

MARION: "Team practice" was there, or "interprofessional practice," and I kept juggling it between the two, because interprofessional has particular connotations. I knew that I wanted to know what people thought influenced or shaped the way they practiced. I knew I would have to unpack the ideologies. I needed to read around those areas. I did that in a multidimensional way from the perspective of professional literature, sociological literature, management organizational structure health reform literature, as well as the methodology literature.

Marion's description of engaged reading, reading widely, reading across disciplines and paradigms reflects the way of multiperspectival thinking to see both the influences and the mindsets. There is an investigative nature to such thinking-as-research, holding everything open and problematic, searching for what lies between the lines.

DEBBIE: Foucault's writing really makes me think, because it is something that I just cannot gloss over. It requires going back, and back, and back to make sense of what he writes. So I have to think, really look at his work quite closely, and then I have to think, "Well, how, in making sense of this, how do I see it fitting my world? How do I see this concept coming alive in my data?" It is a moving back between his writings and my data, backwards and forwards, trying to gain an understanding of both and recognizing what people were talking about.

Understanding Foucault is not a one-read-through thinking experience. Rather, it is a dialogical thinking that is a going-back-and-back-again commitment. At the same time the gleanings of understanding are taken to the data to see if the same notions lie within the accounts of the participants. This thinking as research is conversational. It is a process of dwelling, wrestling, watching, and waiting. Thinking cannot be ordered. It rather is embodied, lived through, awaiting the moments of insight. Deb offers the term "reflexivity" to describe a similar journey:

DEB: The word that describes how I worked with Gadamer's writing is "reflexivity." I would do some writing, think in terms of questions, do some reading. I always had to keep coming back, coming back, coming back. There were times when I would try to read a particular chapter in *Truth and Method*, or I would read again from a whole range of Gadamerian literatures. Depending on how much concentration you could give to something, I would select, pretty much at random. Or if there was a word—thinking for me is very much around words and possible word meanings, what someone says about a word—I would be off on a tangent looking at something like "commitment" or "compassion" or "paradox." That would give another tangent of possible ideas to bring back to what I was finding. Once I had the transcript, the thinking initially was relatively superficial. Things would jump out as seeming important and I would underline them or make a comment in the margin, but it was still pretty small thinking. Then I would turn the interview over so that I could not see it, and I would brainstorm the main things that seemed to be talking to me. I would write about a page, pretty superficial. But it showed me what I noticed first. I would record that in a certain color with the date, so that I knew the levels of thinking that I was coming to with each subsequent rereading. There is lots of backwards and forwards reflexivity between the thinking and the writing and the reading, but it is also between one interview and all of the interviews, and then from a fairly embryonic idea to a development of an idea that does not lose the embryonic idea but takes it further. The thinking goes in quite a lot of different directions. I don't think that you can control that and I don't think that you ought to control it. I think it happens and you have to realize it is happening and capture that it is happening. That is where you are keeping on writing. The journaling that I did helped me to capture those fleeting thoughts. I tried to impose a little bit of order on it so that I would be reasonably able to keep track of "what needs to be done now." It wasn't in the sense of trying to constrain the thinking. It was trying to not lose the good ideas that you might not have time for now because you are doing something else.

Deb attempts to capture in language her experiences of thinking-as-research and offers the notion that in her research thinking there is superficial-thinking and deeper-thinking, little-thinking and big-thinking, specific-thinking and whole-thinking. Always in thinking there is a to-and-fro: between reading and data, between one idea and another, between a word and all the meaning that lies behind. One cannot but wonder how a new hermeneutic researcher learns the art of circular reflexive thinking. Perhaps in contrast to the researchers who are always planning ahead, Deb is always reflecting in cycles to see the thinking that has emerged in the present and is awaiting and holding open a future of new possibilities for thinking the as-yet-unthought. Annette describes such cycles:

ANNETTE: I can remember moments of thinking, "This is it, I have got my thesis," and then reading the next story and thinking, "Oh no, I haven't." I remember that a lot. I haven't ever had a great flash, but I have had, "Well this could be something, and maybe I should think about that area a little bit more or go in a slightly different direction." It felt a bit like a building block process. I learned not to read too much of what other people had written about the area while I was doing it. I remember falling into that trap a few times and thinking, "Oh, I should go and look at trust," and then thinking, "Oh, hold on, I don't want to do that," so I kept on with the building blocks. I am a write-down person, a visual person, so it was the rewriting of the stories. That is where I started to learn how much was hidden in there. Taking the stories out of the transcripts and having to prepare them to send back to the participants, that was really useful. And I think the writing, and having all those comment clusters all over the place—it helped curb my need to go on and do the next thing, because by doing the writing I was doing something, and thinking in the writing.

Reading and writing are practices that co-occur with thinking (Diekelmann, 2001). Thinking is circular and does not come easily. Just when Annette imagines she's "got it" the thought loses itself again. There are dangers to be avoided. For example, there is a temptation to take the ready-made thinking of someone else before her own data has had the opportunity to reveal the meanings within. Knowing that meanings are hidden initially is both the quest and struggle of interpretive thinking-as-research. Learning the method of writing and rewriting is not as easy as it sounds. It is only when she comes to see that writing is thinking, that they co-occur and shape one another, that Annette begins to be content to let the writing show the way to thinking-as-research. Learning, writing, reading, and thinking become intertwined as one, each informing the other. Barbara describes similar learning using grounded theory:

BARBARA: Getting my first transcripts was both terrifying and exhilarating. I took three months with the first three transcripts, because it was holidays. I didn't quite know how to put pen to paper, and I moved between pencils and computer, and books, and my untidy writing. They ended up looking very written on, very used. I would write myself all that, and then I would come up with a code. And I went back constantly, and I learned to go back and see if I had done it properly: "Is that really what they are saying, or is it what I am putting on to what they are saying," and those sorts of things. I thought about process. I thought about dimensions. I knew what to do in the sense that I had begun to read Lenny Schatzman's work on dimensionalising, and to teach myself how to ask questions of the data, how to see movement in the data, how to see the meaning that people have given. There is some debate about whether there is a right way and a wrong way. Some people, who do a particular type of grounded theory tell me, "But you just lift the codes out," and other people believe that certain ways of doing grounded theory forces the data. Lenny Schatzman believes that the dimensional analysis is based on the way people solve problems anyway. And I went back to symbolic interactionism too, looking for ways in which people were giving meaning and constructing their world.

Reading and writing are important common practices of thinking as research. Reading can be both to seek content and a path to thinking. There is a language to be learned before one can understand the directions of method. Then there are the debates about the right and wrong ways to grapple with the data. The first transcript arrives, pristine and vast. Reading the books about how to code the data is not the same as thinking about and doing the coding. Barbara lives through her "learning" phase, and through interpretive thinking develops a sense of what it means to "do" grounded theory. It is a back and forth thinking experience between pencil and computer, reading and thinking, trying and checking, deciding and wondering again. Methodologies are "ways" that are deeply immersed within everything. Melinda shares her learning about trying to combine approaches:

MELINDA: When we were first doing this, and Sherry was a grounded theorist and I was a student phenomenologist, we thought, Wouldn't it be cool if I had a transcript that I had done an interpretation on and she had a transcript that was part of her grounded theory, and we traded transcripts and tried to do the opposite analysis, and then put it forward to show students how the analysis looked different? And it was so hard. It was just hard. I didn't know what to do with the kinds of data. It was all wrong. The data for the grounded theory study did not lend itself to interpretation, and what I had, which was very rich in narrative and all over the place, there was no process to be made for Sherry either.

Methodology and method as paths to thinking as research cannot be pulled apart and uplifted. The data collected for a grounded theory study do not offer enough description for a phenomenologist to even begin an interpretation. And similarly, the grounded theory method becomes overwhelmed with rich narrative. There are ways of thinking particular to methodologies that arise from the philosophical underpinnings, breathe through the data collection, and are reflected in the data analysis.

Perhaps each researcher makes a journey congruent with his or her methodology. Imagine the research-thinking in terms of journey. The more quantitative researchers do not leave home until they are confident they have everything in their suitcases that might be needed. They know that once traveling there will be no opportunity to re-equip. In contrast, the more interpretive researchers set out with fairly empty suitcases. They will have a philosophical text to be read, again and again. The journey takes them deeper and deeper into thinking. They stop many times along the way to repack, adding to their luggage to extend their thinking. Should a rendezvous of all these travelers be called at the two-thirds point of their journey, we would likely find the quantitative people on firm signposted territory, collecting, measuring, and following the preset plan. They are at their prechosen destination. In contrast, their interpretive friends are likely to report being lost in thought, unsure of their circular path, overwhelmed with possibilities. Perhaps the key difference in thinking across the methodologies is the extent to which the researcher is "free to think." Each methodology seems to me to have its own thinking spaces where one must dwell. Some methodologies allow thinking-as-research to flow freely, while others prescribe how and where the thinking will be focused.

There is a difference between thinking that is focused and follows, and thinking that plays and follows the movement of showing. Heidegger's (1959b/1966b) notions of calculative and meditative thinking describe thinking that rushes ahead, more likely to follow predetermined design, as opposed to that which stops and contemplates, more likely to play and keep open the possibilities of anything to show itself as itself. Research as thinking either opens or shuts down possibilities of play. There is a danger in becoming too reductive and labeling the different kinds or experiences of thinking, for thinking-as-experience is always contextual, evolving and ever-changing. The thinking of the researcher cannot help but play with ideas, with questions, toying, wondering, for it is the nature of being human. Perhaps the question then is, "Can the way of thinking reflected in each methodology be articulated to enable the newcomer to try it out, grasp the approach to thinking, and make an informed decision about goodness of fit?" Ways of thinking are ways of being. It is not easy to try to be someone other than self. Self simply thinks. To think in a new way requires conscious thought about thinking, which perhaps weighs heavy and burdens the free flow of ideas. In "forced thinking" I sense the shoulders tensing, the brow furrowing, a headache brewing until enough is enough, and the person walks away. To think as self is to not even think about thinking. It is rather to be in thought.

Thinking as Being in Thought

Thinking is a language experience that is ineffably nonlinguistic. All that has been written above comes together as in-thought experience, leading to the thoughts of the research study. How hard it is to give voice and find the words to describe "in thought" experience. Sherry and Melinda use metaphor:

SHERRY: It is like making a quilt, really. We have an overall pattern for this quilt, and because we have taken data apart, and we have separated it into these big ideas, now we are going to try to put these ideas back together. You kind of stitch them together with your words and your thoughts. If you look at a quilt, your eye moves across the pattern, however the pattern moves you through the quilt.

MELINDA: That you are piecing together the ideas, not in a haphazard way, but in a way that represents the pattern of ideas, and each idea is unique but it does not stand by itself, you know, it has got to be connected to the next idea and the next, so that you get this whole picture.

SHERRY: I always feel like I have basted it together first, big stitches first, and then as we get more, the stitches between the pieces get refined and smaller.

MELINDA: Or you can cut them. You can say this has got to go. Yes, we have got that wrong.

This is a picture of thinking as reciprocity between thinking and thoughts. The eye of the researcher moves across ideas that have been put out on the table, but at the same time the ideas on the table gather together to show themselves in a new way. In thinking, no one idea ever stands by itself but rather has its own place within the complex whole. In thinking experiences, there is no predesigned pattern for the quilt. Rather, the researchers trust that as the ideas come together the new and unique pattern will emerge. Their eyes are attuned always to glimpsing the pattern as it begins to show itself. Through thinking, the bigger picture reveals an idea in the wrong place, an assumption that is unwarranted, or a plan that will not work. The quest in thinking is always in movement and flux until a quiet sense of knowing says: "This is looking good." Then comes a more settled holding together. It is an experience of trust-in-thinking that can still hold itself open and problematic. Thinking, seeing, moving, and fixing all co-occur and are within the experience, almost without awareness.

Thinking as being in thought is about letting go of the sense that there is a known way, and trusting that the way, like the pattern of the quilt, will reveal itself amidst the thinking. It might be only after disengaging from a time of research-thinking that the researcher sees how far the study has moved. In the midst of the experience there is little thinking about "how." There is only thinking about the thoughts that come to invite thinking. How can a new researcher come to know the experience that simply happens unless she or he is open to await the happening? How can the researcher learn to trust the pattern will reveal itself without the stories of those who know?

Hearing the call to thinking is akin to awaiting the emerging pattern. It comes when thinking is watchful and alert. It is known not because it is familiar, but rather because it has a uniqueness and clarity that speaks above the busyness and noise. The self sees and hears: the self in context of time, place, and mood. The self, already in-shape, opens to embrace a new shape (idea), reshaping both self and idea. All this is thinking and all this is research.

Thinking as Thinking Itself

Heidegger says: "We come to know what it means to think when we ourselves try to think" (1954/1968, p. 3). How has my own thinking traveled through the thinking about thinking? Have I come any nearer to understanding that nature of thinking? Certainly we are going through the motions, enacting designs, embodying theoretical frameworks, but are we truly thinking? I turn to my collection of Heidegger's writing and am drawn to *The End of Philosophy and the Task of Thinking* (1993).

Heidegger talks of the clearing. Imagine walking through a dense forest and suddenly coming upon a place without trees. Because it is clear, the light shines in and takes away the darkness. He reminds us that the light is not the clearing. It can only shine in because there is a clearing, a space to take away the darkness. Imagine standing in that clearing and seeing for the first time the beauty of the trees surrounding the space. Previously they had merely been trunks with a vast shared canopy of leaves. Now perhaps we can see a tree in itself, and make comparisons about different trees. Even though we may have tramped for many hours through the forest, now we have a unique opportunity to come to understand the trees without which there would be no forest. Yet the clearing is not the forest.

Melinda describes her thinking as finding the best perspective to help her see:

MELINDA: As a person of extreme near-sightedness, the world to me looks like an impressionistic painting, or more like a Monet. If you are too close you cannot see it very well, and if you are too far away you cannot see it very well, so there is a place where the focus is as good as it can get. I am always feeling like this. You can change your stance forward and back, and if you look at it closer or back up farther away it kind of looks different. But it is always still an impression.

Thinking is about a circling forward and standing back in the place of clearing, trying to catch the view that speaks and shows. Heidegger argues that "the quiet heart of the clearing is the space of stillness from which alone the possibility of the belonging together of Being and thinking, that is presence and apprehending, can arise at all" (1993, p. 445). He goes on to ask should the task of thinking read "Clearing and Presence"?

Let me play with these thoughts in the context of this study. When we are in the midst of what is already thought to be known, and are engaged in research activities that are predetermined with pre-ordained expectations and rules, then perhaps in thinking we have not yet reached the place of clearing. We could still be tramping somewhat thoughtlessly in our thinking toward our destination, guided by markers, following a map. There may not be a call to think. That is my joy of tramping with a group where other people plan and I simply engage my body in keeping up. If everything goes according to plan, we will arrive safely at the hoped-for destination. Our world of research, as Heidegger agrees, calls for such pre-planned journeys. This approach to thinking is necessary but not sufficient. The tension arises, if those are the only journeys of thinking that ever get made, we are not moving forward into virgin territory where the way is unknown and the hazards unpredictable, and the destination is known only on arrival.

Everybody in this study described thinking experiences, times of not knowing, times of searching for insight. I suggest that those are the times we need to learn to value more, for that is where we approach the clearing of thinking the as-yet-unthought. I remember arriving at a clearing on the top of a ridge. The view was spectacular, but the wind cut to the bone. Suddenly I realized I had no idea where I had left the path. That is the danger I sense we experience when we reach the clearing of the thinking space: a scary sense of being lost, of being exposed, of having no next step to move on to. Yet, we need to still ourselves from the drive to rush backwards to known ground. It is only in our lostness that we have the time to look around, to take in the presence of what is there to be seen, heard, smelt, felt. It is only then that unthought possibilities may "upwell" and show themselves.

Thinking is about dwelling in the mess, living with the chaos, holding fallible, stepping back until the picture becomes clear, going forward and then retreating again in cycles. Thinking is trying to grasp that which has not yet been thought. It is more than remembering, more than asking,

more than finding. Thinking is hard work, bringing both angst and de-
light. It is transforming and harnessing. It is also awaiting the insight that
simply comes.

Nietzsche once said: "Thoughts, which come on the feet of doves, guide the
world." People today have largely given up listening to what Nietzsche is talking
about here. Just as one only listens to what makes noise, so one only counts as
being what works and leads to a practical, useful result. (Heidegger, 1987/2001,
p. 117–118)

What is the call-to-thinking for the experienced researchers within the
domain of healthcare and the human sciences? Is it a call to thinking to
guide the world, or to provide practical useful results? If it is both, then
amid the busyness, one must also await the dove that comes with the insight that will guide. Among us, there are those more attuned to awaiting
doves, and those who need to keep busy. Knowing the researchers of this
study, and having dwelt with their stories, I have come to see that no matter what the methodological stance, there is a thinking that comes to us
all that is part of our humanness. Perhaps the key is "comes to us." It is
beyond methodology. Methodologies such as phenomenology demand
meditative, transformative, insightful thinking, just as quantitative research demands analytic and calculative thinking, but I do not believe
that any successful research can enact the process without a healthy
mix of both. *Many paths are necessary to thinking and none is sufficient.*
The mindsets that have been built up about the nature of the different
methodological approaches can blind us to the human experience of
thinking. There are skills we can learn from each other once we acknowledge the call for many paths and kinds of thinking.

From Thinking to Acting: Listening and Responding
to Research Education and Research Practice

I recently attended a workshop discussing the supervision of postgraduate research. On reflection I saw that so much of our conversation is pre-
organized into the discourse of supervision, methodology, ethics, time
lines, progress, and examination. It is about dealing with "things," the content of thinking rather than the experiences of thinking. The path is laid
down; the expectations, congruent to the research design, are already in

concrete. It was only as stories were told of personal experience that glimpses of the thinking-as-thinking, embodied, lived experiences of thinking were revealed. Thinking as listening reveals insights of phenomena in quite a different way to thinking as telling (Diekelmann, N. & Diekelmann, J., forthcoming).

How are researchers educated and how do they practice research? The unanswered questions that arise call for more studies. The questions are about how the tutor (teacher) of research can

- Help someone be attuned to the call of a research idea.
- Uncover the "ways of thinking" a person brings to the chosen methodology.
- Hold open the tension of all that is unknown to prevent a premature closedown on thinking-an-idea, method, or design issue.
- Explore the opportunities for meditative thinking, for playing with ideas, within a particular methodology.
- Help create an understanding of how central "creating a place in one's life" is to practice research thinking.
- Show how the busy world can be put on hold to bring the researcher to the still place of thinking.

Instead of talking mainly about the steps of research, implying that the experience is about getting efficiently from one step to the next, we need rather to spend time dwelling with stories of being-amidst each step in thinking. Perhaps indeed to cast aside the metaphor of a progressive step-like journey and talk instead about thinking as "to and fro," "circling, spiralling," "being with others, being alone," "going ahead and looking back." In such conversations of thinking the myths are more likely to be exposed, turning the "oughts" into honest declarations of personal experience. Teaching, learning, and practicing thinking raises questions of pedagogy. Narrative pedagogies (N. Diekelmann & J. Diekelmann, forthcoming; Ironside, 2001) open a way for interpreting stories as paths to thinking. Conversations in the clearing of open listening have much to teach us all. Listening to language can show us how words shape and confine, opening possibilities to reshape. So often we only hint at the thinking that underpins research. Seldom do we deliberately pause to "talk thinking."

How is it that researchers create a place in their professional lives to practice thinking? What kinds of research activities encourage a focus on thinking as an experience and not an outcome? How can researchers

- Recognize the limits of any path to thinking; for example, thinking that follows prescribed ways?
- Identify embodied taken-for-granted thinking as experienced and bring it to question?
- Find the conversations where ideas, methodologies, and professional disciplines are free to play together in thinking with each other?
- Expose thinking to multiperspectival critique in a climate that seeks to strengthen and grow rather than squash and destroy?
- Learn to manage the tension of understanding that thinking never comes to an end, yet there needs to be "ends" to allow work into the public domain?

This study has opened up several conversations about the thinking of research. I invite each researcher to try to put into words the nature of their own thinking experiences. I encourage all teachers of research to share their own stories of thinking in their ongoing engagements with research students. I ask journal editors to look favorably on submissions that offer a narrative describing how thinking happened in a particular study and what called it forth. Let us together, locally and globally, collectively engage in articulation of the "how" of thinking as a skill, a process, a practice, and an experience (Ironside, 2004). It will not be a tidy conversation. I hope it will not try to put thinking in boxes. Rather, it will create dynamic synergies of insight, leading the way forward. Thinking can only ever be itself in experiences. All we need to do is tell our stories of thinking to each other. Our understanding comes from both telling and listening. It is that easy, and that hard.

Closing Thoughts

The thinking that comes from the feet of doves can be waited upon, but it cannot be demanded. Reading, writing, talking, listening, and questioning may prepare the ground of thinking but in themselves will not bring deep understanding. It is rather "living with," being immersed in a thinking experience that takes us to the clearing. To be a thinking researcher is to open oneself to being lost, taking paths that go nowhere, circling again and again, having the wisdom to pursue feelings and the courage to expose tentative thoughts to critique. It is to struggle and wrestle, and then to walk away trusting that insight will come. It is to attune one's eye, watching for the emerging pattern. It is to play, returning to the thinking of childhood when the unknown called us to adventure. It is exciting, scary, exhausting, and exhilarating. The thinking of research is the being of research. Without "thinking," what is known is merely repackaged and recycled. To research is to search again for that which has been lost or not yet been found. It is thinking, and to be thoughtful, to follow and to play.

> Thinking takes us beyond known ways,
> into the clearing,
> of un-formed understanding.
>
> It is of ourselves, in ourselves and beyond ourselves.
> Uniquely our own, common to us all.
> private, precious
> only be deemed worthy
> when the knowing is "said."
>
> The world of method/methodology
> can confine thinking to pre-made boxes
> with no escape.
>
> In the open place
> trees show themselves
> light shines
> and in both seeing and not-seeing
> thinking comes
> up welling within.
>
> Smythe (2005)

Acknowledgments

I thank the participants who graciously let me shine the light of my thinking into their stories of research, Pam Ironside for her words of helpful encouragement, and Professors Nancy and John Diekelmann for enthusiastically joining with me in "thinking some more," bringing new depth to my writing.

References

Arendt, H. (1978). *The life of the mind.* New York: Harcourt Brace Jovanovich.

Caelli, K. (2001). Engaging with phenomenology: Is it more of a challenge than it needs to be? *Qualitative Health Research, 11,* 273–281.

Diekelmann, N. (2001). Narrative pedagogy: Heideggerian hermeneutical analyses of the lived experiences of students, teachers and clinicians. *Advances in Nursing Science, 23*(3), 53–71.

Diekelmann, J. (2005). The retrieval of method: The method of retrieval. In P. Ironside, ed., *Beyond Method: Philosophical Conversations in Healthcare Research and Scholarship*. Madison: University of Wisconsin Press.

Diekelmann, N. & J. Diekelmann (forthcoming). *Schooling, learning and thinking: Toward a narrative pedagogy.*

Gadamer, H. G. (1982). *Truth and method* (R. Sullivan, Trans.). Berkley: University of California Press (Original work published 1965).

Gadamer, H. G. (1994). *Heidegger's ways* (J. Stanley, Trans.). New York: State University of New York Press.

Heidegger, M. (1966a). Conversation on a country path about thinking. In M. Heidegger, *Discourse on thinking* (pp. 58–90). (J. M. Anderson & E. H. Freund, Trans.). New York: Harper & Row. (Original work published 1959).

Heidegger, M. (1966b). *Discourse on thinking*. (J. Anderson & E. Freund, Trans.). New York: Harper & Row (Original work published 1959).

Heidegger, M. (1968). *What is called thinking?* (J. G. Gray, Trans.). New York: Harper & Row (Original work published 1954).

Heidegger, M. (1993). *Basic writings*. San Francisco: HarperSanFrancisco.

Heidegger, M. (1995), *Being and Time*. (J. Macquarrie & E. Robinson, Trans.). Oxford: Blackwell (Original work published 1927).

Heidegger, M. (Ed.). (2001). *Zollikon Seminars*. Evanston, IL: Northwestern University Press (Original work published 1987).

Ironside, P. M. (2001). Creating a research base for nursing education: An interpretive review of conventional, critical, feminist, postmodern, and phenomenologic pedagogies. *Advances in Nursing Science, 23*(3), 72–87.

Ironside, P. (2004). Covering content and teaching thinking: Deconstructing the additive curriculum. *Journal of Nursing Education, 43*(1) 5–30.

Rilke, R. M. (2002). *Sonnets to Orpheus with letter to a young poet* (S. Cohn, Trans.). New York: Routledge (Original work published 1929).

Smythe, E. A. (2003). Preserving "thinking" in the thesis experience. *Focus on Health Professional Education: A Multi-Disciplinary Journal, 5*(1) 54–65.

Van Manen, M. (1990). *Researching lived experience*. Albany: State University of New York Press.

7

Beyond the Methods Debate
Toward Embodied Ways of Knowing

NANCY JOHNSTON

Challenging us to move beyond our methodological preoccupations and preferences, the title of this volume encourages us to search out new and fruitful avenues of thought—ways of thinking that will breathe new life into health science and healing practices. Yet, it is also true that our ability to envisage these new possibilities arises only in consideration of the frailty of current methodological structures to accommodate and address the problems we currently face in the health sciences.

Struggling with questions about which methods will best advance our fields, practitioners of all disciplines within the health sciences and beyond also face the challenges of how to interact as we work together on interdisciplinary clinical and research teams. Directions for research sketched in by policy-makers and funding bodies, as evidenced by requests for proposals and systems evolving to support the development of proposals, show clearly the expanding opportunities for interdisciplinary collaboration and multimethod research. These trends seem to manifest a belief that the most effective interventions and compelling research come not only from the capacity to bring together individuals with common interests and similar values but also that the strength of the research enterprise overall can be enhanced by diversity of method and dialogue among views.[1] Given the perceived value of reaching more complete understanding of the complex meanings related to promoting health and containing disease in a pluralistic society, and considering the evident imperatives of looking at these complex meanings from different vantage points and through different lenses, a set of challenges for health researchers arise.

These challenges are related to a consideration of what kind of "evidence" is to be gathered by whom, in what manner, and toward what end.

Reflection on the forces that necessitate working together in multidisciplinary teams as well as the more recently observed receptivity, across disciplines and funding bodies, to quantitatively and qualitatively derived evidence throws into focus a new set of challenges. These are related to finding new places of cohabitation, interdependence, and mutual respect among researchers of diverse perspectives and persuasions.

But, Is Cohabitation Possible?

Cohabitation has not always been considered a worthy objective. Convinced of the irreconcilable differences in world views that were believed to underlie qualitative and quantitative methods, some thinkers such as Moccia (1988) and Phillips (1988) warned of the dangers of collaborative activities among qualitative and quantitative researchers. Without consensus on the nature of reality, they cautioned, the relationship was doomed to fail. In contrast, pragmatic thinkers have chosen to overlook these philosophical conundrums and have focused their thinking instead on the advantages of combining qualitative and quantitative methods. According to these thinkers, qualitative and quantitative research are complementary (Duffy, 1987; Haase & Myers, 1988; Knafl and Breitmayer, 1991; Knafl, Pettengill, Bevis, & Kirchoff, 1988; Mitchell, 1986; Risjord, Dunbar, & Moloney, 2002)—the use of both produces a more reliable and trustworthy result than either approach alone.

Underlying the methodological differences in health sciences are philosophical divergences and paradigmatic tensions. By tracing the history of the health sciences, it is evident that many shifts have occurred as disciplines have carved out particular niches while evolving in the light of new understandings of disease, health, and well-being. The particular orientation taken up by the discipline manifests a particular view of reality and how it is discovered and/or constructed. The biomedical paradigm, focused as it has been primarily on disease and dysfunction, and a product of traditional dualism, asserts that mind and matter (mind and the body) are fundamentally separate (Capra, 1982). This paradigm has given way gradually across most health disciplines to a focus on the person as a composite of physical, psychological, social, and spiritual dimensions. Proponents of this view, although concerned to some extent with the "whole person," emphasize certain aspects of human functioning in keeping with the foci of their disciplines or their subspecialities within a particular discipline. For example, physiotherapy considers the whole person but concentrates primarily on physical functioning.[2] Such approaches draw distinctions between mind and body in order to focus on particular and delimited causal interactions. Other disciplines, such as occupational health, social work, and epidemiology, emphasize the relationship among the personal, social, environmental, and political spheres of life, and seek to address the "determinants" of health and well-being.[3]

Some disciplines, notably nursing, have struggled to retain their commitment to the individual person as the primary recipient of nursing care and to enhance "holistic" approaches in relation to the individual, while at the same time acknowledging the professional obligation to address the broader social and political context that operates to enhance health for some while constraining it for others. The tensions between preserving a unified approach to the person on the one hand, and fulfilling an obligation to society on the other hand, are expressed in a vigorously contested debate. One side rejects any remnant of dualism as unacceptable because of its tendency to decontextualize and fragment an understanding of the whole person (Parse, 1992) while the other side critiques this position as an excessive emphasis on the individual and one which is accomplished at the expense of a necessary and broader social and political scrutiny (Thorne, Canam, Dahinton, Hall, Henderson, & Kirkham, 1998).

Embodiment: Slippery Slope or Firm Footing?

An even closer look at the issues under debate reveals fundamental differences in perspective both in conceptions of health and in the importance of the body as a way of knowing and as an object of concern. Fearing a return to biomedical reductionism and a perpetuation of medical and healthcare practices that have the potential to disempower clients and deprive them of their rights by establishing the expertise of health professionals on matters that pertain primarily to the body, this "unitary" perspective has sought to reduce the risk of reductionism and rectify imbalances in the client-practitioner relationship by de-emphasizing expert knowledge and by emphasizing client choice. Seeing the body primarily as a manifestation of underlying patterns within the person's energy field (Smith, 1991; Schroeder, 1993), proponents of this view emphasize an approach to illuminating the lived experience of clients that virtually excludes the consideration of bodily existence. Their reasons for doing so appear to be based in a belief that a focus on the body risks a descent into biomedical reductionism and a return to the past.

Others critique this brand of lived experience that appears to exclude concern for the body, warning of the dangers of such a view (Kikuchi & Simmons, 1986; Thorne et al., 1998). Such critics assert that holistic health could be jeopardized and the responsibility to address the social conditions that undermine health and trigger disease could be obfuscated by a perspective that fails to address the body.

The challenge for health sciences is thus not only related to developing research approaches that span multiple methods and several disciplines but also are related to negotiating a pathway through the diverging opinions within disciplines on the importance of the body (Thorne et al., 1998). As we consider the multifaceted debate about methods and the philosophical basis for the various perspectives, a fundamental challenge arises. This is to think through our conceptions about the nature of reality and how we have come to draw these conclusions.

I suggest that questions pertaining to whether reality is best understood objectively or subjectively, and whether notions of embodiment enable holism or place us on a slippery slope toward biomedical reductionism, can be resolved by a phenomenological investigation into our everyday experience. Such a return to "the things themselves," can free us from a tendency to mistake an idea of something for our actual experience of it and can, in this way, liberate us from our misconceptions. This is an exploration to which I will return shortly.

Causality or Meaning, or Causality and Meaning?

So far, we have explored the challenges that have arisen in collaborative health research as differences in perspectives, paradigms, and methods. A closer look at these challenges reveals that differences deemed to be irreconcilable, or at least worrisome, manifest an underlying tension between faith in realist notions of causality and belief that the search for meaning in the human experience is of the greatest import. Views of reality range from extreme realist understandings, in which everything takes place in the objective world such that there is no consideration of a subject, to extreme idealist positions that posit absolute subjectivity—a pure interiority, a Cogito whose existence is to think. Part of the tension in the health sciences can be characterized as a division between those who seek to uncover determinate patterns of causation and those who approach health science as an intersubjective and relational enterprise.

Given these divergent views of ends and approaches it seems desirable to find a way to conduct a conversation in which the questions and suppositions of each are considered, thus opening a field in which something new can emerge from the interplay. A possibility arising from such an interplay is a system of thought that lowers the barriers between extreme positions, yet preserves distinctions between inner and outer experience, acknowledges the differences between quantitative and qualitative researchers while easing the tensions between them, and accomplishes all of this without perpetuating reductionist or dualist thinking.

The challenge of developing such a system of thought is taken up by beginning with a fundamental assertion. This is that disparate views of reality as inner—or outer—oriented are not in experience separate or separable. The view is offered that subjective and objective ways of thinking do not disclose separate and mutually isolated realms but are rather two sides of the same dimension—each one dependent on the other for its meaning. It is suggested, furthermore, that the differences that separate thoughts oriented toward subjective experience from objectively oriented thought are, in experience, illusions that obscure a deeper unity. This underlying unity can be seen by considering that each point of view, whether oriented toward subjective or objective experience, depends on the other for the very frame of reference that establishes the parameters of its inquiry as either qualitative or quantitative. By exploring this way of thinking, the two sidedness of the human experience is shown—the subjective that lies at the heart of all objective experience and the so called "objective" that (despite positivist assertions to the contrary) cannot ever be detached from any understanding of subjectivity.

Admittedly, moving beyond a dualist stance while at the same time preserving distinctions between inner and outer experience is difficult. This is because our tendency to engage in binary thinking is deeply entrenched and we continue to want to establish definitional categories (inner or outer) that are absolute. This tendency toward absolutism in our thinking has gained ascendancy in spite of our bodily experience that enables bodily derived impressions based on ambiguity, overlap, and continuity. Consider, for example, that at one moment, I am "inside" my hand experiencing its warmth or coolness and, at another moment, I am "outside" looking at my hand as object. The exact nanosecond of the "crossover" in perception from my subjectively experienced hand to the objectively regarded hand is impossible to determine. Yet, in spite of the continuity of experience in preserving fluid movement from subjective to objective experience, it can be seen that such progression preserves, in spite of its continuity and ambiguity, important distinctions.

Why are such distinctions important? Because the understanding of what it means to be human and to have a world can only be reached through an understanding of that which is both inner and particular to me as one human, and that which is outer and common across my experiences as one human among, and in relation to, many humans. It becomes clearer, then, that what is being proposed here is an organizing structure of reality that preserves the distinctions between internal and external experience while at the same time attempting to loosen the grip of these perspectives in order to recognize them for what they are: different styles or systems of thinking.

The position is taken here that any movement beyond the methods debate requires first a way of noticing how we perform the gestalt shift from inner to outer experience and back again. Just as when I shake hands with another person who is also my friend, I am at once aware of the contact of skin and bones, warmth or coolness, and I am also "in touch" with the joy and comfort of being in the presence of another who cares for me and for whom I care.

To expand upon an example offered earlier, consider that as I look at my hand, I see the hand of a middle-aged female. Some wrinkling and thinning of skin is apparent. As I experience my hand as a part of my body, that is, as I perform a gestalt shift from objective experience to subjective experience, I become aware of slight stiffening of my finger joints and a kind of prickly heat in my hands; perhaps early symptoms of circulatory problems or arthritis. Accounting for such gestalt shifts, from objective to subjective experience and back again to a consideration of how my experience compares with that of others and with extant knowledge related to the ailments accompanying aging, can only be reached through

an embodied understanding of reality. In other words I must first be embodied to be able to establish any connections between what is observed
and what is experienced. This way of thinking establishes the reality of
causal connections based on differences both in sense experience and in
lived experience.

By showing how mind and body are interactive and that the body is a
living experience, this way of thinking establishes the indivisibility of
sense experience and lived experience. In so doing, it provides a clearing
for qualitative and quantitative researchers to work together in a way that
does not privilege either way of thinking. Instead, this way of thinking allows both for patterns of commonality across human experiences to be
observed at the same time as it allows for the particularity of individual
experience to be understood in a new way. These dimensions of experience are understood not as manifestations of separate realities, that is, reality is all "out-there" or the other extreme view that reality is only understood with reference to personal, private, interior experiences but, rather,
reality is understood as inner and outer dimensions of one reality experienced by way of gestalt shifts or border crossings. Such gestalt shifts enable a foreground to emerge at one moment and then for it to dissolve
into its context in the next moment.

Moving from the metaphor of a gestalt drawing to that of a border
crossing, we appreciate that, as with any border, it is difficult to determine the exact point at which we have left one territory and entered another; there is a certain ambiguity, overlap, and continuity to our experience of moving from inner to outer dimensions. Paradoxically, it is the
unity of the experience provided for by the intermeshing and overlapping
territories that creates the conditions for differentiation between inner
and outer experience.

The Unity of Everyday Experience

While researchers struggle with the dichotomies and oppositions that
arise from misapprehensions regarding how reality is experienced and
discovered, the practitioners of care, in their daily practice, encounter no
such oppositions and discontinuities. Rather, they traverse the intersection where objective and subjective ways of knowing meet. Practitioners
of care and their clients co-construct meaning in their engagement

with each other. In this context of human engagement, practitioners perform physical assessments and interpret objective laboratory results using numbers to gain insight into the clients' biological function. Clearly, health practitioners are at once engaged in a holistic dynamic intersubjective interplay and an important objective process.

Those in healing professions draw continuously on personal subjective processes and objective knowledge of the client's physical state. Moreover, they link the knowledge gained by these diverse ways of thinking and experiencing to extant technical knowledge in the form of descriptions of relatively enduring configurations or observable patterns of health and disease. Both tacit knowledge and objective knowledge are integrated in the process of grasping what is important to the client and in planning a judicious course of action. In this way, healers in everyday practice constantly and, apparently, seamlessly experience the flow between subjective and objective experience. It is intuitively understood that healing practices require care of the mind and care of the body. In caring for the whole person, attention is given to the conjoined nature of body and mind, and to the potential for both mind and body to be transformed through the meanings that come to be illuminated during the healing experience.

Meaning cannot be divorced from the body that first, by reason of existing, enables the person to have a world in which meaning is experienced. The body, on the other hand, inhabits a changing landscape that is constantly transformed according to the meanings given to personal experience.

How is it then that the methods used by researchers in the health disciplines are so cumbersome and have so much difficulty moving fluidly back and forth across the subjective and objective borders? Could it be that our diverse understandings of reality and theories of causation lie at the heart of our problems? Are we having difficulty coming to grips with the conjoined nature of mind, meaning, and matter? Is dualistic thought itself a retreat in the face of evidence that shows clearly that all ways of knowing, first and foremost are embodied ways of knowing?

Reality and Causality as Border Crossings

Bringing together the work of Hume and Merleau-Ponty,[4] I will now explore a way of thinking that enables fluid movement from subjective experience to objective ways of knowing and back again such as is clearly evidenced in clinical practice. This way of thinking can be characterized as a phenomenological view of reality and causality. I argue that any view of reality assumes a particular understanding of causality, and I assert, furthermore, that it is not possible to find causal connections aside from an intractable personal component whose basis lies in first-hand, or lived experience. By exploring the relationship between theories of causation and lived experience, I consider next how we as humans come to both construct and discover that which we take for being "real."

Reality as Individuation

David Hume, a Scottish philosopher (1711–1776) who practiced a constructive skepticism, insisted that philosophy cannot go beyond experience and that this is even the case in regard to causality. He said something that had not been noticed before, that individuation (i.e., the process of separating a thing from its context in order to study it) is an overture to the description of causal relations. By using the term overture I mean to say that individuation is not sufficient in and of itself to fully account for reality. It is however, an important gesture in the direction of understanding causal relations. What did Hume mean by positing that individuation is a part of the process of constructing reality?

Consider that all experience is experience of something, and that to experience something as a thing, it must first of all be differentiated from a background. Only once a thing has been individuated (i.e. held to be distinguishable from its surroundings) can the constancy be experienced that taking the thing as a continuing object requires; only then may the relations of constant continuity and temporal sequentiality be ascertained.

To enhance understanding of the meaning of individuation the following vignette is offered. A nurse enters the hospital room of a patient. Family members are talking among themselves in low voices by the window, while the patient's face is turned away from them toward the door the nurse has just entered. A radio is playing in the background, intravenous fluids are infusing, oxygen inhalation therapy equipment hangs from the wall over the patient's bed, and a bouquet of spring flowers graces a bedside table as light streams in through the window. The glance of the nurse takes all of this in but focuses in particular on the facial grimace and the labored breathing of the patient. Moving swiftly to the patient's bedside, the nurse looks into the patient's eyes and asks the patient if he is experiencing chest pain. The patient confirms that he is.

With this vignette we see that a foreground has been differentiated from a background and the foreground has become the continuity around which a set of temporal sequences revolve. The patient's facial grimace, labored breathing and chest pain have been brought forward as a particular constellation of meaningful observations; in other words, particular observations have become the foreground around which a predictable set clinical actions will swirl. Only by maintaining a particular focus—paying attention to certain aspects of the situation, while neglecting others—are we able to put in place a deliberate sequence of actions.

Being able to differentiate foreground from background only takes us a certain distance in terms of grasping important dimensions of the reality of this situation. It does not explain, for example, how or why the nurse takes the action she does.

Reality as Making a Difference

Without the feeling that we make a difference, we could not act. Without the felt relation of conjunction, that is, concurrences of thought and action and the felt relations of causality that certain conjunctions produce, we would be unable to act. This is because those lived feelings are the criteria upon which our assurance and convictions rest. It is precisely these lived feelings and this causality that the objective paradigm standing by itself cannot account for.

The nurse acts to inquire whether the patient has chest pain for at least three important reasons—because her intuition, her lived feeling is that something is amiss; because her own lived experience has enabled her to find concurrences between shortness of breath, facial grimacing, labored breathing, and chest pain; and also because she is relying upon the evidence accumulated by physiologists, physicians, and her own discipline, that chest pain and cardiac insufficiency can be reliably linked. She acts additionally because she believes, on the basis of previous experience, that these observations can be conjoined with a set of actions that have, in the past, promoted other patients' safety and forestalled death.

As actors we are causes. The nurse, by acting in this situation, introduces novelty into the situation. A predictable course of events is thereby changed. Hume realized that an effect cannot invariably be found in the cause, because in the process of unfolding, novelty can be introduced. By merely examining the initial conditions, we are not in a position to predict with accuracy the time, place, and form in which novelty will arrive.

Antecedent conditions cannot account for human agency and the freedom to choose.

Being human consists in part in acting—engaging in processes to transform contingency into fact. In losing sight of this, there is grave danger in conceiving of our selves entirely in objective terms. According to this model, we must think of our perceptual lives as reactions to stimuli or, at best, as eddies in the perpetual flux whose motion is ruled by eternal laws of nature—human subjects as nothing but epiphenomenal ghosts of departing energies.

Yet it could be argued, by returning to consider the vignette, that in responding to the situation at hand, the nurse was drawing on her subjective lived feelings, past experiences, and beliefs in the efficacy of her own action, and she was also drawing on objective knowledge. Was it not this objective knowledge that enabled her to link her intuitive impressions to observations of the patient and then to link these observations to extant knowledge in the form of information regarding the clinical features of cardiac insufficiency? Only by engaging this objective knowledge was the nurse able to decide on a course of action.

This brings us to consider the need, particularly in the health professions, for a paradigm that adequately accommodates the body, self-consciousness, and self-reflection as well as the capacity to link these subjective experiences to a larger sphere of knowledge. The challenge becomes how to safeguard the subjective that lies at the heart of objectivity so that the objectivity itself does not obscure it.

Reality as Doublesidedness

A fundamental and inescapable fact of human existence is that we experience everything from, so to speak, two "sides." Every time I speak, for example, I hear my voice as heard as well as my voice uttered. To put this differently, in speech we feel ourselves creating sounds to hear as well as hearing our voices as sounds having been made. As well, we hear the voice we utter and that voice that reflects back to our ears as it does to those of others. This is a feature of everyday awareness; we notice the difference when we first hear a tape recording of our voices. As well as observing our activities from, as it were, the "outside" as an object among other objects in a world, we also experience the world from, so to speak, the "inside."

We often experience the two sides as linked. The difficulty, as we well know, lies in how the portions of experience that we call "mind" might be understood as connected to portions that we call "body," so that the two sides may be thought as interacting, as they do in experience. Another difficulty lies in finding a way to understand this connection and think through this interaction in a way that does not reduce the one to the other, as is manifestly not the case in experience.

Hume and Merleau-Ponty appreciated this problem, that is, that what happens on the inside is something different from what happens on the outside. It is the bond between that which is an impression or lived feeling and the idea of it that interested them both. Main-line science, on the other hand, has tended to focus on the discrepancy between the inner experience and the outer "reality." Dealing with the dissonance by subjecting the two ways of perceiving to a competition in which the criteria used to assess adequacy have guaranteed the triumph of the objective approach has not, however, resolved the issues. It thus becomes important to move beyond notions of competition for ascendancy of one point of view to notice the interdependency of both points of view.

Hume and Merleau-Ponty saw through the illusions of objectivity by showing that what was assumed to be objectivity and to entirely escape lived experience is in actuality intersubjectivity and wholly intertwined with and dependent on first-hand experience. They also saw that all portions of experience that are conceived of as objective have a subjective lining that is not detachable. As Hume observed at the very outset, "All perceptions of the mind are double, and appear both as impressions and ideas" (1978, p. 160). Although inseparable, the two sides are nonetheless distinguishable. Distinguishability, it is important to add, does not imply duality. Both Hume and Merleau-Ponty wanted to understand how, to borrow Merleau-Ponty's words, "the passage from the self and the world and into the other is effected, at the crossing of the avenues" (1968, p. 160).

Merleau-Ponty builds upon the notion of the double-sidedness of reality to transform experience into "flesh." Why flesh? Because it is the most bodily of terms. Merleau-Ponty says "One must see or feel in some way in order to think" and "every thought known to us occurs to a flesh" (1968, p. 146). The point is that the idea of pure consciousness, entirely free from the messiness of contingency and temporality is something of which we have no experience. At one moment objects in the world demand our attention; at the next we recognize that the colors, sounds, smells, tastes, and textures are the objects of our own perceptions.

An idea is not something that is split off from our experience. It is not the contrary of the sensible but rather its lining and depth (1968, p. 149). Everyday experience is neither entirely subjective nor entirely objective; rather, it moves and jumps and flips between these categories. Understanding causality as a condition of reality and understanding individuation and making a difference as overtures to the description of causal relations, I turn now to consider the felt connection between our attempts to act and the results of our actions.

Causation as Lived Inference

By considering a situation in which one is sitting in the shade and desiring to be warm, it can easily be seen that we cannot use logic to change our condition, we must act to become warm. Thus there is a logos visible in the phenomena themselves. When we pay attention to perception, we can notice the lived association that is the natural relation. Shade is cool while sitting in the direct sun is hot. Therefore, if we wish to be hot rather than cool, we move from a shaded area into one that receives the direct rays of the sun. Lived inference from which the meaning of causality stems is a natural relation in which we feel the connection between our attempts to act and the result of our actions. It is only in the lived inference between events that causality resides.

It is relations of cause and effect that constitute reality, and everything that counts as real has that status as a result of some past experiences, as we have seen, of making a difference. Causality is not a principle of abstract reason; it is not a condition that makes a world possible. Causality is a principle of lived experience that makes the word actual. According to Hume,

all beings in the universe, considered in themselves, appear entirely loose and independent of each other. 'Tis only by experience we learn their influence and connexion; and this influence we ought never to extend beyond experience. (1978, p. 466)

How is it then that we have come to rely upon certain evidence in such a way that it structures our notions of reality?

It is not because truth lies hidden deep within a reason independent of lived experience. Rather, "truth" appears to be "truth" based on ideas that have become ingrained in us as a result of past experience. This means that such "facts" have never been contradicted by experience rather than being what cannot, in principle, ever be contradicted. The event of connection occurs in us after a sufficient number of repetitions. After a sufficient number of repetitions, we feel a determination of the mind to pass from one object to its usual attendant, and to conceive of it in a stronger light upon account of that relation.

The emergence of understanding is neither totally subjective or psychological, nor totally objective since lived experience is not limited to one dimension or the other. The point is that causal relationships are the border crossings from one dimension to another. As such these crossings establish the reality of the connection. Through repetition, we seek reliability in our experience, for only then can we trust actions to the domain of habit, which once achieved, frees our consciousness for other activities. Experience of constancy or regularity in connections makes for the greatest vivacity of the connections of certain ideas and, therefore, fashions our understanding of cause and effect relationships. Causality is the lived association among events that gets incorporated as an assurance about the way the world is; it is the carrying over from past to present of the lived experience of repetition, regularity and constant conjunction. Causality is an existential inference.

Causality as Looseness

Causality does not imply analytic necessity; just because events have proceeded in a certain way in the past is no guarantee that they will always do so in the future. We anticipate that they will but there is no guarantee. This is especially the case in human actions. People constantly surprise us by taking actions that we did not anticipate. Since we cannot see beyond the simple fact of connectedness to some hidden and absolute guarantee of the continuance of any particular relationship, there is in causal relationships—no matter how uncontroverted the experience of conjunction may be—an irreducible and undeniable looseness, a certain slippage and undeniable indeterminacy. James explained this notion of indeterminacy as the idea that

the parts [that we draw connections among] have a certain amount of loose play on one another, so that the laying down of one of them does not necessarily determine what the others shall be. It admits that possibilities may be in excess of actualities, and that things not yet revealed to our knowledge may really in themselves be ambiguous. Of two alternative futures which we conceive, both may now be really possible; and the one becomes impossible only at the very moment when the other excludes it by becoming real itself. Indeterminism thus denies the world to be one unbending unit of fact. There is a certain ultimate pluralism in it; and so saying, it corroborates our ordinary unsophisticated view of things. To that view, actualities seem to float in a wider sea of possibilities from out of which they are chosen; and somewhere, indeterminism says such possibilities exist, and form a part of truth. (1977, p. 591)

This looseness, slippage, and indeterminacy, rather than being a reason for despair is actually reason for hope, a theme that we shall return to later in our discussions of the implications of this way of thinking for research within the health disciplines.

Reality and Causality by Agreement

The lifeworld is first and foremost a way of agreeing. James expressed the idea of the lifeworld as agreement in this way:

Although "A feeling only is as it is felt," there is still nothing absurd in the notion of its being felt in two different ways at once, as yours, namely and as mine. It is, indeed "mine" only as it is felt as mine, and "yours" only as it is felt as yours. But it is felt as neither by *itself*, but only when "owned" by our two several remembering experiences, just as one undivided estate is owned by several heirs. (1977, p. 231)

As undivided estate, the lifeworld is owned by all and it is the common object of all of our ideas. As such the lifeworld is a *locus communis* for further agreements, about, for example what things or events count as being correlated or constantly conjoined. Agreeing about similarities in our experience permits agreement about constant conjunctions that are the basis for agreement about causal relationships. We may then say that our understanding of causality and hence reality is reached by agreement. Madison makes the point concisely:

Reality is limitless, but it is reduced to manageable proportions when it is viewed in the light of [not only] our own experience [but our common human experience]. As far as our ability to understand goes, Protagoras was right in saying that man [*sic*] is the measure of things, our [common] experience is the only means we have for sounding out the depths of being.[5] (1982, p. 307)

Just as the lifeworld is constituted by our agreeing on that which is held to be common experience, so hermeneutical interpretation is subject to the same "test" of what may be counted to be reasonable and "true." Madison (2001) states that:

> An interpretation will be held to be true (and thus will count as true) if it meets with general, intersubjective agreement or assent. If an interpretation does not meet this test, it will be considered an idiosyncratic, subjective "fantasy" bearing no connection to "reality." (p. 147)

Ways of Thinking and the Pursuit of New Possibilities: Contingency on the Other Side of Necessity and Mystery as the Cause for Hope

The fact that we cannot attain "truth" through individual and isolated introspection, as well as the fact that we can never get to the bottom of either freedom or necessity need not surprise or dismay us; rather, these are reasons for hope. Understanding that we as humans are neither determined nor are we radically free to pursue our own course in life, unbounded by others' perspectives and what has come before, has implications for resolving the methods debate. This is because understanding our ultimate inability to fully penetrate either our freedom or our necessity (that which constrains us by virtue of the fact that we were born into particular families, have inherited a set of genetic endowments and enjoy, or are deprived of, certain resources) means that while strong, vivid, and enduring patterns over wide expanses may present themselves to us, there is nothing deterministic about these patterns.

Here, I wish to assert that there is nothing inherently wrong in noticing strong and vivid patterns, even if these patterns are arrived at mathematically. What is established after all by statistics is a language of facts. "The questions these facts answer and which facts would begin to speak if other questions were asked are hermeneutical questions" (Gadamer, 1976, p. 11). Hermeneutics challenges us to be aware of danger in the tendency to mistake the statistical "languages of fact" for evidence of a deterministic pattern—a kind of given, unchanging, and subterranean reality, detectable only by means of our own ingenious methods. If we are not careful, the tendency to mistake findings for reality will diminish choice rather than open up possibilities in the human experience, that is, it will operate to constrain our freedom.

Loosening the Constraints and Becoming Free

To illustrate how human possibilities could be diminished rather than enhanced by how we interpret research, let us consider a study (Kools, 1999) that reports that adolescents in foster care tend to engage in self-protective strategies to deal with their perceived devaluation and lack of consistent attachments by keeping relationships superficial, maintaining an attitude of defensiveness and distancing themselves from others. In considering the impact of this study on our thinking, practice, and ways of being, we might notice that it helps us to understand the reasons for the behavior and thus disposes us to engage with such individuals in a patient and compassionate manner. A less positive and more pernicious influence might be recognized if the findings lead us to begin to expect psychological damage, defensiveness, and distancing in adolescents living in foster care and if this expectation leads us, in a purely self-protective manner, to withdraw from them. We need to be careful that research, which has demonstrated strong patterns based on many repetitions of comparable experiences, does not lead us to overlook exceptions and in so doing to come to see only what we have come to expect to see.

When interpretations (and that is all any and all findings can ever be) are transformed into expectations, we risk accepting as determined patterns that have within them a certain looseness, slippage, and indeterminacy. Statistical analysis of data that yields "significant" relationships among variables is, I argue, a form of fallibilistic interpretation. In establishing the validity of this statement consider that contemporary postpositivistic thinking in the philosophy of science has acknowledged the impossibility of pure, theory-neutral observation, entirely detached from the experience of the observer (Kuhn, 1970; Popper, 1963). Hanson (1958) has given a detailed argument against the notion of theory–neutral observations, showing instead that what one "observes" depends on perception rather than simply on retinal images. Furthermore, it has been argued that what stands out as "relevant and significant" is a function of one's prior knowledge and experience, which in turn influences how one conceptually organizes sensory experience (Schumacher & Gortner, 1992). Popper (1963) has, moreover, proposed a conception of knowledge that is nonfoundational. That there are no ultimate sources of knowledge has now been accepted. Instead, contemporary science progresses through its critical attitude and its ability to detect error, rather than by the certainty conferred by "brute facts."

Given the view that all findings or interpretations offered by contemporary scientists are fallible, that is, subject to falsification at some time and under some conditions, a further need for caution arises. This is that in failing to understand the freedom that individuals have to choose, even in the most coercive of circumstances, we dampen our ability to be alert to the possibility that some individuals can and will "beat the odds." Moreover, such thinking manifests fatalism, a way of expecting the worst or of anticipating merely more of the same. Our way of being with those whose life stories disclose these "patterns" can then be a way of expecting and producing diminished possibilities rather than having faith in a fecundity of new beginnings and perhaps even altered causal relations.

Johnston (2003), in a hermeneutical phenomenological study of how meaning is found in adversity, described how people are free (although not radically free) to choose the meanings they give to their experience. A sense of doom, inevitability, and diminishment was pervasive for some in the study, while others described seeing themselves, with the passage of time, as wounded but wiser, flawed but more compassionate, and limited but able to live life more authentically. What becomes clear from this study is that circumstances and events that appear on the surface, and in the short-run, to be injurious to health and well-being can, for some, be the portal through which they arrive at life-altering interpretations. Adversity, for some, ushers in a life of deeper meaning, purpose, and satisfaction.

It is in confronting the limitations of quantitative research to explain those infrequently arising situations in which strong patterns do not hold true or are reversed that some of the greatest opportunities for qualitative research arise. Consider, for example, extant qualitative research through which a relationship between early childhood experiences of loss and the inability to maintain strong, satisfying relationships in adulthood was posited (Bowlby, 1979). This observed relationship was subsequently "confirmed" by longitudinal quantitative research (Werner & Smith, 1993). Of particular interest were the "outliers" in this quantitative research, that is, those individuals who, despite early experiences of loss and trauma, were resilient in the face of adversity. Questions pertaining to how some people come to be resilient in the face of circumstances that lead many others to despair subsequently spawned a whole new field of qualitative and quantitative research on resilience (Glantz and Johnson, 1999).

How do these examples help us to maintain hope as well as move beyond the methods debate to create a new clearing for collaborative ventures between quantitative and qualitative researchers? By holding up two pictures—one of a frequently appearing pattern of early childhood loss and depression in adulthood and the other of a significantly less frequently appearing pattern of resilience in the face of comparable circumstances—we can take hope. Why? Not because these frequent and infrequent patterns occur and have been noticed but because they show us something fundamentally important; *there is no overarching determinate pattern.* Novelty as true change is always possible. To be embodied is to have a world, to be party to the lifeworld that is fundamentally and inescapably shared and therefore cannot be usurped by another.

From a philosophical point of view we may conclude that while, as we may experience ourselves as "objects"—that we have been placed in situations that are not of our choosing where we feel that we are controlled and dominated by external forces—we remain free as "subjects" to reflect upon and manage the causal relationships that we discover among objects. To illustrate this point consider the personal story told by a young woman to an older female confidant:

When I told my live-in boyfriend of five years that we had made a mistake and I was pregnant, he became livid. He beat me up and told me to get an abortion. When I said I wasn't sure I wanted that, he called me some unprintable names and told me basically that the relationship was over. Within a week he had moved out, leaving me no way of contacting him or getting him to pay his portion of the bills. I was very depressed and even considered an abortion just to try to get him back. Ultimately though I decided that I would do what was right for me. This was the first time in five years that I actually thought about what I wanted. I decided to keep the baby. . . . My son [the baby] has provided the reason for me to turn my life around. For his sake, and a better life for both of us, I have persevered through school and now I am graduating with honors. Soon I will have a good career of my own. When I look back on things, I see that getting pregnant was the best thing that ever happened to me. If it hadn't happened I might be still with my boyfriend, still unhappy, still being abused and still thinking there was no other alternative in life for me.

The fact that when we feel ourselves to be oppressed by forces experienced as being external to us, and when we experience our freedom as being constrained, does not negate the fact that as subjects we do remain free to reflect upon these forces and to manage the causal relationships that we discern among these objects. Altered interpretations of ourselves, that is, the refusal to see ourselves as objects, and our circumstances as beyond our control, introduce novelty in our situation and in so doing the causal chain is revised.

This philosophical insight has also been borne out by empirical investigation. Brown (1994, 1997) showed, for example, in a study of depressed women that the number of external adverse events alone did not predict depression. Rather, it was a negative kind of meaning for the self that was given to these external events that was most strongly associated with depression. According to this understanding, it is not the objective "fact" that a woman's husband abandoned her but, rather, the self-understanding that she has reached in which she views herself as a person who is unlovable and who is without resources that constitutes the link to depression.

Explanation and Understanding

Thus, it can be seen with reference to these empirical studies that whereas the value of quantitative research resides primarily in explaining the influence exerted by dominant and relatively decontextualized forces, qualitative research searches for a situated understanding of how humans come to dwell amidst the circumstances that they inherit, are thrown into, and choose. Qualitative research helps us to understand how humans handle (i.e., the manner in which they interpret their circumstances and themselves, and the way in which their understanding does, or does not, introduce novelty into) the causal relationships that they discover among these objects and circumstances.

Finding Freedom in the Search for Causal Relationships

In practice, freedom and causality are mutually reinforcing; the more causal relationships we ascertain the freer we become. For example, the more that I am able to notice that a habit of interrupting people while they are talking results in a situation where people withdraw from me or talk over me, the more able I am to choose whether or not to continue this way of relating. Our freedom is dependent upon our understanding of causal relationships, and our understanding of causal relationships is dependent upon our freedom to investigate them; freedom and causality are thus mutually reinforcing. Causal relationships are inventive discoveries: they emerge in the active interaction between ourselves and the world.

This understanding has implications for how we think about the objectives of research, both qualitative and quantitative, and the purposes and uses to which our studies are put. The purpose of finding a statistically significant pattern as an inventive and creative discovery is to not only to illuminate exterior dimensions of causal relationships but, more importantly to offer choice, that is, to free humans to think about these patterns in the light of an understanding of what it means to be human and to have choice. The intent in uncovering how humans manage the relationships that they find among themselves and objects, such as is the scope of qualitative research, is also to question whether and in what ways the meaning of human being is revealed. Thus, neither quantitative research nor qualitative research is subject to discrete criteria by which to judge its ultimate value.

Not Either/Or but Both/And

This new style of thinking cannot rightly be called realist or idealist. The notion of the flesh as double-sided and border-crossing avoids both of these extremes. The process of creating reality is reciprocal between self and the world. This way of thinking permits us to think "object" and "subject" as interrogating one another in a two-sided process of "creation that is at the same time a reintegration of Being" (Merleau-Ponty, 1968, p. 197). By extending this thought to a consideration of its implications for research can we begin to allow our objective and subjective approaches to interrogate each other in a two-sided process of creation? Can we look toward the objects of each methodological disclosure to consider both what is both revealed and concealed? By identifying that which is concealed by our own approaches and interpretations, bearing in mind that every revelation, is at the same time a concealment, can we begin to appreciate the opportunities that lie at hand to effect a border crossing? Can we really begin to grasp that we do not inhabit separate realities but rather that in noticing our own methodological limitations (an idea that comes close to Gadamer's notion of hermeneutical humility/charity) we are in a place that holds the greatest promise for interdependence and collaboration?

Oppositions Imply Wholeness

Since flesh is fundamentally two-sided, we can expect subject and object and all of the oppositions following upon this distinction to arise interdependently. As much as distinctions serve to separate, the fundamental contact between oppositions is never entirely lost. A thing can be best understood for what it is by considering it in the light of what it is not. We cannot experience light without familiarity with darkness. In a similar vein, intimacy cannot be appreciated without an experience of reserve and aloofness. Recognizing the underlying unity or intersection between subjective and objective experience and between qualitative and quantitative approaches does not suggest that we have now found an overarching, all encompassing method per se. It does, however, provide a reason to continue to search, amidst the apparent paradoxes and contradictions of objective and subjective ways of knowing, for an understanding that can encompass and create space for both.

By this I wish to make the point emphatically that I do not endorse ways of thinking that seek to blend qualitative and quantitative methods so that the unique perspective of each is lost. Nor do I endorse any approach that would relegate qualitative work to a kind of research underclass in which the role of the subservient is to generate confirmatory evidence to support realist pretensions and aspirations. Rather, by stepping away from the realist paradigm to embrace a phenomenological view of reality and causality, I aim to establish a position of relational equity between quantitative and qualitative researchers. Recognizing that our distinctiveness does not imply duality or separation, and establishing that it is our very differences that first define us and present the possibility for a unity among differences, we can come to see ourselves as inter-related and interdependent.

Shifting Landscapes

Times are changing. Interpretive research in the health sciences needs to continue to be critical of the main-line, empirical paradigm, that is, to identify the questions that its facts answer and more importantly, as Gadamer has said, "to address which facts would begin to speak if other questions were asked" (1976, p. 11). It is also important, as Gadamer reminds us, to bring to bear on all of our scientific undertakings, an attitude of openness and respect for the other—an approach characterized by hermeneutical humility, that is to say to accept that all interpretations (even our own) are fallible and incomplete. He advises that:

In human relations the important thing is, as we have seen, to experience the Thou truly as a Thou—i.e., not to overlook his [*sic*] claim but to let him really say something to us. Here is where openness belongs. But ultimately this openness does not exist only for the person who speaks; rather anyone who listens is fundamentally open. Without such openness to one another there is no genuine human bond. Belonging together always also means being able to listen to one another. When two people understand each other, this does not mean that one person "understands" the other. Similarly, "to hear and obey someone" does not mean simply that we do blindly what the other desires. We call such a person slavish. Openness to the other, then involves recognizing that I myself must accept some things that are against me, even though no one else forces me to do so. (1999, p. 361)

Scientism has spawned a strong and well-deserved reaction to its overweening arrogance. At the same time, interpretive researchers need to remember that not all empirical scientists are scientistic in their approach. Some are sincerely searching for newer and better approaches. A few even admit to grave doubts about the central "truths" of empirical doctrine.

A recent experience of the author helped to confirm the presence of some of these undercurrents as reason for hope. That experience is now shared with you the reader.

Gathered together recently in Ottawa to consider how research could play a stronger role in reducing health disparities and promoting equity in Canadian society, was a large group of researchers.[6] The mood after days of discussion was pensive, introspective, and very self-critical. One scientist commented that, to date, research has not been effective in revealing to Canadians the opportunities that lie at hand to become a better, stronger, more just society; "As researchers, we are," he said, "so easy to ignore." "Why," he continued, "is our research so powerless to bring about change? Could we achieve our objectives more successfully by bringing stories into our research rather than relying primarily on numbers to speak for us? Would stories bring the public and policy markers into more direct contact with human suffering? By this would they be persuaded to seize every opportunity to ameliorate it?" Other comments had to do with the dawning recognition that research is not value free. One scientist questioned the validity of his training that had instructed that the proper stance to approach a research question was one of value-free neutrality.

He noted that he is never value-free. To the contrary, he emphatically emphasized, he is engaged in his work because of his belief in social justice as a cause worth striving for. Subsequent discussion revealed a suspicion of research driven by personal agendas, yet at the same time it was admitted that researchers cannot persuade without reference to explicit values, transparent assumptions, and alternative visions for the future.

Where does consideration of these public confessions of some scientists take us as we return to think about the need to move beyond the methods debate? For hermeneutic understanding there is no blank screen, no anonymity, no neutrality. According to Gadamer we understand by standing under or within, not by standing outside. In other words, to understand we try to enter the whole predicament that confronts us as researchers in the health sciences at this particular point in our history. This is that we in the health sciences have not found a philosophy of science that enables us to move back and forth across the borders of subjective and objective experience fluidly and in a manner that resonates with our everyday experience. Thus, we live in a perpetual state of estrangement from each other. The smooth movement observed in clinical practice exists not because of the presence of a coherent, guiding philosophy of science but in spite of its absence. Qualitative and quantitative researchers live in a state of philosophical dissonance as they continue to be "encouraged" to work together by research funding bodies who are apparently ignorant of, or indifferent to, the philosophical chasm spawned by dualistic thinking.

Does interpretive phenomenology and the way of thinking that I have outlined in this paper have anything to offer in terms of a way to confront these concerns? I suggest that it does and I have sketched in a way based on philosophical phenomenology of moving beyond debate toward respectful dialogue. Reaching this place of dialogue is afforded by a realization that dualism is an illusion not born out in lived experience. Lived experience is rather an embodied understanding of reality that establishes the reality of causal connections based on continuities between, and differences in, both sense experience *and* in lived experience. By showing how mind and body are interactive and that the body is a living experience, I have established, with reference to the thinking of Hume and Merleau-Ponty, the indivisibility of sensed experience and lived experience. In so doing I have provided a philosophical clearing or border crossing for qualitative and quantitative researchers. This border crossing is a way of thinking that preserves the subjectivity, the meaning and the values that live at the heart of objectivity and the objectivity/commonality that lies at the heart of subjectivity. According to this view, and assuming this mutually held understanding, interpretive phenomenologists can work confidently with objectively oriented scientists. This is because a philosophical basis has been constructed that respects each point of view, not as competing views of reality but as two sides of the same reality. Accordingly, this way of thinking does not require the sacrificing of values and commitments that inspire those whose orientations are different, rather, it asks that these be highlighted, respected, and affirmed.

Lingering Dilemmas: Local Consensus or Liberating Dialogue?

By urging movement beyond the methods debate as well as active, diligent, and thoughtful engagement in the search for places of cohabitation, interdependence, and respect among qualitative and quantitative researchers, it could be argued that I am actually advocating a form of philosophical pragmatism.[7] It could additionally be surmised that I am promoting a position in which world views are called into question and the search for "truth" is abandoned in favor of developing certain politically inspired commitments and formulating localized and situated consensus statements about what "works" in the context of what appears to be necessary, expedient, and useful. Moreover, it could be argued that, in describing the thinking of Risjord, Dunbar, and Moloney (2002) and others who suggest that quantitative and qualitative research is complementary and that the use of both produces a more reliable result than either approach alone, I am deliberately disregarding, or at least papering over, the differences in the values and foci of qualitative researchers of interpretive persuasions and quantitative researchers who adhere to the realist paradigm. Furthermore, it could be construed that in telling the story about the self-scrutiny and methodological doubt admitted to by some researchers of realist persuasions, and by arguing for open dialogue and collaboration among persons of diverse philosophical and methodological traditions, I have called off the search for any overarching philosophical metanarratives or normative theory and have concluded instead that what most matters are the fallibilistic and "for the time being" adjudications of what is "helpful" by those who have entered into dialogue at a certain time and in a particular place.

In addition, it might be inferred that since strong practical reasons for overcoming dualistic thought have been described (such as the expectations of research funding bodies for multimethod research) and, given that it has also been affirmed that there is now agreement among realist and interpretive researchers that there is no longer any metaphysical foundation for value-free observation and epistemological certainty, it might reasonably be predicted that I might gravitate toward the pragmatism of such philosophers as Richard Rorty, for example. If such conclusions were drawn, they would be true to some extent but also partially false. Obviously further clarification is necessary!

To establish which of the above conclusions are endorsed in this paper and which are not, it will first be necessary to deal very briefly with philosophical pragmatism as a lens through which to examine the exigencies of resolving the methods debate. Since a full exploration of pragmatism's central tenets and numerous permutations is beyond the scope of this paper, I shall confine my discussion to a very brief exploration of how Rorty's thought helps to move us away from the fallacy of decontexualized theoretical reasoning and authoritative iteration to find value instead in contextualized narrative. From there I will go on to point out some the weaknesses of Rorty's thinking. Having identified these, I will then be in a position to outline an approach based on Gadamer's thought that holds promise for escaping theoretical foundationalism[8] on the one hand, and moral relativism on the other, while engaging diverse traditions (including those adhered to by qualitative and quantitative researchers) in liberating dialogue that expands our freedom rather than constraining our human possibilities.

In concluding this paper, I will return to the discussion of the double-sidedness of reality as a feature of our everyday human experience and I will argue that it is this very feature that necessitates an ongoing dialectic between that which is individual and unique in the human experience and that which is discovered, through dialogue, to be common and widespread. Moreover, I will argue that understanding that doublesided nature of our experience, that is, the subjective and objective that can never be detached (because they are by their very nature constitutive of reality), offers us a certain assurance that we cannot go astray by thinking in this phenomenological manner. This is because our appreciation of, and for, the doublesided nature of reality ensures that there will always be a place in our thinking for differentiation between the particulars of our individual, subjective experience and the commonalities and concerns (objective experience) that we share with other humans as common heirs of one undivided estate, the lifeworld. In so doing, I will show that both subjective and objective dimensions are integral to a system of thought that aims for a greater unity—a liberating unity of interdependence and belonging rather than a hegemonic and totalizing whole.

Having outlined the sequence for these explorations, I return at this point to consider the relevance of the philosophical pragmatism of Richard Rorty. Being perhaps the most noted opponent of normative theory on this side of the Atlantic, Rorty urges us to give up all talk of philosophical foundations, of theoretical reasoning, and of grounding our practices in anything outside of, or transcending, our practices themselves. Offering a description of Rorty's view, Fairbairn asserts that:

> It is no more necessary (nor are we able) to step outside of our local ethical and political commitments by means of theoretical reason than it is to somehow step outside of our language to verify its resemblance to a reality which obtains objectively. The criteria that are available to critical reflection are in no sense axiomatic, but are instead never more than the platitudes which contextually define the terms of a final vocabulary currently in use. The only constraints on moral action, as well as what comes to pass as truth and justice, are conversational ones. They are not universal principles deduced from foundational premises, but local and historically contingent commitments that have managed to generate consensus within a particular culture at a particular time. (1999, p. 141)

Two questions arise in consideration of Rorty's position. First, if the best we can hope for are mutually agreed upon platitudes, can there be any basis at all by which to judge whether overcoming the problems caused by dualistic thought is a worthwhile venture? Second, in the end, is there any way of assessing whether or not this new way of thinking has potential to strengthen the health sciences and in turn to advance the society that the health sciences are intended to serve?

As Fairbairn points out, the problem with Rorty's philosophical pragmatism comes when we ask what the philosophical basis is for a constellation of values and a set of practices. Abandoning the foundationalists' quest for value-free observation and epistemological certainty based on methodological rigor does not absolve scientists nor health practitioners from giving an account not only of their clinical choices, but also of the moral choices upon which their practices rest. Thus it can be seen that a dilemma presents itself when we try to respond to the imperative to provide such accounts without resorting to metaphysical foundationalism and objective grounding on the one hand, and when we try to do this in a way that prevents us from losing our bearings in a nihilistic quagmire brought on by moral relativism[9] (the notion that one view and set of practices is as good as the next, since there is no longer any way to form judgments about which practices are superior and which should be abandoned) on the other.[10]

One way out of the quagmire offered by Rorty is to appeal to consensus and to justify this approach through appeals to local, ethnocentric, and historically situated community-based narratives. While the strength of this approach lies in finding some basis of commonality for justifying our actions, there are serious problems with this solution. The limitations present themselves in consideration of how community consensus often works. As we all know, communities are not without their notable and even nefarious failures in arriving at just solutions. Medical, scientific, and philosophic communities are not dissimilar to naturalistic communities in that these clinical and academic communities can be considered no more immune to dogmatism, intolerance, and self-interest than other communities. The members and representatives of many communities, Fairbairn (1999, p. 144) points out,

may (and frequently do) become so enamored with what comes to pass within their borders, or on their membership lists, for the truth that their concern for justice and human well-being may well take a back-seat to furthering an agenda, clinging to an outmoded belief system or retaining power. Basing moral claims upon local consensus, as any number of historical examples would illustrate, faces serious difficulties when an appeal to justice becomes crude majoritarianism or a strategy for excluding unwelcome opinions.

A further problem arises in consideration of the notion of pragmatic justification. Rorty describes how the way in which we lend support to our final vocabulary is by showing how it favourably compares with others in terms of its practical advantages. Yet Fairbairn (1999, p. 145) also notes that this comparative strategy overlooks the fact that:

what is regarded as a practical advantage is only intelligible when evaluated in the light of a set of prior values and interests, which in turn function as the final vocabulary that one has already adopted. . . . The circularity of pragmatic justifications and ethnocentric appeals, in short, severely limits the force of critical reflection and provides little reason for those who do not share our vocabulary and think as we do to reform their practices and institutions.

Given the need to avoid any system of thought that suggests the possibility of autonomous, a priori, unconditioned rationality on the one hand, and the dangers of pragmatic circularity and ethnocentric justification on the other, the question becomes whether it is possible to develop a way of thinking that allows us to examine not only the questions we are asking and the kind of "evidence" we are accumulating, but one that also enables us to critically examine the ends to which our research is directed. Is it possible, in other words, to develop a way of thinking that takes its bearings from practice itself yet does not end up being dead-ended by circular pragmatic justifications?

A review of the challenges we are currently facing in developing a vibrant philosophy to guide the health sciences helps us to grasp the dimensions of an acceptable solution. These challenges are: the need to overcome the barriers posed by theoretical reasoning and dualistic thought detached from lived experience, the various subsets of practices that appear to be generally problematic within the research enterprise overall, such as methodologies that obstruct rather than afford smooth passage between subjective and objective ways of knowing, and the difficulty we are experiencing in finding ways of determining the ends to which our research is directed.

What becomes obvious is that the acceptable solution we are looking for is a hermeneutical approach which takes up the practical character of reasoning while having as its aim the comprehension, cultivation and reform of our social practices. Clearly, some way of making reasonable judgments about the social practices that should be retained and those that should be abandoned is desirable. Moreover it could be argued that the liberal virtues of universal freedom, mutual recognition, openness and respect inherent to the practice of dialogue oriented toward human understanding, should be apparent. If these qualities appear to be insufficiently developed in Rorty's work to handle the task of recovering principles and clarifying the meaning of our norms and approaches, where then can we look?

Not Philosophical Pragmatism but Communicative Understanding

Warnke (1993, cited in Fairbairn, 1999, p. 147) expresses a viewpoint consistent with Gadamerian thought in which hermeneutics is understood to be the facilitation of dialogue and conversation among opposing viewpoints:

The idea behind the notion of hermeneutic conversation is the idea that an interpretive pluralism can be educational for all the parties involved. If we are to be educated by interpretations other than our own, however, we must both encourage the articulation of those alternative interpretations and help to make them as compelling as they can be. And how can we do this except by assuring the fairness of the conversation and working to give all possible voices equal access? If we are to learn from our hermeneutic efforts, then no voice can retain a monopoly on interpretation and no voice can try to limit in advance what we might learn from others. Democracy thus turns out to be the condition for the possibility of an enriching exchange of insight. Democratic conditions act against the entrenchment of bigoted interpretations by offering others a fair fight as equals and hermeneutic conversation itself acts against the reduction of diversity by allowing that more than one rational interpretation might "win."

While it could be argued that Warnke, in emphasizing the need for conversation among opposing views, over consensus among local forms of self-understanding and settled convictions, affords us some passage beyond mere self-contemplation toward a basis for critical reflection and social reform, a firmer footing is needed. We are still left with the question of, as Fairbairn points out, how to determine why we should believe "x" and not "y."

Invoking the thinking of Heidegger and Gadamer, Fairbairn (1999, p. 155) suggests that the solution lies in grasping understanding not as a methodological problem but as the "fundamental mode of being of human existence." He points out that:

Understanding is not something we do, but rather what we "are." It represents the basic mode in which the human being orients itself and finds its way about in the world. It belongs to the very constitution of human subjectivity and of the world in which we live. Along similar lines Gadamer speaks of interpretive and dialogical understanding as belonging to the ontological condition of human beings. It is through the practice of dialogical understanding that human beings reflectively cope with our experience of the world in general. As linguistic beings, our manner of gaining familiarity with, and orienting ourselves within the world involves articulating it in language. While human experience is never without a certain prereflective comprehension . . . the "universal human task," (as Gadamer describes it) is to bring to speech the phenomena that confront us—to find the words that allow us to reflectively understand and speak of what confronts us, in dialogue with others. Gadamer in speaking of "the conversation that we ourselves are" recommends that we regard the practice of dialogue oriented toward intersubjective understanding as, in a sense constitutative of our humanity. Not merely a form of behaviour one voluntarily undertakes, dialogical understanding is a practice the scope of which is universal, and the import of which is best described as ontological.

With this exposition of Heidegger's and Gadamer's thought, Fairbairn has offered a way to move from the particulars of individual experience and local agreement to a wider sphere—one that can be considered to be ontological and universal in scope. Considering that any normative practice should first demonstrate its universality, Fairbairn identifies communicative understanding as practice that is universal in scope. In so doing, he clears the way for a discussion of dimensions of this universal practice that can now be legitimately deemed normative. What then constitutes the normative core of communicative understanding?

Communicative understanding is more than advancing our preconceived opinions on a given subject matter. It revolves around recognition of the other as one who truly has something to say. It presupposes an orientation of receptivity and openness, and it remains attuned to the possibility that there is something to be learned from another—even and especially one who retains an opposing view. Within the to and fro of an open dialogue, of question and answer, of assertion and rebuttal, it is assumed by both parties that neither are sole posessors of the truth but rather that both are sincerely engaged in the search.

Conclusion

From the foregoing discussion, which has dealt with what might be considered lingering questions regarding my own viewpoint, it becomes clearer that what has been attempted here is an exegesis of a philosophical system of thought that, it has been argued, has the potential to overcome several problems that have plagued research in the health sciences for the past two decades. These problems have had to do with obsolete ways of thinking as well as strained, competitive, and intolerant ways of engaging with each other as qualitative and quantitative researchers in the health sciences. At this juncture, and by way of summarizing and concluding the paper, I will review the problems in a little more detail and I will outline the solutions that have been proposed.

Part of the tension in the health sciences, as we have seen, can be characterized as a division between extreme positions taken by those who seek to uncover determinate patterns of causation based on realist notions of causality in which everything takes place in the objective world such that there is no consideration of a subject, and those who approach health science from an idealist position, positing an absolute subjectivity—a kind of pure interiority, a Cogito whose existence is to think.

In dealing with this problem, and with reference to Hume, a theory of causation, which is an indeterminate theory, and one that is founded squarely on lived experience, has been proposed. This theory affirms the impossibility of finding causal connections aside from an intractable personal component whose basis lies in first-hand, or lived experience. In exploring the relationship between theories of causation and lived experience and by bringing Hume's ideas together with Merleau-Ponty's notion of the flesh, an embodied understanding of reality and causality has been elaborated. This way of thinking, it has been argued, has potential both for uncovering objective patterns and for illuminating intersubjective and relational human understandings. These dimensions of experience are understood not as manifestations of separate realities, that is, reality is all "out-there" or the other extreme view that reality is only understood with reference to personal, private, interior experiences. Rather, reality is understood as inner and outer dimensions of *one* reality experienced by way of gestalt shifts or border crossings. In differentiating the phenomenological understanding of causality from realist explanations of it, I have strongly stated that causality is not a principle of abstract reason nor is it a condition that makes a world possible. Instead, I have asserted emphatically and with conviction in this paper, that causality is a principle of lived experience—one that makes the word actual.

Another tension in the health sciences, as we have seen, emanates from the hotly contested debate on the role of the body in research in the health sciences. As was discussed, there are diverse views on the extent to which its consideration enables holism or whether it places us on a slippery slope sliding helplessly toward biomedical reductionism.

The way of thinking that has been offered here, by highlighting the insights of Hume and Merleau-Ponty, offers assurance with its phenomenological view of reality and causation, which has the potential to calm the fears expressed in relation to the body becoming the site for the unwelcome return of biomedical reductionism. Through his notions of the "flesh" and the doublesided nature of reality it has been shown that Merleau-Ponty unites (while distinguishing) both mind and matter/body. In so doing, he enables us to see that it is not a matter of approaching our research questions from the point of view of lived experience *or* sense experience but rather that there is a place for both. This is because lived experience always, already is, sense experience; in other words, no idea can ever be detached from the bodily impression of it. By showing how mind and body are interactive and that the body is a living experience, this way of thinking establishes the indivisibility of sense experience and lived experience in a way that privileges neither the qualitative nor the quantitative way of thinking. Instead, patterns of commonality across human experiences can be observed at the same time as the particularity of individual experience is encouraged to emerge and to be understood afresh.

As touched on briefly and earlier, some intriguing thoughts arise in relation to the evident doublesidedness of reality, which we experience at the same time as a continuity of distinction. One wonders at the manner in which a dialectic appears to have been built into our existence, that is, the inescapable existential imperative for an intersubjective conversation to take place in order to move from the particulars of my experience to the particulars of your experience in order for us together to gain a larger appreciation of what we both might hold in common. Does the meaning of being human exist in safeguarding (but not privileging) the particular within the common, the subjective within the objective?

In the attempt to get to my underlying "rationale" for this new way of thinking and to understand more clearly the ends to which this approach was directed and the manner in which these ends could be sought, it became obvious that the search had moved past the notion of agreement about desirable social practices based on consensus and politically inspired commitment, to ones based on an understanding of what it means to be human and thus why social reform is necessary. In this way, communicative understanding was discovered to be the preferred mode for acknowledging the barriers that our abstract reasoning has imposed upon us. Moreover, this recognition was seen to necessitate a return to the

practice of learning directly from our manifest experience and listening
to each other as persons coming together in solidarity to discuss, debate,
understand and improve the world in which we live.

Notes

1. An example of such a trend, which is supported by Canada's leading health research funding body, CIHR (Canadian Institutes of Health Research), is a major report
highlighting the roles of the social sciences and humanities in health research. This report,
being developed by R. Lyons and colleagues at Dalhousie University is entitled Understanding and Improving the Health of Canadians: Contributions from the Social Sciences
and Humanities. This project is intended to facilitate interdisciplinary research. The resource will serve as a guidebook, with a major section comprising an extensive list of disciplines highlighting each field's relevance to health research, and providing examples of
methodological approaches used and key references for each discipline.

2. According to the Australian Physiotherapy Association, "the primary focus of
physiotherapy is the restoration of function. Physiotherapists assess and diagnose the
problem, then plan and administer treatment programs that aim to restore function or
minimize dysfunction after disease or injury. Physiotherapists strive to improve an individual's quality of life by physical means. A combination of manual therapy, movement
training and physical and electrophysical agents is used to achieve this." Retrieved from
the website of APA at http://apa.advsol.com on January 3, 2004.

3. The American Association of Occupational Therapists outlines their professional
domain as one that offers skilled treatment that helps individuals achieve independence in
all facets of their lives. It gives people the "skills for the job of living" necessary for independent and satisfying lives. Retrieved from http://www.aota.org on January 3, 2004.

The Canadian Association of Social Work asserts that social work is a profession concerned with helping individuals, families, groups, and communities to enhance their individual and collective well-being. It aims to help people develop their skills and their ability
to use their own resources and those of the community to resolve problems. Social work is
concerned with individual and personal problems but also with broader social issues such
as poverty, unemployment, and domestic violence. Human rights and social justice are the
philosophical underpinnings of social work practice. Retrieved from http://www. casw.org
on January 3, 2004.

4. I am deeply indebted to Dr. Ingrid Harris for the philosophical framework used to
organize this section of the paper. This framework derives substantively from her doctoral
dissertation "A Natural History of Causality" (1996). The essence of this thesis will be published under a new title: "Causal Knowledge and Causal Emptiness" in T. S. K. (Time,
Space, Knowledge) Perspectives (Berkeley, CA: Dharma Publishing).

5. Brackets added with consent of the author, Dr. G. B. Madison.

6. International Think Tank on Reducing Health Disparities and Promoting Equity
for Vulnerable Populations. September 21–23, 2003. Fairmount Chateau Laurier Hotel,
Ottawa, Canada.

7. In offering some background on philosophical pragmatism, I rely on the description of its development offered by Geddes MacGregor (1991, p. 496–497): "C. S. Pierce,
the founder of pragmatism introduced the term in 1878. He adapted it from Kant, who
had distinguished the practical (related to acts of the will) from the pragmatic (related to

consequences). Pierce developed the concept of the pragmatic into a theory of meaning and truth expressed in the following way: 'Consider what effects, that might conceivably have practical bearings, we conceive the object of our conception to have.' These effects we conceive will constitute our entire conception of the object. Truth may be defined, on Pierce's view as a set of beliefs that a community . . . would hold in the long run after a long and exhaustive process of inquiry. Truth is what issues from such an exhaustive inquiry. . . . William James whose name is also very much associated with philosophical pragmatism, expounded it in a somewhat more general way to the effect that the meaning of any proposition can always be boiled down to the practical consequences that will issue from it in practical experience. . . . John Dewey, beginning with pragmatic views developed a system he called 'Instrumentalism' perceiving truth as 'warranted assertability.' . . . Pragmatism has been very influential in molding aspects of 20th century philosophy, more especially in inquires into the nature of meaning and truth. It has a ready popular appeal in as much as it can be easily treated in loose terms along the following lines: instead of telling Tommy, whose behaviour is deplorable, how objectionable his conduct is, one says instead, 'I know we can count on you to be a good boy, because that is what you want to be.' The statement on the face of it, is by no means indisputably true, to say the least; nevertheless to the extent that through such encouraging words Tommy's behavior is in fact temporarily transformed for the better, it becomes true, i.e., the consequences demonstrate its truth."

8. The debate between foundationalism and antifoundationalism according to Fairfield (2000) turns on the issue of what kind of rational warrants are required in order for moral and political judgments to be considered justified. Simpson (1987, p. 2–3) describes the most basic point of contention between foundationalists and nonfoundationalists as their relationship to epistemology: "The one seeks and the other dismisses the notion of, criteria defining conditions in which some beliefs are finally justified. Few deny that beliefs need foundations, that is the more or less secure grounds which make the conclusions of argument as solid as they can be. Any pure foundationalism, however supposes that genuine grounds for judgment are not merely confident assumptions but absolutely secure and which are not subject to amendment, or are amendable only in the direction of greater accuracy. Only in this way could they serve as arbiters of rational judgment. This is the notion of a single over-arching, ahistorical, standard against which any claim must be tested, so that it is possible in principle to decide between rival points of view."

9. MacGregor (1991, p. 532) defines relativism in ethics as: "the doctrine that criteria for ethical judgment do not exist; therefore one cannot lay down absolute standards of 'right' conduct. The rightness of an action depends upon the agent, upon the cultural milieu, upon the circumstances, and many other factors."

10. Madison (2001, p. 17) succinctly addresses the "consequences" of Rorty's postmodern pragmatism: "I think they can be summed up in two words: relativism and nihilism." Rorty, has to be sure protested the charge of relativism but his responses are evasive and his arguments lack the power of conviction (which I suppose is only fitting in the case of someone who no longer believes in philosophical argumentation). We are inevitably condemned to relativism when, rejecting like Rorty the metaphysical notion of Truth, we also reject all metanarratives, when that is, we reject the legitimacy of theory, which always seeks some form of universal validity. And, similarly we find ourselves in a state of nihilism when, rejecting the metaphysical notion of Reality, we go on to assert as well that everyone's "truths" are merely their own private "fictions," when, that is, we equate fiction with mere semblance (simulacrum) and deny it the power to recreate or refigure, and thus enhance, what is called "reality."

References

American Association of Occupational Therapists. *What is occupational therapy?* Retrieved from website http://www.aota.org/featured/area6/index.asp on 3 January 2004.

Australian Physiotherapy Association. *About physiotherapy.* Retrieved from website https://apa.advsol.com.au on 3 January 2004.

Bowlby, J. (1979). *The making and breaking of affectional bonds.* London: Tavistock Routledge.

Brown, G. W. (1994). Life events and endogenous depression. *Archives of General Psychiatry 51,* 525–534.

Brown, G. W. (1997). Loss and depressive disorders. In B. P. Dohrenwend, *Adversity, stress and psychopathology.* Washington, DC: American Psychiatric Press.

Canadian Association of Social Work. *About us.* Retrieved from website http://casw.org on 3 January 2004.

Capra, F. (1982). *Science, society and the rising culture.* Bantam: Toronto.

Duffy, M. E. (1987). Methodological triangulation: A vehicle for merging quantitative and qualitative methods. *Image: Journal of Nursing Scholarship 19,* 130–133.

Fairbairn, M. (1999). Hermeneutical ethical theory. In G. B. Madison & M. Fairbairn (Eds.). *The ethics of postmodernity: Current trends in continental thought.* (p. 141–155). Evanston, IL: Northwestern University Press.

Fairfield, P. (2000). *Moral selfhood in the liberal tradition: The politics of individuality.* Toronto: University of Toronto Press.

Gadamer, H-G. (1976). *Philosophical hermeneutics* (D. E. Linge, Ed. & Trans.). Berkeley: University of California Press.

Gadamer, H-G. (1996). *The enigma of health: The art of healing in a scientific age.* Stanford, CA: Stanford University Press.

Gadamer, H-G. (1999). *Truth and method* (2nd Ed.). (J. Weinsheimer & D. Marshall, Trans.). New York: Continuum. (Original work published 1960.)

Glantz, M. D., & Johnson, J. L. (1999). *Resilience and development: Positive life adaptations.* New York: Kluwer Academic/Plenum Publishers.

Haase, J. E., & Myers, S. T. (1988). Reconciling paradigm assumptions of qualitative and quantitative research. *Western Journal of Nursing Research 10,* 128–137.

Hanson, N. R. (1958). *Patterns of discovery.* Cambridge, England: Cambridge University Press.

Harris, I. (1996). *A natural history of causality: Philosophical principles toward a more human sciences.* Dissertation Abstracts International. McMaster University.

Harris, I. (forthcoming). *Causal knowledge and causal emptiness.* In Time, space, and knowledge: Perspectives. Berkeley, CA: Dharma Publishing.

Hume, D. (1978). *A treatise of human nature* (2nd Ed.). L. A. Selby-Bigge (Ed.). Oxford: Oxford University Press.

James, W. (1977). *The writings of William James.* J. J. McDermott (Ed.). Chicago: University of Chicago Press.

Johnston, N. E. (2003). *Finding meaning in adversity.* Dissertations Abstracts International: McMaster University.

Kikuchi, J. & Simmons, A. (1986). Nursing: A science in jeopardy. In K. King, E. Prodrick, & B. Bauer (Eds.). *Nursing research: Science for quality care* (pp. 28–31). University of Toronto, School of Nursing, Toronto.

Knafl, K. A., & Breitmayer, B. J. (1991). Triangulation in qualitative research: Issues of conceptual clarity and purpose. In J. M. Morse (Ed.). *Qualitative research: A contemporary dialogue* (pp. 236–239). Newbury Park, CA: Sage.

Knafl, K. A., Pettergill, M. M., Bevis, M. E., & Kirchoff, K. T. (1988). Blending qualitative and quantitative approaches to instrument development and data collection. *Journal of Psychosocial Nursing 4*, 30–37.

Kools, S. (1999). Self protection in adolescents in foster care. *Journal of Child and Adolescent Psychiatric Nursing 11*, 139–142.

Kuhn, T. S. (1970). *The structure of scientific revolutions* (2nd Ed.). Chicago: University of Chicago Press.

MacGregor, G. (1991). *Dictionary of religion and philosophy.* New York: Paragon House.

Madison, G. B. (1982). *Understanding: A phenomenological-pragmatic analysis.* Westport, CT: Greenwood Press.

Madison, G. B. (2001). *The politics of postmodernity: Essays in applied hermeneutics.* Dordrecht, The Netherlands: Kluwer Academic Publishers.

Madison, G. B., & Fairbairn, M. (Eds.). (1999). *The ethics of postmodernity: Current trends in continental thought.* Evanston, IL: Northwestern University Press.

Masten, A. S. (1994). Resilience in individual development: Successful adaptation despite risk and adversity. In M. C. Wang, & E. W. Gordon (Eds.). *Environmental resilience in inner city America: Challenges and prospects.* Hillsdale, N.J.: Lawrence Erlbaum.

Merleau-Ponty, M. (1962) *Phenomenology of perception.* (C. Smith, Trans.). London: Routledge & Kegan Paul.

Merleau-Ponty, M. (1968). *The visible and the invisible: Followed by working notes.* (C. Lefort, Ed., A. Lingis, Trans.). Evanston, IL: Northwestern University Press.

Merleau-Ponty, M. (1983). *The structure of behaviour.* (A. L. Fisher, Trans.). Pittsburgh, PA: Duquesne University Press.

Mitchell, E. S. (1986). Multiple triangulation: A methodology for nursing science. *Advances in Nursing Science 18*, 18–26.

Moccia, P. (1988). A critique of compromise: Beyond the methods debate. *Advances in Nursing Science 10*, 1–9.

Parse, R. (1992). Human becoming: Parse's theory of nursing. *Nursing Science Quarterly 5*, 35–42.

Phillips, J. R. (1988). Diggers of deeper holes. *Nursing Science Quarterly 1*, 149–151.

Popper, K. R. (1963). *Conjectures and refutations: The growth of scientific knowledge.* New York: Harper and Row.

Risjord, M. W., Dunbar, S. B., & Moloney, M. F. (2002). A new foundation for methodological triangulation. *Journal of Nursing Scholarship 34*, 260–275.

Schroeder, C. (1993). Nursing conceptual frameworks arising from field theory: A critique of the body as manifestation of underlying field. *Nursing Science Quarterly 4*, 146–148.

Schumacher, K. L., & Gortner, S. R. (1992). (Mis)conceptions and reconceptions about traditional science. *Advances in Nursing Science 14*(4), 1–11.

Simpson, E. (1987). Colloquimur ergo sumus. In E. Simpson (Ed.). *Antifoundationalism and practical reasoning: Conversations between hermeneutics and analysis.* Edmonton: Academic Printing and Publishing.

Smith, M. C. (1991). Response: Affirming the unitary perspective. *Nursing Science Quarterly 4*, 148–152.

Thorne, S., Canam, C., Dahinton, S., Hall, W., Henderson, A., Kirkham, S. (1998). Nursing's metaparadigm concepts: Disimpacting the debate. *Journal of Advanced Nursing 27*, 1257–1268.

Warnke, G. (1993). *Justice and interpretation.* Cambridge: MIT Press.

Werner, E. & Smith, R. (1993). *Overcoming the odds: High risk children from birth to adulthood.* Ithaca, NY: Cornell University Press.

Contributors

John Diekelmann, MSLA, is an architect and landscape architect, and an interpretive phenomenological scholar deeply interested in philosophical issues. Throughout his career as an architect and landscape architect, he has taught courses at the University of Wisconsin–Madison and given papers on the relation of interpretive phenomenology to nature, architecture, and landscape architecture. Recently, his international activities include teaching the works of interpretive phenomenologists such as Martin Heidegger to graduate students in the United States and New Zealand. His current research, with Nancy Diekelmann, focuses on an interpretive phenomenological exegesis of schooling, learning, and teaching, and in explicating a regional ontology. This work has been widely published in journals such as *Nursing Inquiry* and the *Journal of Pediatric Nursing*. The Diekelmanns are co-authoring a book, *Schooling Learning Teaching: Toward a Narrative Pedagogy*.

Kathryn Hopkins Kavanagh, BSN, MS, MA, PhD, is a medical anthropologist. Prepared as a psychiatric/mental health clinical nurse specialist, she has taught for many years in the University of Maryland system. Her interests in healing and cross-cultural healthcare led her to conduct a series of summer field schools on the Pine Ridge Reservation in South Dakota. She also taught for Northern Arizona University, for which she directed a baccalaureate program on the Navajo and Hopi Reservations. Happiest as an independent and somewhat itinerant scholar, she currently teaches courses in medial anthropology, indigenous healing traditions, American Indian cultures, and the anthropology of foodways. Widely published in cultural aspects of health and healthcare, she continues to write on various diversity-related topics.

Pamela M. Ironside, PhD, RN, received her BA from Luther College, MS from the University of Minnesota, and her PhD from University of Wisconsin–Madison, where she is currently an assistant professor. Her research program includes using interpretive phenomenology to explicate a) the ways new pedagogies influence the practices of thinking in classroom and clinical courses, b) the reforming practices nursing faculty, and c) the experiences of teachers and students in nursing doctoral programs. She chairs the Nursing Education Advisory Council Executive Committee for the National League for Nursing. She has served as an invited member of the National League for Nursing's think tanks on Graduate Preparation for the Nurse Educator role and on Standards for Nursing Education. Her work is widely published in journals such as *Journal of Qualitative Health Research, Journal of Nursing Education, Journal of Advanced Nursing, Advances in Nursing Science*, and *Nursing Education Perspectives*.

Nancy E. Johnston, PhD, RN, is an Assistant Professor in the Department of Nursing in the Atkinson Faculty of Professional and Liberal Studies at York University, Toronto, Ontario, Canada. Her current interpretive scholarship explicates the contribution of hermeneutical, phenomenological thinking to research and practice in nursing and the human sciences, and it examines the construction of meaning and the lived experiences of people who are resilient in situations of overwhelming extremity. She has been President of the Canadian Federation of Mental Health Nurses and Vice-President of Nursing at the Clarke Institute of Psychiatry (now the Centre for Addictions and Mental Health) in Toronto.

Rosemary A. McEldowney, RCompN, PhD (Nursing), is a Senior Lecturer in the Graduate School of Nursing and Midwifery at Victoria University of Wellington, New Zealand. She is a Fellow of the College of Nurses Aotearoa New Zealand and was recently voted best supervisor by postgraduate students in the Faculty of Humanities and Social Sciences at Victoria University of Wellington. For the past 15 years she has been in the forefront of developing and sustaining cultural safety programs in nursing education and practice. As a former dean of a nursing school, she has been working in partnership with Maori nurse educators to develop undergraduate and postgraduate programs for indigenous students. In June 1995 she was Helen Denne Schulte Visiting Professor at the University of Wisconsin–Madison School of Nursing, where she presented a paper on developing and implementing a bicultural curriculum. Her doctoral research used life story as a method of inquiry into the lived experiences of nurse educators who teach for social change.

Philippa Seaton, PhD, RN, is presently a postdoctoral research fellow at the Research Centre for Clinical Practice Innovation at Griffith University, Queensland, Australia. She has a background in both undergraduate and postgraduate nursing education. Her research interests are in nursing education, particularly online teaching and learning in nursing. Her methodological interests are in the use of the philosophies of Heidegger and Gadamer in research, and the uses of multiple methodologies.

Elizabeth Smythe, PhD, RN, is an Associate Professor at Auckland University of Technology, New Zealand. Her background was first nursing and then midwifery. Her current teaching focus is within interdisciplinary postgraduate programs, introducing students to philosophical paradigms to equip them with wider skills to think through the issues of practice. Her interest in "thinking" has been pursued in research related to the call to thinking in education and thinking of leadership. She embraces the philosophical writings of Heidegger and Gadamer in her understandings of hermeneutic research.

Christine Sorrell Dinkins, PhD, received her BA with Honors from Wake Forest University and her MA and PhD from the Johns Hopkins University. She is an Assistant Professor in the Philosophy Department at Wofford College in Spartanburg, South Carolina, where she teaches courses in Ancient Greek philosophy, 19th- and 20th-century German philosophy, philosophy of law, and philosophy through literature. Dr. Dinkins's primary interests are the philosophical methods of Plato and Heidegger. Her current research includes employing Heideggerian hermeneutics in a non-doctrinal contextual interpretation of Plato's works. She is also exploring hermeneutics in music, and her chief hobby is composing choral music, both sacred and secular. In her work with undergraduates, Dr. Dinkins encourages philosophy students to engage in interdisciplinary research with students in other humanities fields and the sciences.

Index

Abram, D., 59, 60, 66
absence, 3, 9, 13, 34; dynamic of, 48, 49
absolutism, 264
Adorno, R. D. C., 204
Ahern, K., 197, 216, 217
Albrecht, G. L., 73
Alterio, M., 160
American Association of Occupational
    Therapists, 292
analogies, 131–132
Anderson, K., 164
anthropocentrism, xii, 6, 10, 60, 66
Anti-Stigma Project, 74
Appignanesi, R., 195
Apple, M., 152
Appleton, J. V., 203
Arendt, H., 223
Arias, A., 101
Aristotle: and gender, 61
Armitage, S., 164
Atkinson, P., 68, 93, 101
Atkinson, R., 153, 161, 162
audit trail, 211
Australian Physiotherapy Association, 292
autobiography, 153, 155
Ayres, L., 198

Bailey, P., 154, 159
Baker, B., 159
Baker, C., ix, 195, 204, 205, 212, 213
Baker, L. D., 79, 91, 92, 97
Banks-Wallace, J., 159
Barbour, R. S., 197, 209, 210, 211, 212,
    213, 214, 216
Barkan, E., 82
Barroso, J., 192, 212, 213
Barth, F., 98

Basso, K., 71
Bataille, G., 64, 97
Bateson, M. C., 70, 87, 101
Bathgate, M., 175
Beck, C. T., 205, 221
Becker, H. S., 73
Beech, I., xv
Begley, C. M., 195, 197
being-with: of being, 44; in experience, 47
Benhabib, S., 87
Benner, P., 112, 113, 114, 128, 136, 146, 204
Bergbom, I., 154, 159
Berkhofer, R. F., Jr., 84
Bern-Klug, M., 160
between: as invisible, immeasurable phe-
    nomenon, 35–36; as a relationship, 35
Bevis, M. E., 260
Bhabha, H. K., 76
Billings, C., 175
Bloom, L., 164
Blumenfeld-Jones, D., 158
Bochner, A. P., 68, 71
Boone, M. S., 92
border crossing, 265–269, 270, 272, 282–
    283, 290
boundaries, 3
Bowlby, J., 276
Bowman, G., 92
Brace, C. L., 83
Breitmayer, B. J., 198, 260
Brewer, J., 202
Brooks, R. L., 92
Brown, E. R., 92
Brown, G. W., 278
Brown, K., 87
Bruner, J., 153
Bunkle, P., 157

Interpretive Studies in Healthcare and the Human Sciences

Series Editor
Nancy L. Diekelmann, PhD, RN, FAAN, Helen Denne Schulte Professor
Emerita, School of Nursing, University of Wisconsin–Madison

Series Associate Editor
Pamela M. Ironside, PhD, RN, Assistant Professor, School of Nursing,
University of Wisconsin–Madison

Volume 1
First, Do No Harm: Power, Oppression, and Violence in Healthcare
Edited by Nancy L. Diekelmann

Volume 2
Teaching the Practitioners of Care: New Pedagogies for the Health Professions
Edited by Nancy L. Diekelmann

Volume 3
Many Voices: Toward Caring Culture in Healthcare and Healing
Edited by Kathryn Hopkins Kavanagh and Virginia Knowlden

Volume 4
*Beyond Method: Philosophical Conversations in Healthcare Research and
Scholarship*
Edited by Pamela M. Ironside